VULVOVAGINAL INFECTIONS

WILLIAM J LEDGER, MD
Professor and Chairman Emeritus
Department of Obstetrics and Gynecology
Weill Medical College of Cornell University
New York, NY, USA

STEVEN S WITKIN, PHD
Director and Professor of Immunology
Division of Immunology and Infectious Diseases
Department of Obstetrics and Gynecology
Weill Medical College of Cornell University
New York, NY, USA

MANSON PUBLISHING

DEDICATION

To our beloved wives, Jacque and Iara.

Fulfilled scientists are more productive scientists.

We were able to conceive and author this book because you complete our lives.

Dr. Witkin also lovingly acknowledges the lifelong support and encouragement of his father, Bernard Witkin, in all his endeavors.

Please note the following text change – on page 69 substitute the last 15 lines with:
Finally, prevention is the mainstay of care in any infectious disease. A monovalent preventive HPV 16 vaccine and quadravalent HPV 6, 11, 16, and 18 vaccines had successful trials and the quadravalent vaccine was approved for use in the United States by the FDA in 2006. The advantage of this vaccine is that protection against HPV 6 and 11 reduces the incidence of condyloma, as well as CIN1 and CIN2, VaIN1 and VaIN2, and VIN1 and VIN2. Protection against HPV 16 and 18 reduces the incidence of CIN1, CIN2, CIN3, AIS, VaIN1, VaIN2, VaIN3, VIN1, VIN2, and VIN3 (Villa, *et al.*, 2006). Over time, it should also reduce the incidence of invasive cancer of the cervix, vulva, and vagina. A bivalent HPV 16 and 18 vaccine has also been approved in Europe (Harper *et al.*, 2004). It produces higher antibody levels when measured after the third injection, and there is preliminary evidence that it might offer some cross-protection against other high-risk HPV strains. Currently, decisions about which vaccine to use are largely based upon the cost of the vaccine. Long-term follow-up studies of clinical outcomes, including the frequency of physician interventions by colposcopy and conization, and the incidence of pre-cancers and cancers of the cervix, vulva, and vagina, will be the true clinical measure of effectiveness.

Harper DM, Franco EI, Wheeler C, *et al.* Efficacy of a bivalent L1 virus-like particle vaccine in prevention of infection with human papillomavirus types 16 and 18 in young women: a randomised controlled trial. *Lancet* 2004;**364**:1757–1765.

Villa LL, Ault K, Giuliano AR, *et al.* Immunologic responses following administration of a vaccine targeting human papillomavirus types 6, 11, 16, and 18. *Vaccine* 2006;**24**:5571–5583.

Softcover edition 2010

ISBN: 978-1-84076-138-2

A CIP catalogue record for this book is available from the British Library.

For full details of all Manson Publishing Ltd titles please write to:
Manson Publishing Ltd, 73 Corringham Road, London NW11 7DL, UK.
Tel: +44(0)20 8905 5150
Fax: +44(0)20 8201 9233
Website: www.mansonpublishing.com

Commissioning editor: Jill Northcott
Project manager: Ruth Maxwell
Copy-editor: Ruth Maxwell
Cover design: Cathy Martin
Book design and layout: Cathy Martin
Colour reproduction: Tenon & Polert Colour Scanning Ltd, Hong Kong
Printed in Spain and the UK

Contents

Abbreviations 5

Preface 6

Acknowledgements 8

Chapter 1
Microbiology of the Vagina 9
- Background 9
- Vaginal pH 10
- *Lactobacillus* species 10
- Menstrual cycle changes in vaginal flora 11
- Sexual intercourse, conception, and vaginal flora 11
- Vaginal flora in post-menopausal women 11
- A word of caution 11

Chapter 2
Vaginal Immunology 12
- Background 12
- Vaginal epithelial cell immunity 12
- 'Danger' signalling by heat shock proteins 13
- Intracellular innate immune system components 14
- Phagocytic and natural killer cells 14
- Dendritic cells: interface between innate and acquired immunity 14
- Acquired immunity 15
- Antibody production in the lower genital tract 15
- Sexual intercourse and vaginal immunity 15

Chapter 3
Diagnosis of Vulvovaginal Disease 16
- Current state of medical knowledge 16
- Physician focus on the patient 17
- History 17
- Equipment requirements for a diagnosis 17
- Physical examination 18
- Pelvic examination 18
- Laboratory testing with delayed results 22

Chapter 4
***Candida* Vulvovaginitis 25**
- Background 25
- Microbiology 25
- Immunology 26
- Diagnosis 27
- Treatment 32

Chapter 5
Bacterial Vaginosis 35
- Background 35
- Microbiology 36
- Immunology 37
- Diagnosis 37
- Treatment 40

Chapter 6
***Trichomonas vaginalis* Vaginitis 43**
- Background 43
- Microbiology 44
- Immunology 44
- Diagnosis 44
- Treatment 47

Chapter 7
Desquamative Inflammatory Vaginitis 49
- Background 49
- Microbiology 49
- Immunology 50
- Diagnosis 50
- Treatment 52

Chapter 8
Genital Herpes 53
- Background 53
- Microbiology 54
- Immunology 54
- Diagnosis 55
- Treatment 57

CHAPTER 9
HUMAN PAPILLOMAVIRUS INFECTIONS **61**
Background 61
Microbiology 62
Immunology 63
Diagnosis 63
Treatment 67

CHAPTER 10
OTHER SEXUALLY TRANSMITTED DISEASES OF THE VULVA AND VAGINA **70**
Background 70
Microbiology and immunology 72
Diagnosis 73
Treatment 77

CHAPTER 11
STAPHYLOCOCCUS AUREUS AND GROUP A STREPTOCOCCAL INFECTIONS OF THE VAGINA AND VULVA **81**
Background 81
Microbiology 82
Immunology 82
Diagnosis 83
Treatment 85

CHAPTER 12
ALLERGIC VULVOVAGINITIS **86**
Background 86
Microbiology 87
Immunology 87
Diagnosis 88
Treatment 90

CHAPTER 13
MENOPAUSAL VULVOVAGINITIS **93**
Background 93
Microbiology 94
Immunology 94
Diagnosis 94
Treatment 101

CHAPTER 14
VULVODYNIA **103**
Background 103
Microbiology 105
Immunology 106
Diagnosis 106
Treatment 108

CHAPTER 15
DERMATOLOGIC DISORDERS CAUSING VULVAR DISEASE **111**
Background 111
Immunology 112
Diagnosis 113
Treatment 117

REFERENCES 119

INDEX 126

Abbreviations

5FU 5-fluorouracil

AGUS atypical glandular cells of undetermined significance

ASCUS atypical squamous cells of undetermined significance

BCA bichloracetic acid

BV bacterial vaginosis

CDC Centers for Disease Control

CLIA Clinical Laboratory Improvement Amendment

CMV cytomegalovirus

DIV desquamative inflammatory vaginitis

FDA Food and Drug Administration

FTA-ABS fluorescent treponemenal antibody absorption (test)

FUO fever of undetermined origin

GI gastrointestinal

H_2O_2 hydrogen peroxide

HGIL high-grade glandular intraepithelial lesion

HIV human immunodeficiency virus

HPV human papillomavirus

HRT hormone replacement therapy

HSIL high-grade squamous intraepithelial lesion

HSV herpes simplex virus

I&D incision and drainage

Ig immunoglobulin

IL interleukin

IL-1 ra interleukin-1 receptor antagonist

IVIG intravenous immunoglobulin

KIR killer cell immunoglobulin-like receptor

KOH potassium hydroxide

LEEP loop electrosurgical excision procedure

LGIL low-grade glandular intraepithelial lesion

LSIL low-grade squamous intraepithelial lesion

MBL mannose-binding lectin

MHC major histocompatibility complex

NIH National Insitutes for Health

OTC over-the-counter

PCR polymerase chain reaction

PGE_2 prostaglandin E_2

RVVC recurrent vulvovaginal candidiasis

SF seminal fluid

SLPI secretory leukocyte protease inhibitor

SSRI selective serotonin uptake inhibitor

STD sexually transmitted disease

TABM T cell-derived antigen binding molecule

TCA trichloracetic acid

TGF-β transforming growth factor β

TLR Toll-like receptor

TNF tumor necrosis factor

TP-PA *Treponema pallidum* particle agglutination (test)

TSS toxic shock syndrome

TSST toxic shock syndrome toxin

UTI urinary tract infection

VIN vulvar intraepithelial neoplasm

VIP Vaginal Infection in Pregnancy (Study)

VLP virus-like particle

VVS vulvar vestibulitis syndrome

WBC white blood cell

PREFACE

We hope the reader will be as convinced of the significance of vulvovaginal infections as are the authors. These problems are an important consideration for any doctor caring for women. On a volume basis alone, they account for one-third of patient complaints in an outpatient gynecologic practice. More relevantly, the current standard of care needs to be improved. Too often, patients with vulvovaginal symptomatology are ignored, misdiagnosed, or mistreated. One glaring example of current medical care shortcomings is the failure of physicians[1] and patients[2] to diagnose *Candida* vaginitis correctly. This book will address these inadequacies and offer practical solutions.

There are many reasons for current physician misadventures in the diagnosis and treatment of vulvovaginal infections. This area of clinical practice receives scant attention in contemporary medical school and residency training. Physicians in practice have not had adequate instruction in the use of the microscope. Basic office diagnostic testing and laboratory screening are not emphasized. These are the realities of a busy office practice. Most gynecologists in the United States, Great Britain, and the European Union have a high-volume practice with tightly consigned short time intervals for each patient visit. To deal with overwhelming patient numbers, many practices have a triage system that avoids an office visit by the symptomatic woman and assigns patients with vulvovaginal symptoms to phone management by a nonphysician member of the medical care team[3]. The errors of this system of patient management have been documented[3].

In this text, we will attempt to provide a scientific rationale for the care of patients with vulvovaginal symptomatology. To paraphrase Euclid's counsel to Ptolemy I, there is no royal road to the care of patients with these problems. Each patient has an individual problem that often will require an investment of time and attention to assign a diagnosis properly and provide adequate and appropriate care. Our aim in this book is to provide suggestions for accurate diagnosis and care that will avoid ineffective treatments and discomfort and stress for these women.

This text will offer a unique approach to the subject matter. Physicians are biologists and use classification as a means to achieve order in their patient contacts. Figure **1** of an uncultivated forest glen serves as an example of the lack of order in the presentation of patients with vulvovaginal symptomology. It is an undefined picture with no clarity. In medical textbooks, this vague picture of nature's disorder becomes transformed to the pattern of a geometrically planted nursery in which each row of seedlings and trees represents a defined clinical entity such as bacterial vaginosis, *Candida* vaginitis, and *Trichomonas* vaginitis (**2**), each with proscribed symptoms, diagnostic findings, and treatment. Too often the time-constrained physician arbitrarily assigns the patient to one of these three entities without proper testing. When the misdiagnosed patient fails to respond, she is assigned again to another of these three categories. In addition to these misclassifications, these three infectious categories do not account for all patients with vulvovaginitis. This text will expand the list of diagnostic possibilities and

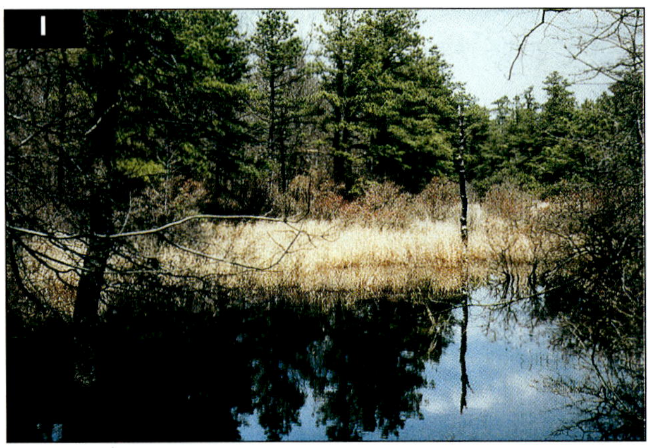

1 A forest glen. The disorder of nature reflects the random signs and symptoms in the diverse population of women with vulvovaginitis.

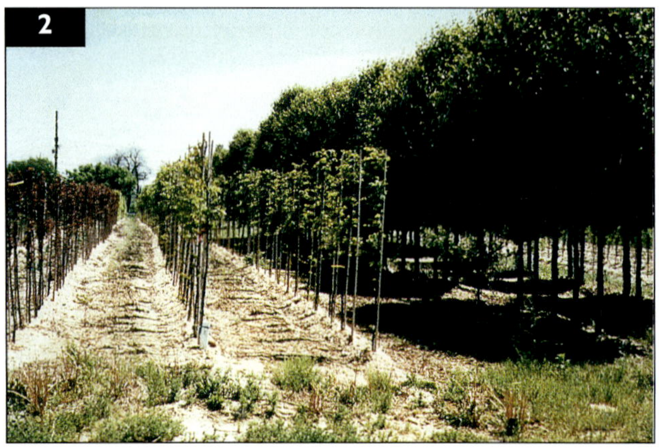

2 The order of a cultivated nursery. Each row of similar plantings reflects the classifications of a vulvovaginal disease textbook in which one row represents bacterial vaginosis, another *Candida* vulvovaginitis, and another *Trichomonas* vaginitis.

provide techniques to achieve a correct diagnosis as well as treatment options. Finally, we will de-emphasize the classical signs and symptoms of various vulvovaginal disease entities. These classical presentations do not apply to the majority of patients with vulvovaginal problems and they take attention away from the growing number of asymptomatic women who have a sexually transmitted infection. In each of the chapters on vulvovaginal disease entities detailed treatment options are presented. Details of therapy are provided, with particular emphasis on the nuances that can be applied in women who fail to respond to the original medication prescribed or who respond and then become symptomatic again after the treatment has ended.

Finally, in this new century of increasing numbers of HIV-infected women, it is important to note the double quandary this presents to physicians. These women are more likely to get the vulvovaginal infections that are described in this text[4] and, when infected, they are more likely to transmit this HIV infection to others[5]. It places a special burden of responsibility on the doctors who care for these women.

Be aware of the shortcomings of these insights. Chronic vulvovaginitis has been a stepchild of medical research around the world. In many cases, the pathophysiology of disease and optimal therapy are not yet established. Each research clinic has a distinct patient population and is likely to make independent observations and establish unique practices. Opinions and practices not referenced in this text either to a specific author or to some other publications simply reflect the authors' research clinic experience of more than two decades. Now, we invite you to read on.

William J Ledger
Steven S Witkin

Acknowledgements

Both Dr. Ledger and Dr. Witkin are aware that this book would not have been completed without the contributions of many people. At Manson Publishing, we had Jill Northcott, who encouraged us through our early stumbles during our first manuscript drafts, and Ruth Maxwell, a dedicated editor with a passion for accuracy. We welcomed their efforts, which markedly improved the book's quality. This book required a wide range of illustrations, some beyond the scope of our vulvovaginitis clinic in New York. Dr. Iara Moreno Linhares of Brazil and Dr. Paul Summers of Salt Lake City were kind enough to fill these voids with outstanding pictures of vulvovaginal pathology. We especially appreciated Paul's careful reading of our first drafts. His suggestions always improved the syntax, and we adopted them in nearly every instance. Our secretaries Anthony Flood and Sandra Green labored away on first drafts and multiple revisions, and Tony's Internet skills made us feel as though Manson Publishing House in London were across the street from our offices in New York City.

CHAPTER 1

MICROBIOLOGY OF THE VAGINA

BACKGROUND

Much confusion and over-simplification exists about the composition of the vaginal flora in healthy asymptomatic women, and what constitutes 'normal' microbial flora (*Table 1*). The microorganisms that colonize the vagina are in dynamic equilibrium with the environment and can change daily. Vaginal microorganisms fluctuate with a woman's age, hormonal status, immune status, sexual activities, use of medications, presence of vaginal blood, mode of contraception, and exposure to a variety of vaginal products (*Table 2*). Therefore, there is a good probability that a single microscopic examination is not representative of an individual

Table 1 Microorganisms detected in the vagina of healthy, asymptomatic reproductive age women

Lactobacilli	Predominantly *L. crispatus*, *L. jensenii*, or *L. gasseri* both producers and non-producers of H_2O_2
Cocci	*Staphylococcus aureus*, Group B and D streptococci, peptococci, peptostreptococci
Bacilli	*Gardnerella vaginalis*, diphtheroids, *Escherichia coli*, propionibacteria, clostridia, *Bacteroides* species, *Prevotella* species, fusobacteria
Mycoplasmas	*Mycoplasma hominis*, *Ureaplasma urealyticum*
Yeast	*Candida albicans*
Virus	Human papillomavirus

Table 2 Endogenous and exogenous factors influencing the composition of the vaginal microbial flora

Vaginal estrogen concentration	Decreases vaginal pH and fosters lactobacilli predominance
Genetics	Individual variations in production of immune activators or inhibitors influences the capacity of the host to eliminate specific microorganisms
Immune status	Vaginal immediate hypersensitivity reactions or immune tolerance to specific microbial antigens effect the ability of the immune system to control microbial proliferation
Sexual activities	Deposition of semen, saliva, or foreign objects into the vagina alters vaginal pH and immune functions and elicits the direct deposition of exogenous microorganisms. The ability of H_2O_2-producing lactobacilli to inhibit growth of *E. coli* is inhibited by semen
Oral or vaginal medications	Alter local immune status, vaginal pH, and ability of select microorganisms to survive and replicate (*Candida* species)
Vaginal blood	Increases vaginal pH, alters microbial ecology by providing nutrients for a select group of microorganisms
Contraception	Oral contraceptives alter vaginal estrogen levels, diaphragm and condom usage are associated with increased vaginal levels of enterobacteria, intrauterine devices have been associated with increased levels of *Bacteroides* species and group B streptococci
Vaginal products	Douches, deodorants, pads, tampons can alter the vaginal ecosystem

woman's vaginal flora. The influence of genetic factors on variables that facilitate or inhibit vaginal colonization by specific microbes is also becoming increasingly apparent[1,2]. Ethnic differences in the composition of the vaginal flora have not received sufficient attention, but recent investigations using gene amplification technology indicate that there can be pronounced differences between white and black women.

A multitude of microorganisms have been isolated by culture from the vagina of asymptomatic women. However, any attempt to culture vaginal microflora in a medical office will have only limited success. The majority of vaginal bacteria require special culture media and incubation conditions. When utilized for collection of vaginal bacteria, the standard culture swab that was originally intended for cultures of the oropharynx may identify lactobacilli, streptococci and staphylococci, as well as some Gram-negative bacteria and yeast but will fail to identify many vaginal microorganisms. Gene amplification technology has resulted in identification of additional nonculturable vaginal microorganisms, some present in relatively high concentrations[3]. Each microbial species influences the ability of other microbial species to persist and thereby contributes to the uniqueness of the vaginal ecosystem in different women.

Despite an acknowledgement of the probable uniqueness of the microbial flora in each woman due to her individual genetic and immunologic makeup and environmental exposures, it is necessary and unavoidable to make generalizations about the composition of the vaginal microbial flora in relation to several distinct variables.

VAGINAL pH

A major influence on the microbial composition of the vagina is the vaginal pH. This in turn is dependent upon the woman's hormonal status, specifically the vaginal concentration of estrogen. Estrogen stimulates glycogen deposition on the surface of vaginal epithelial cells. Both epithelial cells and microbial enzymes degrade the glycogen to glucose. Lactobacilli, and perhaps also the vaginal epithelium, then metabolize glucose to yield lactic acid. This results in a vaginal pH <4.5 in most asymptomatic, reproductive age women with normal menstrual cycles. The lactobacilli have a selective advantage and constitute the major microbial species under these distinctly acidic physiological conditions. It has been estimated that there are approximately 10^8–10^9 lactobacilli in the vagina of healthy cycling women. Other microorganisms, such as the yeast *Candida albicans* and aerobic streptococci, are also tolerant of this acidic pH.

LACTOBACILLUS SPECIES

Over the years it has become almost dogma that *Lactobacillus acidophilus* is the predominant species of lactobacilli in the vagina of healthy, reproductive age women. This has led to numerous attempts to treat a variety of vaginal disorders by the introduction, either by mouth or directly into the vagina, of *L. acidophilus* or *L. acidophilus*-containing products such as yogurt. There has been a notable lack of success in these attempts due to a variety of factors. Recent refinements in the ability to differentiate *Lactobacillus* species have lead to the realization that *L. crispatus*, *L. jensenii*, and *L. gasseri*, and not *L. acidophilus*, are the predominant vaginal lactobacilli[4]. These three *Lactobacillus* species have been shown to be predominant in the vaginas of women residing in North America, South America, Europe, and Asia. Furthermore, the vaginal strains were significantly different in their DNA sequences than lactobacilli isolated from food or the environment.

In addition to determining the acidic pH of the vagina, lactobacilli influence the vaginal microbial ecosystem by at least two additional mechanisms. Some strains of lactobacilli produce hydrogen peroxide (H_2O_2), a product with potent antimicrobial activity *in vitro*. Whether H_2O_2 is also antimicrobial in individual women *in vivo* will depend on the rate of catalase production by other microorganisms also present at this site. The majority of *L. crispatus* and *L. jensenii* clinical isolates appear to be H_2O_2 producers. Some lactobacilli also release bacteriocins, compounds that inhibit the growth of other vaginal microorganisms.

The persistence of lactobacilli in the vagina varies among different women and in the same woman over time. Recent studies of asymptomatic women demonstrated the dynamic changing quality of *Lactobacillus* vaginal colonization[5–7]. In one study, while 95% of subjects were culture-positive for lactobacilli at least once over an 8-month time period, two-thirds of the women tested fluctuated between being culture-positive and culture-negative for *Lactobacillus* species during this time interval. H_2O_2 production was observed in 70% of the *Lactobacillus* isolates. It appeared that vaginal *Lactobacillus* colonization was most likely to persist in women who were colonized with H_2O_2-producing *L. crispatus* or *L. jensenii*. The loss of vaginal lactobacilli was associated with having engaged in sexual intercourse at least once a week or with taking antibiotics. It is interesting to note that while persistent colonization with H_2O_2-producing *L. crispatus* or *L. jensenii* was associated with a decreased acquisition of bacterial vaginosis as compared to women only transiently colonized with these *Lactobacillus* species, 26% of those with persistent colonization nevertheless developed bacterial vaginosis. Thus, H_2O_2 production by itself appears to be insufficient to inhibit growth of anaerobic bacteria and mycoplasmas in the vagina.

There are ethnic differences in *Lactobacillus* vaginal colonization. White and Hispanic women of reproductive age are far more likely to harbor lactobacilli in the vagina than are black women. Conversely, black women are more likely than other women to be positive for *Mobiluncus* species in their vagina. This remains true after controlling for other possible influencing factors. The relative lack of vaginal lactobacilli in black women may explain the observation that black women in general have a higher vaginal pH than do other women. Whether genetic or other yet undetermined variables are responsible for this ethnic difference in *Lactobacillus* vaginal colonization still remains to be determined. Possible genetic factors to be examined include variations in vaginal epithelial cell membranes that influence the adherence of different microbial species, and the extent of production of pro-inflammatory cytokines and immune mediators.

It is becoming increasingly clear, due to the changing dynamic nature of *Lactobacillus* vaginal colonization and ethnic variations in physiological conditions, that it is impossible to determine by a single microscopic examination of a vaginal wet mount in an asymptomatic woman whether or not her vaginal flora is 'normal'. Similarly, in women with vaginal symptoms the finding of seemingly 'normal' flora on a single microscopic examination may not give an accurate picture of the vaginal milieu. The vaginal bacterial flora of some women may be 'normal' even though lactobacilli may be absent or present only in low concentrations. Antibiotic treatment of healthy women based only on a microscopic examination is, therefore, inadvisable. Disturbing the endogenous flora that is typical for a given woman by administration of antimicrobial compounds may only serve to increase susceptibility to development of abnormal and potentially harmful vaginal microorganisms.

MENSTRUAL CYCLE CHANGES IN VAGINAL FLORA

It is not surprising that the vaginal flora changes over the course of the menstrual cycle due to variations in hormone levels, glycogen concentration, vaginal pH, and availability of sloughed cells and menstrual blood as microbial substrates[6]. Vaginal pH is lowest at mid-cycle and is greatly elevated during menstruation. The vaginal glycogen content is maximal the week prior to menstruation. In general, vaginal levels of non-*Lactobacillus* bacterial species, excluding the mycoplasmas, are highest on days 1–5 of the menstrual cycle. *Lactobacillus* species, *Ureaplasma urealyticum*, and *Mycoplasma hominis* remain at nearly constant levels throughout the cycle, while vaginal concentrations of *C. albicans* tend to increase towards menstruation. Specimens obtained at menstruation typically contain the greatest number of different bacterial species.

SEXUAL INTERCOURSE, CONCEPTION, AND VAGINAL FLORA

Oral contraceptives cause only a slight decrease in the level of estrogens and so their use is associated with only minor variations in vaginal flora. In general, the levels of *Lactobacillus* species, either producers or nonproducers of H_2O_2, remain relatively constant as do concentrations of facultative and anaerobic microorganisms, *C. albicans*, and mycoplasmas. In contrast, usage of depo-medroxyprogesterone for a 6-month period is associated with decreased vaginal colonization with lactobacilli, including H_2O_2-producing strains.

The relationship between unprotected sexual intercourse, enteric vaginal colonization, and bacteriuria is well known. Condom use reduces the frequency of *E. coli* vaginal colonization while diaphragm use has been associated with increased vaginal colonization with *E. coli* and a consequent increased frequency of urinary tract infections (UTIs)[8]. Possibly, diaphragm insertion or anatomical changes associated with diaphragm usage increases the capability of microorganisms to enter the vagina from the perirectal region. Vaginal *E. coli* colonization after sexual intercourse is not inhibited by the presence in the vagina of H_2O_2-producing *Lactobacillus* species. It has been suggested that a component of semen interferes with the ability of H_2O_2-producing lactobacilli to effectively inhibit growth of *E. coli*. The much trumpeted ability of H_2O_2-producing lactobacilli to inhibit growth of other microorganisms, as well as human immunodeficiency virus (HIV) infectivity, under *in vitro* conditions must therefore be viewed with caution since *in vivo* these microbes are present in semen.

VAGINAL FLORA IN POST-MENOPAUSAL WOMEN

After the menopause, vaginal estrogen levels are markedly decreased and the consequent reduction in vaginal glycogen concentration leads to a marked change in the vaginal flora. *Lactobacillus* species are absent or present at only low levels and the vaginal pH becomes elevated. There is a concomitant increase in colonization by Gram-positive cocci and coliforms in the vagina. In contrast, the use of hormone replacement therapy (HRT) by post-menopausal women results in the return to a *Lactobacillus*-dominated vaginal flora[9]. The absence of lactobacilli also applies to prepubertal females. As estrogen production is initiated during the beginning of puberty, the vaginal epithelail barrier is enhanced and the concomitant increase in vaginal glycogen promotes colonization of the vagina with lactobacilli from the colon.

A WORD OF CAUTION

It is just beginning to be appreciated that the 'normal' vaginal microbial ecosystem is quite variable. It is almost completely unknown what factors contribute to the composition of the vaginal microorganisms in individual women and how the development of a unique flora contributes to protection of each specific woman from vaginal pathogens. To label mistakenly vaginal flora as abnormal that which is not dominated by lactobacilli and treat with antibiotics or other antimicrobial preparations carries the risk of interfering with that woman's vaginal ecosystem and increasing her susceptibility to growth of microorganisms that are normally suppressed. In addition, the use of probiotic lactobacilli-containing vaginal preparations in women where that particular *Lactobacillus* species is normally absent also may upset homeostatic mechanisms and do more harm than good. It is incumbent upon the practitioner first to determine carefully what is 'normal' for each individual patient before embarking on a course of treatment to change the vaginal microbial milieu.

CHAPTER 2

VAGINAL IMMUNOLOGY

BACKGROUND

Invasion of the vagina by a multitude of microorganisms is undoubtedly a daily occurrence. Sexual activities (masturbation, sexual intercourse, receptive oral sex), nonsexual touching, contamination from the rectum, and environmental exposures all result in deposition of various microorganisms onto the vaginal epithelia. Concomitantly, sub-pathological levels of a number of different microbes colonize the vagina of healthy women. The prevention of clinical symptom development in response to this constant microbial incursion is the responsibility of the normal endogenous microbial ecosystem, an intact epithelial cell barrier, and the local genital tract immune system.

The epithelial barrier consists of a keratin layer on the surface of the vulva and a thin coating of mucus in the vagina. The keratin prevents microbial adhesion to the epithelium while vaginal mucus traps microorganisms and prevents them from coming into contact with vaginal cells.

The immune system in the vagina can be divided into two branches. The innate immune system provides an initial and immediate defense against microorganisms. This system recognizes molecules common to many different microbes and is, therefore, not specific for any given microorganism and does not have to be 'learned'. Components of vaginal epithelial cells, as well as phagocytic and natural killer cells, and genital secretions comprise this innate system. In contrast, the specific (acquired) immune system is characterized by a delayed response of several days and is uniquely specific to a single microbial antigen or product. The innate immune response sends out signals that alert cells of the specific immune system, T and B lymphocytes, to become activated and produce microbe-specific cell-mediated or antibody-mediated immunity.

VAGINAL EPITHELIAL CELL IMMUNITY

It has only recently been recognized that epithelial cells in the vagina are major components of the local immune defense against pathogens[1]. These cells are the initial surface that exogenous microorganisms come into contact with upon entering the vagina. In healthy women, cells of the immune system are usually not present in the vaginal lumen in significant concentrations. It is perhaps not surprising, therefore, that vaginal epithelial cells have evolved mechanisms for recognizing microbial invaders and for providing signals to attract and activate immune cells to the source of 'danger'.

The vaginal epithelial cell surface contains molecules called Toll-like receptors (TLRs) that function in the recognition of specific microorganisms. Eleven TLRs have been identified to date that recognize what are called pathogen-associated molecular patterns, or specific structures present only in unicellular microorganisms[2,3]. For example, TLR2 in association with either TLR1 or TLR6 recognizes lipoprotein and peptidoglycan from Gram-positive bacteria as well as yeast cell wall mannan and glycosylphosphotidylinositol lipid of *Trypanosoma cruzi*; TLR3 recognizes double-stranded viral RNA; TLR4 recognizes the lipopolysaccharide of Gram-negative bacteria; TLR5 recognizes bacterial flagellen; TLR9 recognizes the unmethylated cytosine-guanine dinucleotide, CpG, present only in bacterial and in many viral DNAs. In humans, CpG is typically methylated. TLR11 recognizes uropathogens. Attachment of the specific microbial component to its corresponding TLR induces the activation of transcription factors that travel from the cytoplasm to the nucleus and induce the transcription of genes coding for pro-inflammatory cytokines and chemokines. The subsequent release of these cytokines triggers the activation of immune cells in the underlying lamina propria while the chemokines induce their migration to the vaginal lumen. The repertoire of epithelial cell innate immune defense mechanisms is illustrated in Figure **3**.

A second component of epithelial cell innate immunity is the protein secretory leukocyte protease inhibitor (SLPI). SLPI, which is produced and released by epithelial cells in the vagina and uterus of reproductive age women, was initially characterized as a serine protease inhibitor. Further studies identified SLPI as being bacteriocidal for both Gram-positive and Gram-negative bacteria. SLPI also has been shown to interfere with the entry of human immunodeficiency virus (HIV) into susceptible target cells. Recent investigations have identified a new immune-related property of SLPI – inhibition of TLR2 and TLR4 activation in monocytes/macrophages.

Epithelial cells also release peptides that are capable of rapidly killing a broad spectrum of bacteria, fungi, and enveloped viruses upon contact[4,5]. Antimicrobial peptides, called defensins, have a cationic charge and bind to anionic-charged molecules on the surface of microorganisms. The resulting membrane disruption leads to lysis of the affected cell. Even those microorganisms that have developed

3 Epithelial cell innate immune defense mechanisms.
A: Epithelial tissue releasing interleukin (IL)-1, IL-6, IL-8, and tumor necrosis factor (TNF); **B**: epithelial cell with surface receptors for toll-like receptor (TLR)-2, TLR4, TLR5, and TLR9; **C**: Gram-positive bacterium associated with TLR2; **D**: Gram-negative bacterium associated with TLR4; **E**: bacterium bound by its flagella to TLR5; **F**: DNA helix with an unmethylated cytosine-guanine (cpG) dinucleotide binding to TLR9.

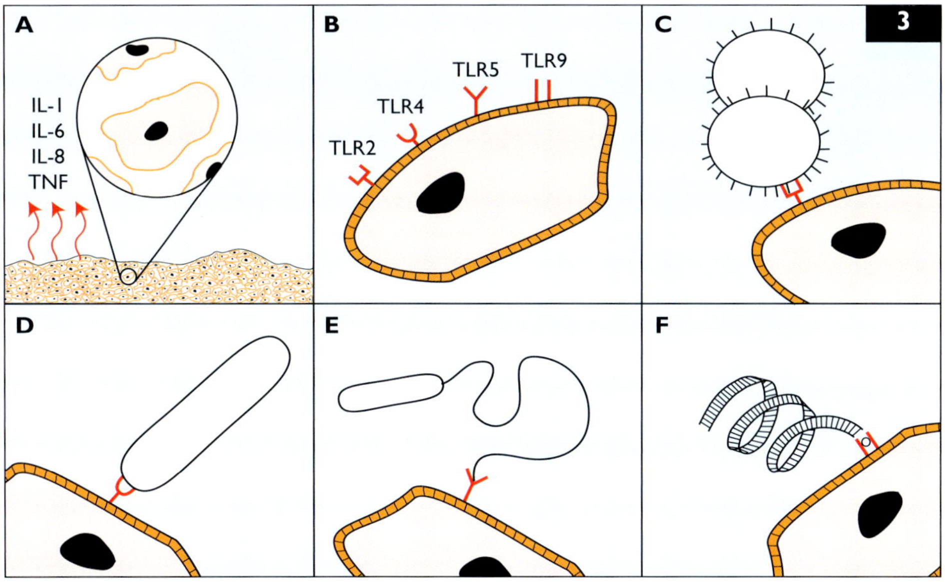

antibiotic resistance remain sensitive to defensins. At least eight defensins have been identified in humans.

Mannose-binding lectin (MBL) is an innate immune system component present in the circulation and in vaginal secretions. It binds to mannose, N-acetylglucosamine, and fucose residues on microbial surfaces. This results in complement-mediated microbial destruction and/or opsonization via MBL receptors on phagocytic cells[6]. MBL has recently been shown to bind to immunoglobulin A (IgA) and the resulting complex has complement-activating activity. This provides a novel mechanism for MBL-mediated killing of microorganisms to which MBL does not directly bind, but in which vaginal IgA immunity is present. A deficiency in MBL production due to a genetic polymorphism has been associated with recurrent vulvovaginal candidiasis[7].

Two other antimicrobial products produced by epithelial cells in the vagina are lysozyme and lactoferrin. Lysozyme acts primarily on cell membranes of Gram-positive bacteria and may also inhibit the growth of *C. albicans*. Lactoferrin, a nonheme iron-binding glycoprotein, sequesters uncomplexed iron from biological fluids, thereby removing it from potential utilization by microorganisms. It is inhibitory to the growth of a wide range of bacteria as well as *C. albicans* and viruses such as cytomegalovirus, adenovirus, HIV, and hepatitis C virus. Soluble components of vaginal innate immunity are shown in Figure **4**.

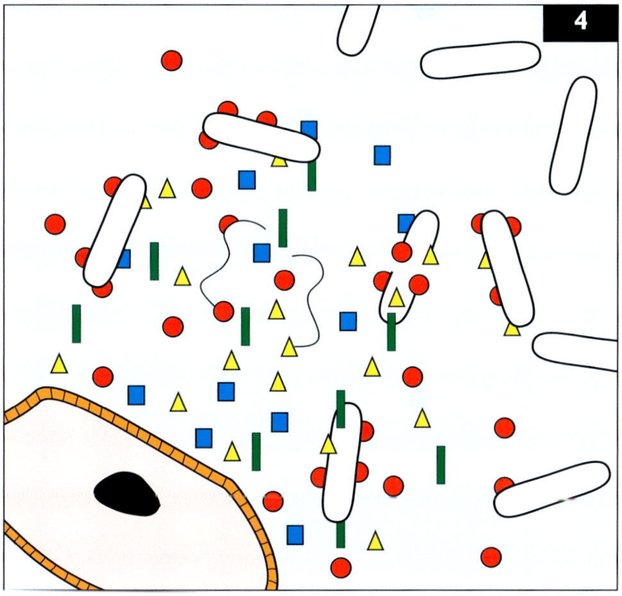

4 Soluble components of vaginal innate immunity: secretory leukocyte protease inhibitor: ●; defensins: ■; lactoferrin: ▲; lysozyme: ▌.

'DANGER' SIGNALLING BY HEAT SHOCK PROTEINS

Heat shock proteins, or stress proteins, comprise several protein families that are essential to life and are present in every known organism including bacteria, plants, and humans. When a cell finds itself under nonphysiological 'stressed' conditions such as elevated temperature (heat shock) or invasion by microorganisms, the biosynthesis of heat shock proteins is greatly up-regulated. It has been amply demonstrated that the release of heat shock proteins from infected cells serves as an initial warning to the immune system that cells are in danger and that immune cells should migrate and concentrate in the region of heat shock protein release[8]. Several members of the heat shock protein family bind to specific receptors on the surface of phagocytic cells. This results in the release of cytokines and chemokines from these cells and the initiation of immune system activation. The complement system is also activated by cell-free heat shock protein. The deposition of activated complement components on the surface of bacterial cells results in cell lysis or phagocytosis by cells possessing complement receptors. Cell-free heat shock proteins have been identified in the vaginal lumen of women with a history of recurrent vulvovaginal candidiasis. The mechanism of heat shock

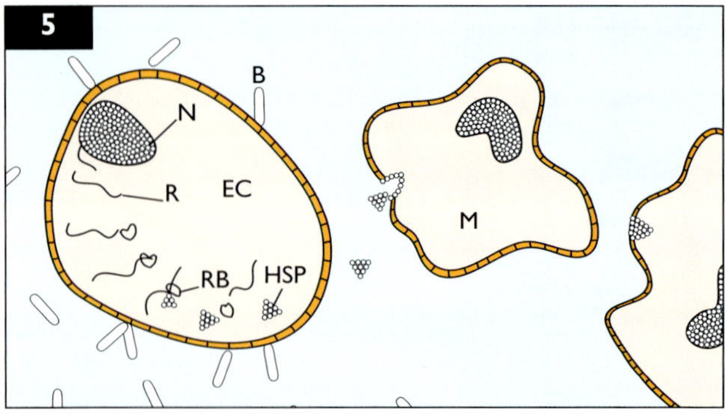

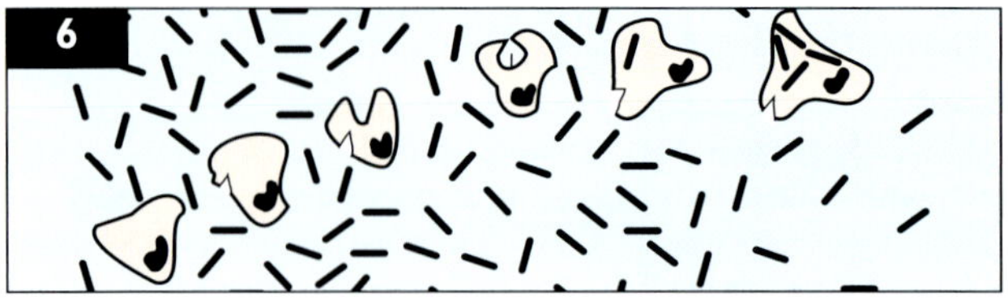

5, 6 Mechanism of heat shock protein-related immune system anti-bacterial activation. **5**: Several bacteria (B) attach to an epithelial cell (EC). Inside the cell RNA for heat shock protein (R) is released from the nucleus (N) into the cytoplasm, where heat shock proteins (HSP) are produced on ribosomes (RB). HSP are released from the cell and bind to receptors on the surface of macrophages; **6**: macrophages with HSP ingesting the bacteria.

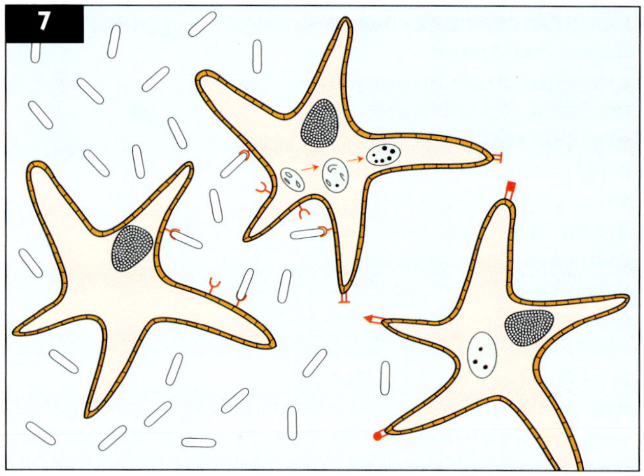

7 Pattern recognition and binding of toll-like receptors to a microbial surface antigen or bacterial unmethylated CpG-containing DNA rapidly induces dendritic cell maturation.

protein-related immune system anti-bacterial activation is shown in Figures **5, 6**.

The inducible 70kDa heat shock protein (hsp70) is also a highly effective adjuvant and is capable of potentiating immune responses to microorganisms. Thus, vaginal hsp70 production in response to infection results in hsp70 binding to microbial antigens. This complex is many times more efficient than the microbial antigen alone in inducing specific antimicrobial immunity.

INTRACELLULAR INNATE IMMUNE SYSTEM COMPONENTS

Components of innate immunity also are present within the cell cytoplasm. A protein kinase known as PKR is activated by double-stranded RNA, an intermediate produced during intracellular viral infections. Activated PKR blocks viral protein synthesis and induces cellular production of interferon alpha, an antiviral protein. Another family of intracellular proteins, known as NOD proteins, are also able to recognize intracellular bacterial infections by pattern recognition.

PHAGOCYTIC AND NATURAL KILLER CELLS

Components of innate immunity are present on a variety of cells of the immune system, mostly those with phagocytic or lytic functions[2]. Macrophages, dendritic cells, neutrophils, natural killer cells, mast cells, and eosinophils all have innate immune functions.

Natural killer cells are capable of recognizing and destroying cells that are infected with microbial pathogens. This activity is not learned and is not microorganism-specific and so is a component of innate immune defenses. The natural killer cells are inhibited under physiological conditions by specific receptors on their surface, called killer cell immunoglobulin-like receptors (KIR)[9]. The recognition of major histocompatibility complex (MHC) class I molecules on healthy cells by KIR prevents cell lysis. Infection, however, results in a marked down-regulation of MHC class I cell surface expression, and under these altered conditions natural killer cell binding is no longer blocked and lysis occurs. Cytokines such as interferon gamma that are capable of activating the acquired immune system are also released from activated natural killer cells.

Macrophages possess multiple TLRs and nonspecifically recognize a variety of microbial pathogens. They also possess membrane-bound receptors for complement and immunoglobulins, and opsonize and destroy microorganisms that contain these components on their surface. Similar to what occurs in epithelial cells, the association of TLRs with its appropriate ligand also results in activation of the macrophage genes coding for pro-inflammatory cytokines and chemokines. This leads to recruitment of T lymphocytes and the induction of pathogen-specific immunity. Once within the macrophage, ingested microorganisms are degraded and their components become available for induction of antigen-specific acquired immunity (see below).

DENDRITIC CELLS: INTERFACE BETWEEN INNATE AND ACQUIRED IMMUNITY

Dendritic cells, also known as Langerhans cells, are probably the most important link between innate and acquired immunity in the female genital tract. These cells are potent antigen-presenting cells and have been identified in the vaginal epithelia as well as in cervical squamous epithelia and vulvar epidermis[2]. They are derived from bone marrow and migrate to the skin. The dendritic cell surface contains high levels of several different TLRs. Pattern recognition and binding of these receptors to a microbial surface antigen or bacterial unmethylated CpG-containing DNA rapidly induces dendritic cell maturation (**7**). The mature dendritic cells acquire the capacity to engulf microbial pathogens very effectively, process pathogen-specific antigens, and transport these antigens to their cell surface. Maturation also involves the induction of chemokine receptors and adhesion molecules and reorganization of the dendritic cell cytoskeleton. These changes facilitate migration of the dendritic cells through the lymph to regional lymph nodes. The dendritic cells then come into intimate contact with T lymphocytes and induce them to recognize specifically the microbial antigens processed by the dendritic cells (**8**). The mature dendritic cells also produce pro-inflammatory cytokines and interferon alpha to stimulate immune system activation further.

ACQUIRED IMMUNITY

Acquired immunity, in contrast to innate immunity, takes several days to develop and results in the recognition of a single unique antigen present only on one specific microbial pathogen. Within those dendritic cells and macrophages that have engulfed microorganisms the microbial protein components are degraded into small peptides. These peptides associate with MHC class II molecules and both are transported to the cell surface. In rare instances, microbial-MHC class I complexes can also be produced. In the lymph nodes, MHC-microbial antigen-bearing dendritic cells and macrophages come into contact with naïve uncommitted CD4-positive T lymphocytes as well as B lymphocytes. Both T and B lymphocytes possess receptors on their surface that recognize microbial peptide-MHC molecule complexes. The subsequent binding of lymphocytes to the phagocytic cells results in acquisition by the lymphocytes of the ability to recognize the specific microbial peptide that was presented to it. T lymphocytes also become activated to release the cytokine, interleukin 2 (IL-2). IL-2 induces the replication of T and B lymphocytes, resulting in the formation of a large number of lymphocytes which can recognize and respond to a specific microbial invader. Interferon gamma is also released by the activated T cells which stimulates macrophages to become more efficient in engulfing and processing microorganisms. By this mechanism, a repertoire of T and B lymphocytes is generated (memory cells) which will recognize the specific microorganism if it should ever be present in the vagina in the future and quickly activate a cell-mediated and/or antibody-mediated immune response to prevent its proliferation and ability to cause disease.

8

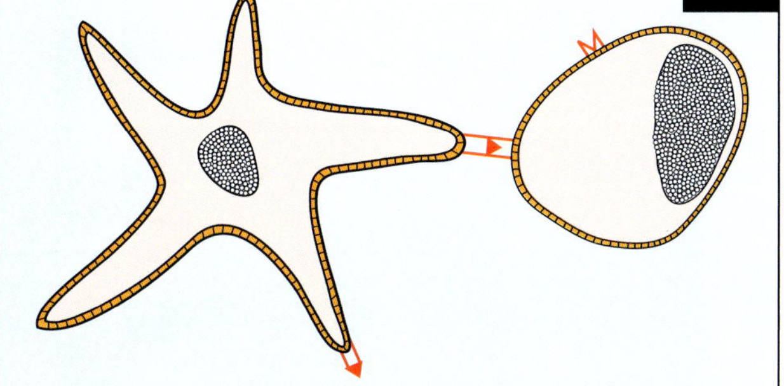

8 Dendritic cells migrate to regional lymph nodes and come into intimate contact and bind with T lymphocytes and induce them to recognize specifically the microbial antigens processed by the dendritic cells.

ANTIBODY PRODUCTION IN THE LOWER GENITAL TRACT

As stated above, the ability of B lymphocytes to produce specific antibodies to bacterial components is dependent upon their interaction with MHC II-microbial peptide complexes on the surface of antigen presenting cells. Antibodies to viral antigens and bacteria that replicate intracellularly are usually generated by B cell interaction with cells that present peptides in association with MHC class I molecules. Once primed to recognize a specific microorganism, subsequent contact with this microbe results in specific antibody production. The female genital tract contains B lymphocytes capable of producing either IgG or IgA antibodies. Most of these antibody-producing cells are located in the endocervix but lesser quantities can be found in the vagina[10].

The vaginal lumen contains a mixture of IgA and IgG antibodies. The majority of IgG antibodies are probably not induced in response to genital tract pathogens and enter the vagina by transduction from the systemic circulation. In contrast, the majority of IgA antibodies probably have their origin in B lymphocytes residing in the endocervix. Unlike systemic IgA which is monomeric, most of the IgA in the vagina is polymeric and contains a secretory component. Polymeric secretory IgA is a product of the mucosal immune system which is distinct from systemic antibody production. B lymphocytes in the cervix, as well as at other body mucosal sites, produce antibodies with different specificities than those found in the blood. Thus, IgA antibodies to microorganisms in the vagina might be present in vaginal fluid while absent from the peripheral circulation.

SEXUAL INTERCOURSE AND VAGINAL IMMUNITY

Sperm-specific components are not produced in females and so spermatozoa are viewed as 'foreign invaders' by the female immune system. However, development of immunity to spermatozoa is clearly not desirable. The presence of anti-sperm antibodies in women is a recognized cause of infertility. Semen deposition in the human vagina does result in an influx primarily of polymorphonuclear leukocytes and low levels of mononuclear macrophages and T lymphocytes. However, in the vast majority of sexually active women, immunity to spermatozoa is never induced. The major component resulting in inhibition of development of anti-sperm immunity appears to be the seminal fluid. Semen is the body fluid with the highest concentration of prostaglandin E_2, a potent inhibitor of IL-2 production by T lymphocytes. In addition, seminal fluid inhibits production of interferon gamma, the major inducer of macrophage activation, while stimulating synthesis of IL-10, an anti-inflammatory cytokine that inhibits induction of cell-mediated immunity.

This potent inhibition of vaginal immunity by seminal fluid is beneficial for maintaining fecundity but may inhibit vaginal immunity from effectively combating pathogenic microorganisms that are present in the male ejaculate. Variations between women in their frequency of sexual intercourse and differences in the extent of immune inhibitory factors in semen from different men may influence the likelihood of sexually transmitted microorganisms being able to evade vaginal immune defense mechanisms.

Chapter 3

Diagnosis of Vulvovaginal Disease

CURRENT STATE OF MEDICAL KNOWLEDGE

To care properly for the woman with genital tract symptomatology, the physician must be aware of the expanding information about the pathophysiology of vulvovaginal disease. An open mind is required. Many contemporary truths run counter to clinical dogma that have been repeated over the years in one edition after another of standard gynecologic texts. There are many obvious examples: the diagnosis of the etiology of these symptoms is neither easy nor automatic. It cannot be accurately determined after a phone conversation in which a patient describes a discharge, an itch, or discomfort. It also cannot be definitively diagnosed by the gross evaluation of the vulva or the vaginal discharge when a speculum is inserted. Figure **9** shows an irritated vulva, coated with a white discharge. Figure **10** shows a typical white curdish vaginal discharge, the *sine qua non* of the gross physical findings of *Candida* vaginitis. Both of these patients had no microscopic evidence of a *Candida* infection, and *Candida* was not confirmed by culture. Too often, physicians focus upon the three most common infectious entities, *Candida* vaginitis, bacterial vaginosis, or *Trichomonas* vaginitis as the only causes of vulvovaginal symptomatology. One example of this oversimplification of diagnostic alternatives is seen in this advertisement of a testing strip for pH and amines (**11**). The message is clear: if a symptomatic woman has a normal pH and negative amines, she must have a *Candida* vaginitis. This narrow view ignores those patients with symptoms due to allergic vaginal or vulvar reactions, those hard to detect but profound alterations in the bacterial flora of the vagina, sometimes related to a new sexual partner, or vaginal changes due to new hormonal imbalances. Physician awareness of this broader range of etiologies will avoid the current all-too-frequent erroneous diagnostic switches from yeast to bacteria to protozoa when patients fail to respond to treatment. These symptomatic women deserve better care.

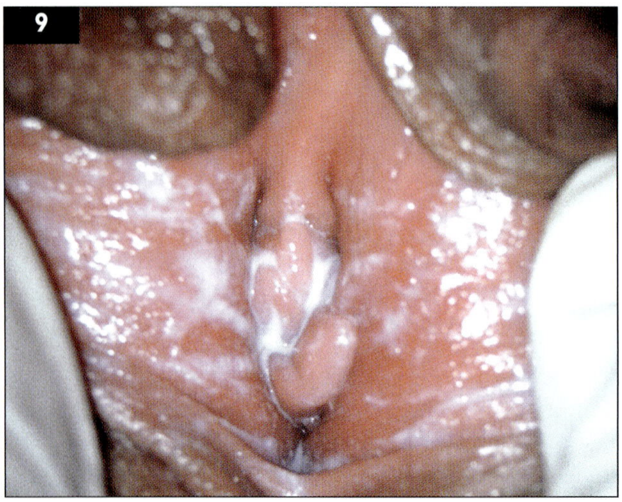

9 An irritated vulva covered by a white exudate. *Candida* was not confirmed by microscopic or culture examination of the exudate.

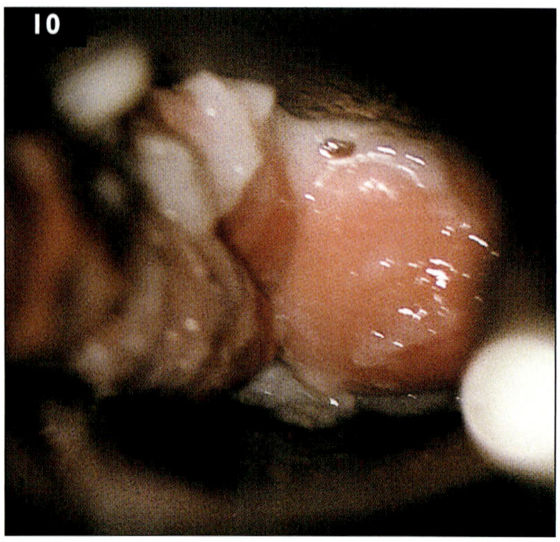

10 An excessive, white, curdish vaginal discharge. *Candida* was not confirmed by microsopic or vulvar examination.

PHYSICIAN FOCUS ON THE PATIENT

Better patient care starts when health care workers acknowledge that vulvovaginal problems are not trivial, but are important and require attention. Persistent symptoms impact unfavorably upon the daily quality of life and they often spawn unspoken concerns about such infections as genital herpes, *Chlamydia trachomatis*, and human immunodeficiency virus (HIV) disease that, if present, could cause major changes in the future life-options for the patient. Part of the job of the physician is to expose these concerns and deal with them appropriately.

HISTORY

The care of these women begins with the history. This requires a private interview environment, which is always important for a sexually active woman, combined with the physician's commitment to nonjudgmental listening. There are two distinct categories of patients to be evaluated: those with a new acute problem and those with a chronic or recurring difficulty. Each requires some differences in the physician's focus. *Table 3* presents an outline for questions to be directed towards patients with an acute problem. *Table 4* presents an outline for questions for the patient with recurrent or chronic problems.

EQUIPMENT REQUIREMENTS FOR A DIAGNOSIS

There are a limited number of diagnostic aids needed to enable the physician to begin the process of accurate diagnosis of vulvovaginitis. Unfortunately, many physicians caring for women have few or none of these available in the outpatient setting where these patients are to be examined.

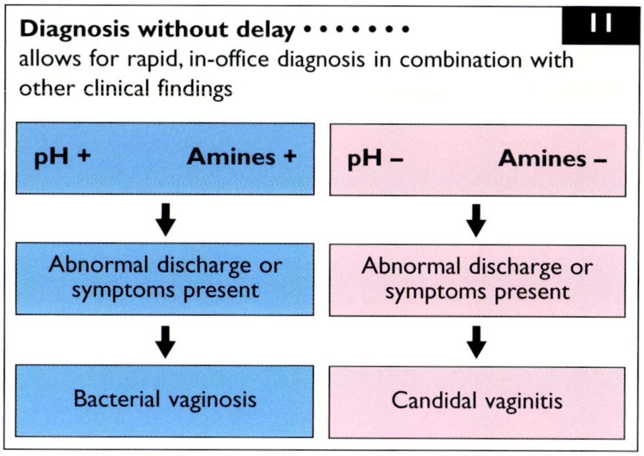

11 An advertisement for a test kit to measure vaginal pH and amines. The implication is clear: if the symptomatic patient does not have bacterial vaginosis, she must have a *Candida* vaginitis.

Table 3 Questions for a patient presenting with an acute problem

1. Where does it bother you?
2. How does it bother you?
3. When did it begin?
4. Do you have a new sexual partner?
5. What type of contraception are you using?
6. What most concerns you?

Questions 1 and 2 provide some clues for the focus of the physical examination, the next three can give some insights on suspected etiologies, and the last question provides the basis for dialogue with the patient after completing the examination.

Table 4 Questions for a patient presenting with chronic or recurring problems

1. Where does it bother you?
2. How does it bother you?
3. Relationship to the menstrual cycle?
4. Any history of allergy or a reaction to local vaginal or vulvar medications?
5. What medications are you taking?
6. Relationship of symptoms to current sexual partner?
7. What type of contraception are you using?
8. Does your sexual partner have any allergies and what medication is he or she taking?
9. What most concerns you?

The first two questions guide the examiner on sites to focus upon at the time of the physical examination. Question 3 can provide a hint of recurrent *Candida* infection. Questions 4 and 5 can give insights on possible causes or a reason for exacerbations of symptoms. Questions 6–8 can provide hints about the causes of the problem. Question 9 provides a starting point for the dialogue with the patient after completing the examination.

For many such doctors, this book's emphasis upon office laboratory diagnostic techniques is at such variance with their current practice that it could elicit a response similar to a damsel receiving an unwanted gift of swords from a soldier. The swords could represent an office microscope and other testing equipment that is not available to them. This is not their reality or presumed need. Anything less than this, however, represents a compromise in patient care. Alternatives to immediate office diagnostic aids will be offered (*Table 5*), highlighting the shortcomings of these alternative approaches.

PHYSICAL EXAMINATION

A general physical examination is an important starting point in the care of these women. A general examination should be done whether or not it is the scheduled time for a periodic health evaluation. It provides a view of the general status of the patient's health and nutrition, gives insights into the extent of body piercing and the use of tattoos, and provides a view of the general health of the skin. All of these observations are important. The questions running through the examiner's mind include: Is there an overall problem of health? Is body piercing or tattooing a marker for personal rebellion against family or societal norms? Is this patient prone to skin afflictions? One should particularly focus upon the porcelain quality of the skin of many women with vulvar vestibulitis who demonstrate marked dermographism when the skin is lightly scratched. A light scratch of the skin will give an idea of skin reactivity. In addition, careful palpation of the inguinal region for nodes is recommended, for this can be a marker for chronic vulvar inflammation and infection.

PELVIC EXAMINATION

An error made by many physicians is to begin the pelvic examination with the insertion of the vaginal speculum. For the woman whose chief complaint is either vulvar burning or itching or the inability to have intercourse because of severe entry pain due to vulvar vestibulitis, this premature use of the speculum removes the possibility of making a diagnosis. Vulvar itching when present can be due to vulvovaginal candidiasis, but this symptom can also be present with new tissue formation from a new growth on the vulva, either benign, or malignant, or another type of vulvar infection, for example, a healing genital herpes lesion. Figure **12** depicts a minor recurrent vulvar irritation (in the view of the patient), annoying, not thought by her to be a problem. This was cultured for herpes and it was positive for herpes simplex virus-2 (HSV-2). Any vulvar lesion with a break in the skin surface should be cultured and screened for HSV-1 and -2. Other lesions will only be found by direct

Table 5 Office equipment for the care of women with vulvovaginitis

- pH paper
- Microscope
- Glass slides with cover slips
- Solutions at room temperature:
  - Normal saline
  - 10% potassium hydroxide
  - 4% acetic acid
- Small cotton swabs
- Plastic spatula
- Magnification system: colposcope or hand-held magnifying glass
- Biopsy set: forceps, scalpel, small scissors, syringe, needle, Monsel's solution (ferrous sulfate), 1% lidocaine without epinephrine
- Specimen tubes for viral, bacterial, and fungal cultures, plus tubes for detection of microorganisms by gene amplification techniques such as polymerase chain reaction

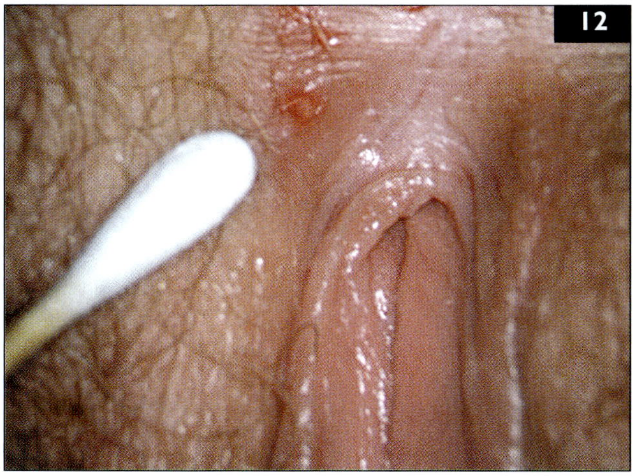

12 A recurrent minor vulvar irritation, disregarded by the patient, found to be culture-positive for HSV-2.

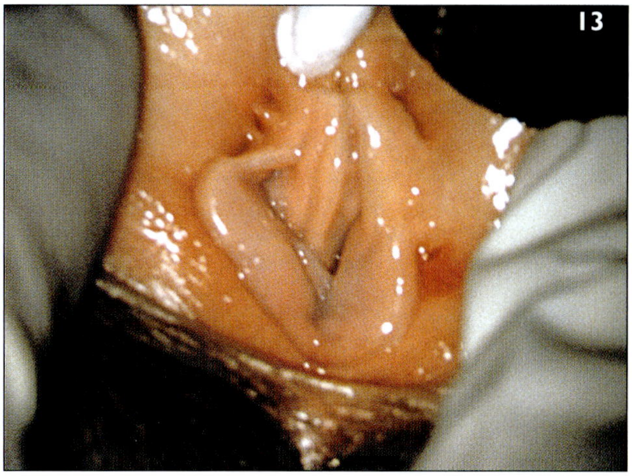

13 Vulvar inflammation and pain with cotton swab tip palpation of vestibular glands in a patient with vulvar vestibulitis.

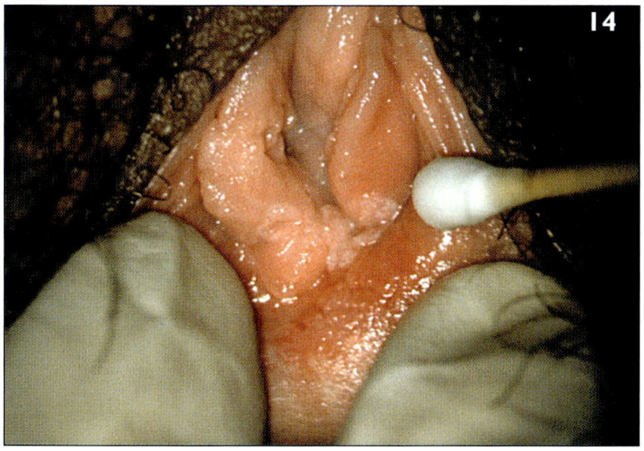

14 Discovery of condyloma acuminata in the introitus of a patient complaining of the recent onset of dyspareunia.

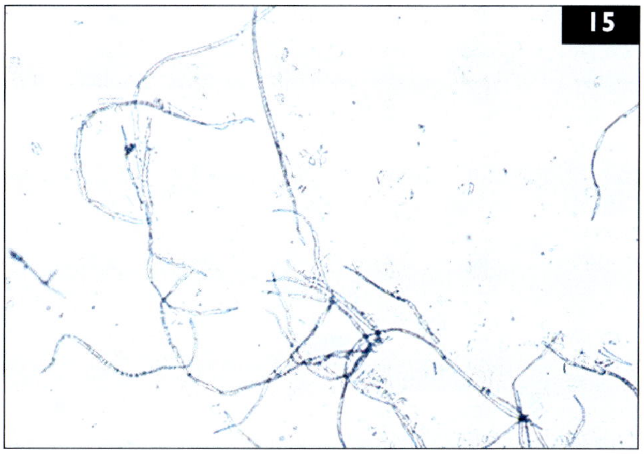

15 Cotton fibers seen on the microscopic examination of a saline preparation.

inspection. Patients complaining of dyspareunia can have vulvar vestibulitis (**13**) or condyloma acuminata at a site where there will be penile contact on attempted intercourse (**14**). If the vulva is not examined, this diagnosis will not be made. A hand-held magnifying glass or a colposcope is an invaluable diagnostic aid.

The vaginal examination is the next step in the examination progression. There is a protocol to be followed to give the physician the best chance of making a correct diagnosis and to make the best use of the available diagnostic aids.

The use of pH paper is a crucial component in the evaluation of a patient with vulvovaginal symptomatology. The vaginal pH is normally acidic, and an alkaline pH can be the first clue of the etiology of the problem. An alkaline pH is usually present in *Trichomonas* vaginitis, bacterial vaginosis, desquamative inflammatory vaginitis, estrogen lack vaginitis, and infections due to *Neisseria gonorrhea*, *Chlamydia trachomatis*, *Staphyloccus aureus*, and Group A streptococcus.

Some procedural guidelines must be followed for diagnostic accuracy. The mucous secretions of the endocervical canal can be alkaline, particularly at mid-cycle, so the lateral vaginal wall should be sampled, not the endocervix. Many physicians use tap water for speculum lubrication; if the pH of the tap water is alkaline, the physician should avoid using it in these patients.

A plastic spatula is a useful tool to gather vaginal secretions; these should be placed immediately on a drop of saline and 10% potassium hydroxide (KOH) on a microscopic slide. This procedure is superior to the use of a cotton swab. The cotton swab absorbs some of the vaginal sample and it increases the chance of cotton fibers being present in the specimen examined under the microscope (**15**). To the uninitiated microscopist, these fibers can be confused with *Candida*. True *Candida* has hyphae with protrusions on the body (**16**). The vaginal sample added to the KOH solution is immediately checked for the presence of a spoiled fish odor, a positive whiff test. Alternatively, samples can be transferred directly onto the glass microscopy slide from the small pool of discharge in the lower blade of the speculum after its removal from the vagina. For those physicians without pH paper or a microscope, there are test kits that can determine the presence of an excess number of *Gardnerella vaginalis* organisms, an alkaline pH, or if aromatic amines are present. These test kits can oversimplify the complexity of the varied pathology of patients with vulvovaginitis (**11**).

Correct use of the office microscope is the most important ingredient in making an accurate diagnosis at the time of the office visit. It can immediately confirm the diagnosis or lead the physician to order appropriate confirmatory laboratory testings. Unfortunately, in the United States, many physicians either no longer have a microscope in their office, because of Clinical Laboratory Improvement Amendment (CLIA) regulation, or seldom use the one that is present. In the United States, physicians are often poorly trained in medical school and residency in the use of the microscope and are poorly compensated for these services. Fortunately, there remains an emphasis on the use of microscopy in the European Union, with medical school, residency, and post-graduate medicine training available. A practicing physician should perform microscopic examinations of vaginal fluids of women with vulvovaginal symptoms and colposcopic examinations of women with abnormal cytology reports. Although the interpretation of the colposcopic examination is much more difficult than the microscopic evaluation of a wet mount smear, residents in the United States master this demanding technical skill because they have one-on-one training with a faculty colposcopist and they will be adequately compensated for this procedure when they go into practice[1].

Concerns about physicians' inability to diagnose infection properly is not limited to vulvovaginal disease. A recent article documented the decline in the quality of microbiology performed in the context of pulmonary infections, and a subsequent reduction in the reported percentage of pneumococcal pneumonia infections[2]. An editorial comment on this article summarized the factors leading to this decline[3]. The CLIA of 1988 in the United States eliminated house staff laboratories and one-on-one staff physician training of the house officers in the use of the microscope. Why has this shortcoming not been addressed? One physician's response summed up this lack of concern: 'If my patient appears to have pneumococcal pneumonia, I generally pick a fluoroquinolone, since this seems to be the best drug at the present time. If the patient does not have a pneumococcoal pneumonia, I usually pick a fluoroquinolone, because that seems to be the most reliably active drug against the other diagnostic possibilities.' The message is clear. The time-costly physician-performed evaluations will not alter the subsequent care of the patient. The same is not true for the physician caring for a woman with vulvovaginal disease. Correct use of the microscope will be an important guidance in the initial and subsequent care of these unfortunate symptomatic women.

The wet mount illustrations available in this book are meant to serve as aids to physicians using microscopes. Most of the microscopic examination can be accomplished by scanning the field under low-power magnification. The microscopist begins by looking at the spaces between the epithelial cells to survey the bacterial flora. Normally, the predominant bacteria are the lactobacilli, which present as long rods (**17**). These are more clearly seen with the KOH preparation, which makes the squamous cells 'ghost' cells (**18**). In contrast, an overgrowth of bacteria with few or no lactobacilli present is obvious in the next slide (**19**). The excessive numbers of bacteria can be more easily confirmed by higher power magnification on the KOH preparation slide, which reduces the background interference of vaginal squamous cells, turning them into ghost cells and eliminating any white cells (**20**). Next, the physician should evaluate the saline wet mount preparation for the presence of white cells. Few are present in uncomplicated *Candida* vaginitis (**21**) or in bacterial vaginosis (**19**). Not all patients

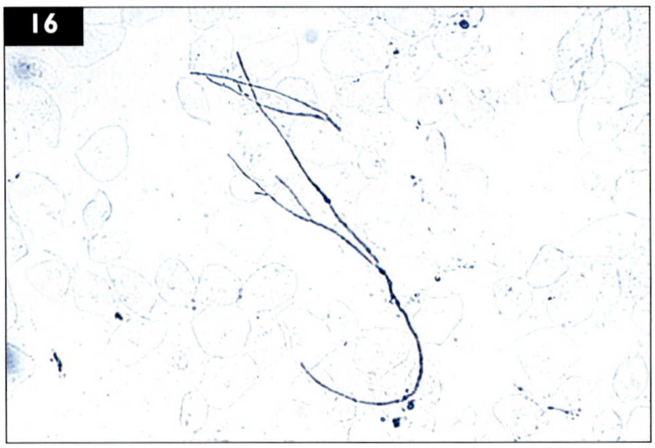

16 Hyphae seen on a potassium hydroxide preparation. Swelling on the hyphae are apparent.

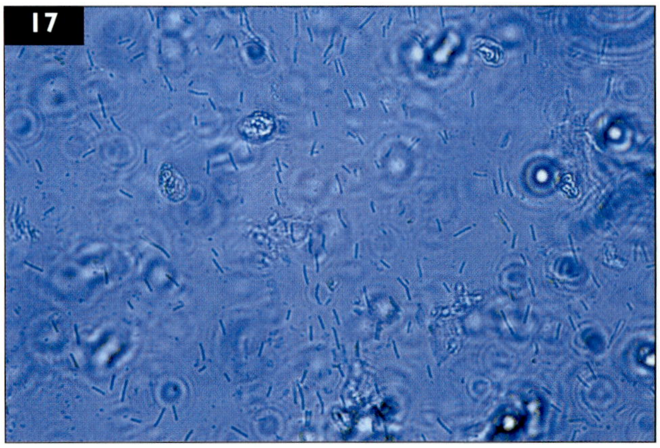

17 High-power view of a saline preparation showing a predominance of lactobacilli.

with a *Candida* vulvovaginitis present with such an easily identified microscopic image.

The symptomatic patient with a *Candida* vulvovaginitis will often exfoliate sheets of cells with hyphae tightly attached to them. This yields the microscopic picture of a scan of the saline preparation seen in Figure **22**. Repeated scans suggest hyphae. In contrast, these hyphae are much easier to detect when scanning the KOH preparation (**23**).

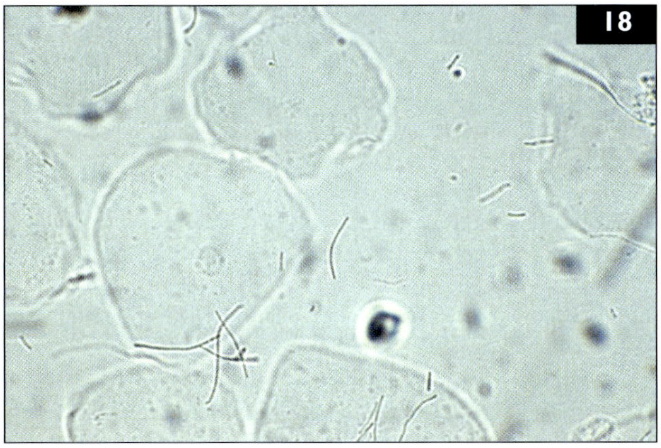

18 Predominance of lactobacilli on the high-power microscopic view of a potassium hydroxide preparation.

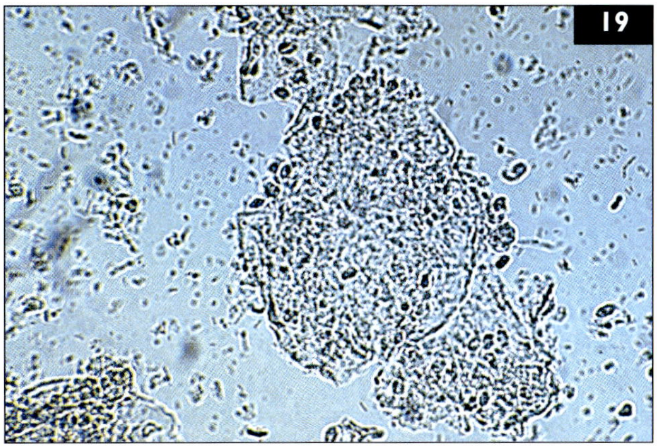

19 Saline preparation with clue cells, overgrowth bacteria, rare white blood cells, and few or no lactobacilli are seen.

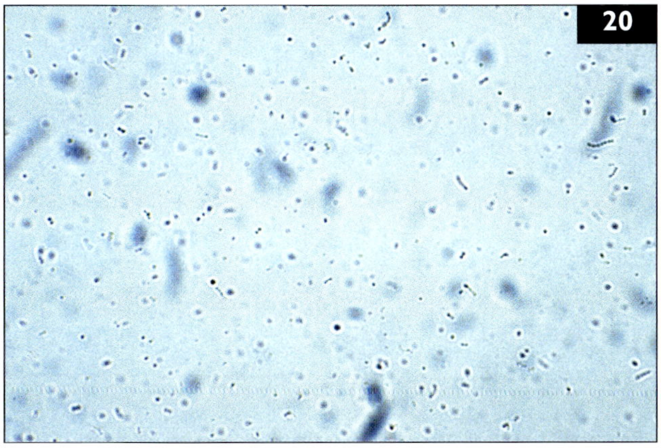

20 A potassium hydroxide preparation with an excessive number of bacteria and no lactobacilli seen.

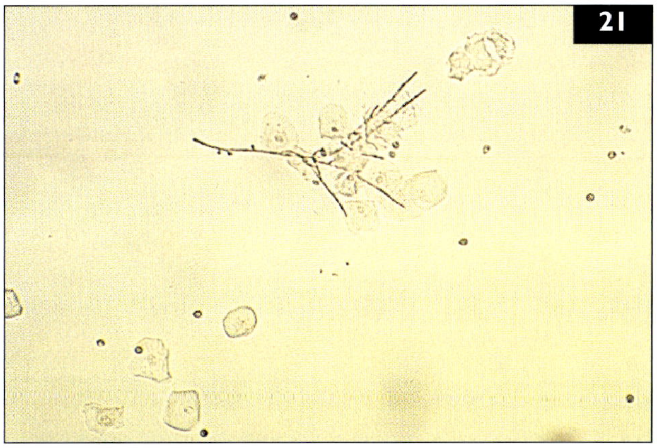

21 Few white blood cells present in a saline preparation of a woman with *Candida* vaginitis.

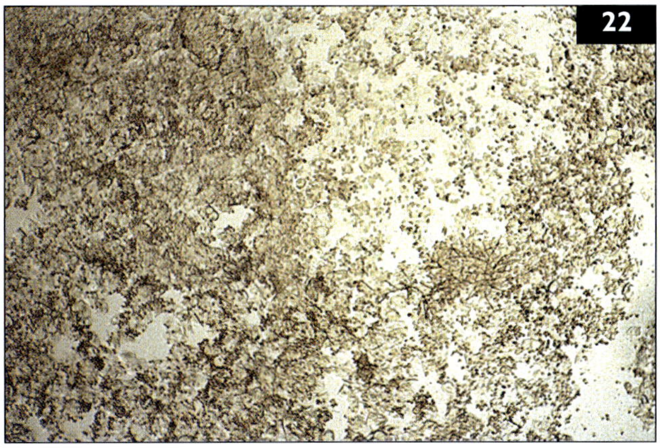

22 Microscopic view of a saline preparation. Sheets of squamous cells with hyphae attached to the cell mass. These can be missed by too rapid a scan by the microscopist.

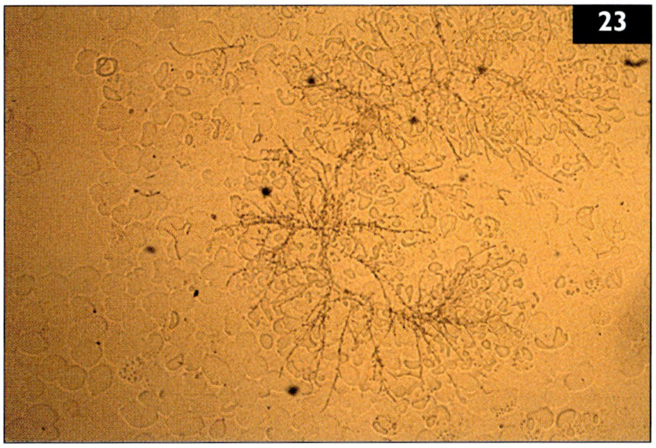

23 Microscopic view of vaginal secretions placed in a potassium hydroxide solution from the same patient as in **22**. The yeast forms are much more apparent.

Candida spores are difficult to detect on the saline preparation (**24**). The suspicion that these indistinct forms might be spores led to the higher-power examination of the KOH preparation (**25**). The spores are clearly seen and the culture grew *Candida glabrata*.

When increased numbers of white cells are present (**26**), the physician should consider the possibility of another infection being present. In this case, bacterial vaginosis plus *Trichomonas* vaginitis, which was confirmed by polymerase chain reaction (PCR).

There are other observations that could be confusing: Figure **27** shows a complex foreign object seen on both the saline and KOH preparations that could be mistaken for a clustered mass of hyphae due to an overwhelming *Candida* infection. In fact, the culture had no growth of *Candida*, and the patient gave a history of using a vaginal estrogen cream the night before this specimen was collected. Figure **28** is a high-power view of elements that could be construed to be spores. Again, there was no growth of any yeast on the culture, and the patient had a history of using an anti-fungal vaginal cream three nights before this specimen was obtained. These were globules of cream, not spores. Other clinical information can be obtained from histologic examination: Figure **29** shows the presence of spermatozoa on the saline preparation. This confirms the fact that a barrier method of contraception had not been employed.

LABORATORY TESTING WITH DELAYED RESULTS

Gram stain

In the past decade, there has been increasing use of the Gram stain to make the diagnosis of bacterial vaginosis. This has been a predictable diagnostic evolution. Many physicians either do not have a microscope available or do not avail themselves of the microscope in the outpatient setting in which they see patients. If this becomes the standard of care, there is no reason to keep KOH solution available and there is little impetus to check the vaginal pH. Three of the four components used to make an immediate diagnosis of bacterial vaginosis have been lost. To fill this diagnostic void, a vaginal smear is obtained and sent to the laboratory to be Gram stained and examined under oil immersion. These smears are

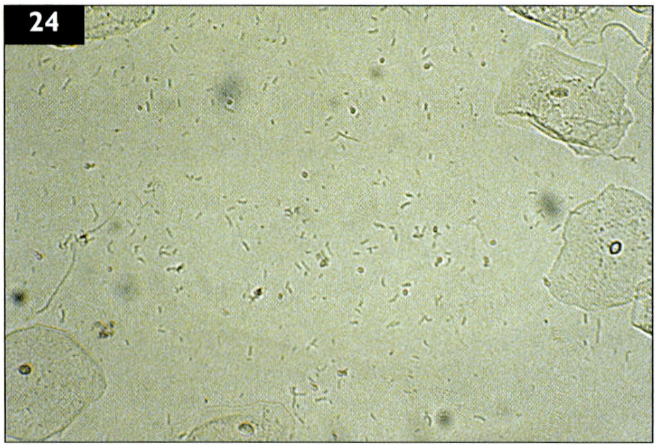

24 Microscopic examination of a saline preparation from a woman with a *Candida glabrata* vaginitis. The spores are barely visible.

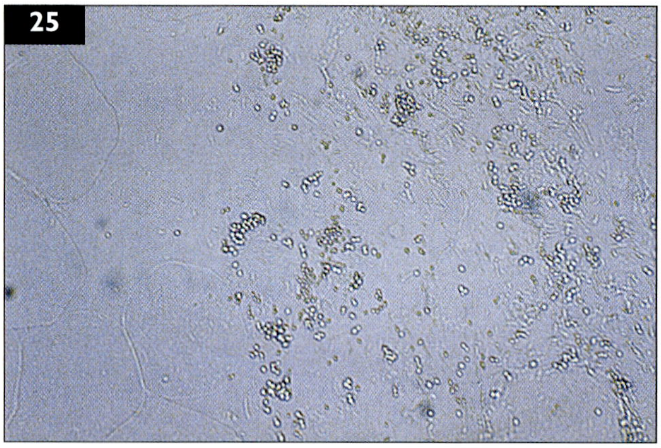

25 Microscopic examination of the vaginal secretions in a potassium hydroxide preparation under higher magnification from the same patient as in **24**. The spores are easily seen.

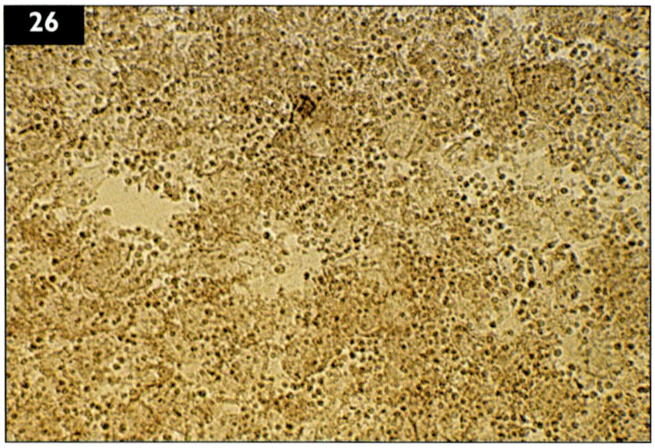

26 Increased number of white blood cells are present in a patient with bacterial vaginosis and *Trichomonas* vaginitis.

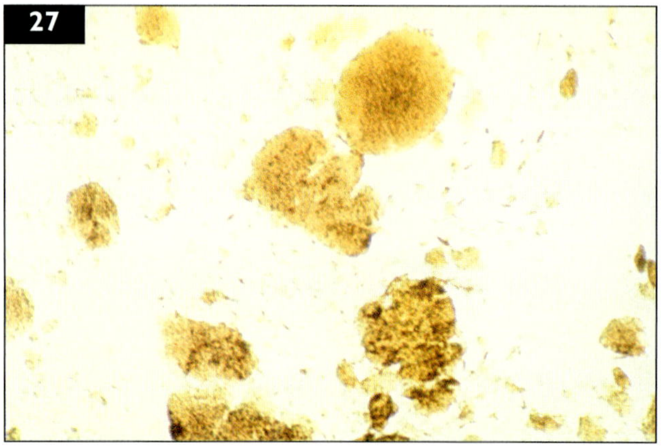

27 A complex foreign object present on the microscopic examination of a potassium hydroxide preparation, found to be the residual from a vaginal estrogen cream used the night before.

scored with a 10-point Nugent system. *Table 6* shows the basis for the system[4]. When the slide has been reviewed, the patients are diagnosed depending on the score: normal, a score of 0–3; intermediate, a score of 4–6; and bacterial vaginosis, a score of 7 or higher.

There are advantages to this system. The slides are read by trained microscopists, relieving the busy clinician of the task of office laboratory diagnosis. The slides can be saved, permitting future quality assessment. However, there are many disadvantages to this system. The primary problem is that the slide will not be read and reported until after the patient has left the outpatient setting. It makes no difference whether the turn-around time for the report is the next day or a week later, it requires either an additional phone call to the patient if the report is positive or, in the case of prenatal care, often a delay until the next scheduled visit. There are other problems: any microscopic scoring system will have variations between observers (witness the lack of uniformity of Pap smear reports with different cytotechnologists). In addition, the population diagnosed with bacterial vaginosis by Nugent criteria varies from those in whom the immediate clinical diagnosis is based upon the Amsel criteria with three of four present, an excessive uniform discharge, an alkaline pH, a positive whiff test, and more than 20% of the vaginal squamous cells noted to be clue cells[5]. In addition, the paucity of lactobacilli in a menopausal woman not taking estrogen raises her baseline score.

CULTURES

Obtaining cultures in women with symptomatic vulvovaginitis can be very helpful, and is important in women suspected of having *Candida* vulvovaginitis. If the physician performing microscopy sees yeast forms, the culture acts as a check to confirm the accuracy of the wet mount evaluation. This is a clinical aid, for studies have shown that practicing physicians have false-positive results for *Candida* with wet mount microscopy[6]. Most laboratories will select colonies growing on the initial blood agar plate and transfer these to Sabouraud's media to confirm the presence of yeast. Identification is usually given as 'albicans' or 'nonalbicans'. If no yeast forms are seen on microscopy in a woman with a chronic or recurrent problem, initial specimen plating can be requested on Sabouraud's agar, with an additional request to identify the *Candida* species.

In the standard vaginal culture on blood agar, a range of bacteria will be isolated and identified. If requested by the physician and there is no delay in transport of the specimen to the laboratory, the laboratory should also plate the specimen on Thayer Martin or equivalent special media so that the pathogen, *Neisseria gonorrhea*, will be isolated. Other Gram-positive aerobic organisms are possible problems and should not be considered part of the normal bacterial flora of the vagina. These include the Group A streptococcus, *Streptococcus pneumoniae*, and the coagulase-positive *Staphylococcus aureus*. Isolation of Group B streptococcus in the culture obtained at 35–37 weeks identifies candidates for the intrapartum use of antibiotics to lower the risk of newborn infection. Group B streptococcus is often recovered in nonpregnant patients, particularly in patients with desquamative vaginitis, but this laboratory finding neither establishes a diagnosis nor dictates treatment. The isolation of *Gardnerella vaginalis* does not confirm the diagnosis of

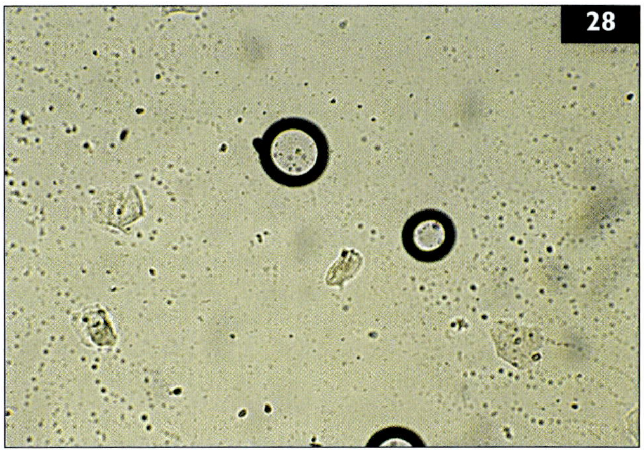

28 Fat globules in a potassium hydroxide preparation, found to be the residual of a vaginal anti-fungal cream used 3 nights before.

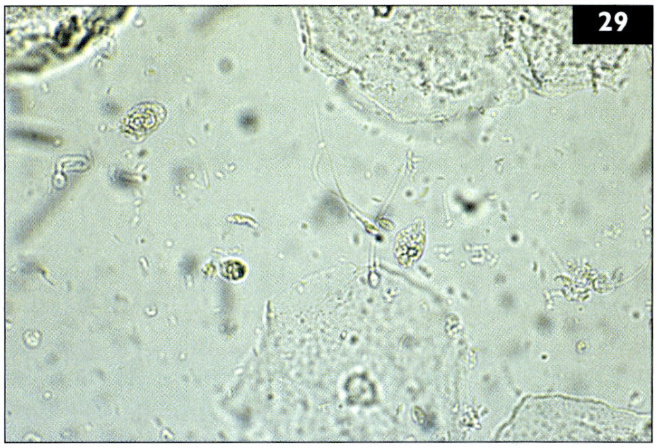

29 Spermatozoa seen on a saline preparation. This confirms a sexual exposure without the use of barrier contraception.

Table 6 Scoring system (0–10) for Gram-stained vaginal smears[a]

Score	*Lactobacillus* morphotypes	*Gardnerella* and *Bacteroides* spp. morphotypes	Curved Gram-negative variable rods
0	4+	0	0
1	3+	1+	1+ or 2+
2	2+	2+	3+ or 4+
3	1+	3+	
4	0	4+	

(Morphotypes are scored as the average number seen per oil immersion field. Note that less weight is given to curved Gram-variable rods. Total score = lactobacilli plus *G. vaginalis* and *Bacteroides* spp. plus curved rods. 0: no abnormal morphotypes present; 1: <1 abnormal morphotype present; 2: 1–4 morphotypes present; 3: 5–30 morphotypes present; 4: ≥30 morphotypes present.)

bacterial vaginosis. Bacteria will always be isolated from the vagina of a normal, healthy, sexually active woman, particularly lactobacilli. A common treatment error in women with recurrent or persistent vulvovaginitis in whom the first treatment trial has failed is to give systemic antibiotics against a species of bacteria that has been isolated. This treatment maneuver usually doesn't help the patient and often makes the clinical symptomatology worse.

Concern about other microorganisms dictates other culture strategies. These different media preparations have to be present in the office for use. Any healing sore of the vulva should have a sample of the exudate placed in transport media to be plated in a cell culture system in the laboratory to determine the presence of HSV-1 and -2. In the patient with an inflammatory vaginitis, a specimen should be placed in Diamond's media to determine the presence of *Trichomonas vaginalis*. These can be done even when trichomonads have been detected on the wet mount saline microscopic examination for quality control of the microscopy.

DNA probe testing

DNA probe test assays utilizing hybridization of a DNA probe with specificity for one of these microorganisms are commonly used to determine the presence of *Neisseria gonorrhea* and *Chlamydia trachomatis*. These are more convenient tests for the clinician to perform. In the case of *Neisseria gonorrhea*, they obviate the problem in the laboratory of special media and specific CO_2 environment levels to promote the best growth of the organism. For the clinician, it also removes the problem of specimen collection delay by the laboratory, which lowers the frequency of a positive culture. The usual microbiologic laboratory sequence is to identify the organism and then to do antibiotic susceptibilities. In the case of *Neisseria gonorrhea*, the frequency of absolute resistance to penicillin is high enough in the United States that the Centers for Disease Control recommendations for treatment do not include penicillin as an option[7]. The situation is different with *Chlamydia trachomatis*. Commercial laboratories do not have the resources available for cell culture, which is necessary to isolate this intracellular organism. For most physicians, DNA probe testing seems the logical answer. A sample for analysis can be easily obtained in the office when the patient is seen and a positive result will dictate therapeutic intervention for the patient and her sexual partner. There are two problems with the test however, sensitivity and specificity. Lessened sensitivity as compared to cell culture means that some women infected with *C. trachomatis* will be negative by DNA probe. Specificity is also a problem. Some women who are not infected with *C. trachomatis* will test positive due to binding of the DNA probe to a related DNA sequence in another microoganism. Since a positive test indicates acquisition of the organism from a sexual liaison outside of the supposedly monogamous couple relationship, a false-positive test puts unnecessary strain on the emotional health of the woman involved.

Polymerase chain reaction testing

Because of this problem, one future choice could be polymerase chain reaction (PCR) testing, because it is more sensitive and specific than DNA probe testing or culture. In the case of *C. trachomatis*, it is the ideal test, because it is the most sensitive and specific test available[8]. This means that infected women will almost always be detected so that treatment can be offered to them. Other organisms can also be identified by these techniques. *Trichomonas vaginalis* can be identified by PCR[9]. PCR can also be used to identify *Candida* species: one test now available can identify seven strains of *Candida*, including *C. albicans*, *glabrata*, *guilliermondi*, *kefyr*, *krusei*, *parapsilosis*, and *tropicalis*. To date, the test systems for *Candida* or *Trichomonas* have not been approved by the Food and Drugs Administration (FDA).

PCR is a more sensitive screen for *Candida* than culture. In one study of women with symptomatic vaginitis, culture was positive in 20 cases, while a PCR for *Candida albicans* was positive in 30[6]. This testing is particularly useful in women with recurrent *Candida* vaginitis when the cultures show no growth of *Candida* during treatment. Finally, PCR testing for *Mycoplasma hominis* and *Ureaplasma urealyticum* is a more sensitive test than the usual culture techniques. Again, this has not been FDA approved. Since these mycoplamas have been implicated in infertility and pregnancy loss, testing women with a history of spontaneous abortions or who are infertile may be warranted. Major concerns with PCR testing include the added costs of the tests and the applicability of this sensitive testing in populations with a low incidence of *Chlamydia* infection. In this situation, a false-positive test would be a problem.

Molecular analysis

Molecular analysis of the bacterial flora of the vagina in healthy women and in disease states provides more complete information of the microbial community[10,11]. The traditional culture methods may not identify the full range of bacteria, only those organisms most easily grown on culture. Cultivation-independent analysis by sequencing of 16S rRNA genes PCR-amplified is the technique now in use. At least one study using this method has identified *Atopobium vaginae*, an only recently described anaerobe resistant to metronidazole, as being present in the majority of patients with bacterial vaginosis[12]. This technology could open new vistas in our understanding of the pathophysiology of vaginal disease and lead to more effective future therapies.

Gene polymorphism testing

Gene polymorphism, the existence of more than one allele at a given specific genetic locus, can have clinical significance in vulvovaginal disease. Polymorphism is a common event. It is estimated that there are approximately 200,000 single nucleotide polymorphisms within the coding region of the estimated 80,000 human genes. To date, the authors have identified two polymorphisms that seem to be related to lower genital tract disease in women. There is a strong association between homozygous possession of allele 2 in intron 1 of the interleukin-1 receptor antagonist (IL1-ra) gene and the inflammatory vulvar condition, vulvar vestibulitis[13]. These women have a net increase in the pro-inflammatory cytokine interleukin-1β. Patients with a mannose-binding lectin (MBL) polymorphism at codon 54 of exon 1 associated with low MBL levels have an increased frequency of recurrent *Candida* vulvovaginitis[14]. Both of these polymorphisms, IL1-ra and MBL can be determined in the laboratory. Their detection could influence future therapies.

Chapter 4

Candida Vulvovaginitis

BACKGROUND

Candida vulvovaginitis is an important medical problem in the United States and other western countries. It is a common ailment. Symptomatic infections of the lower genital tract by *Candida* species are very common in women of reproductive age, and the incidence appears to be increasing. It is estimated that about 75% of women will have at least one symptomatic candidal vulvovaginal infection by the age of 40; 40–50% of these women will subsequently have a second episode, while about 5% will develop recurrent vulvovaginal candidiasis (RVVC), defined as at least four culture-verified symptomatic episodes within a 12-month period. Over the past decade, National Institutes for Health (NIH) investigators, whose study populations were predominantly young, sexually active women, have touted bacterial excess vaginitis or bacterial vaginosis as the number one cause of vaginitis in the United States. For any private practitioner, whose patient population is usually in monogamous relationships, *Candida* vulvovaginitis is a more frequent problem. Using the volume of over-the-counter (OTC) sales of anti-fungal vaginal preparations as a measure, the perception is overwhelming that vaginal fungal infections are the number one cause of symptomatic vulvovaginitis in the United States.

In addition to the frequency, this is a common medical burden to women, whether in the workplace or at home with the family. Although not life-threatening, *Candida* vulvovaginitis diminishes their quality of life with either increased vaginal discharge, itching, or burning. It can be an impediment to spontaneous heterosexual activity and for those women with frequent or persistent *Candida* infections, there is the often unexpressed fear, engendered by an emphasis in many women's magazine articles, that such symptoms could be a symptom of unrecognized human immunodeficiency virus (HIV) disease. *Candida* vulvovaginitis is not a trivial problem to symptomatic patients.

Physicians should be concerned about the presence of *Candida* in the vagina of HIV-infected women who have vaginitis symptoms. One recent study showed this population had an increased number of copies of cell-associated and cell-free HIV-1 RNA in cervicovaginal secretions when compared to HIV-infected women who were symptom-free[1]. This is probably related to the immunologic and inflammatory responses elicited by *Candida* infection on the vagina mucosa. Obviously, this is a population with a higher risk of HIV transmission.

MICROBIOLOGY

Candida albicans is the species that is present in approximately 80–90% of women with vulvovaginal candidiasis; *C. glabrata* is associated with 5–10% of cases, *C. tropicalis* in about 5%, while other *Candida* species (*C. krusei*, *C. parapsilosis*, *C. guilliermondii* and others) are only rarely identified[2]. This predominance of *C. albicans* may be due to the unique ability of the yeast form to undergo germination into a more invasive mycelial form. The other *Candida* species are not dimorphic and exist only in the yeast form.

C. albicans is often classified as a commensal microorganism since it can be readily isolated or otherwise identified using an ultrasensitive detection method, the polymerase chain reaction (PCR), from about 20% of healthy women who do not have any signs or symptoms of infection[3]. The mechanisms favoring *C. albicans* persistence in the vagina and preventing its conversion from a commensal microorganism to a pathogen remain incompletely elucidated. The predominance of *C. albicans* colonization in reproductive age women, and its infrequent occurrence in children or menopausal women who are not using estrogen supplements, strongly suggests that colonization is hormone-dependent. Estrogen promotes elevated glycogen production by vaginal epithelial cells which is the primary nutrient source for *Candida*. Conditions associated with elevated hormone production (pregnancy, diabetes, high estrogen-containing oral contraceptives) are all associated with increased *Candida* growth and a higher frequency of infection. The often-observed conversion of an asymptomatic *Candida* colonization to a symptomatic infection following the ingestion of antibiotics, strongly implicates the vaginal flora, particularly *Lactobacillus* species, in down-regulating the ability of *Candida* to proliferate. An intact cell-mediated immune system also appears to limit *Candida* vaginal proliferation (see below).

Whatever the triggering mechanism, symptomatic *C. albicans* vulvovaginal candidiasis is associated with transformation of the yeast forms into mycelia that are capable of invading the mucous membranes and eliciting clinical symptoms. Mutants of *C. albicans* that are unable to form mycelia are nonvirulent in animal models. However, an important point for clinicians to remember is that there is not necessarily a connection between the concentration of *C. albicans* that is observed microscopically and the extent of clinical symptoms. Some women with a heavy colonization may be totally asymptomatic, while others with just a low number of organisms might have florid symptoms. An explanation for this is that some women are allergic to components of *C. albicans* and manifest an immediate hypersensitivity response upon exposure to even low concentrations of organisms (see below). *Candida* cultures are mandatory to obtain an accurate clinical diagnosis.

Recent DNA fingerprinting of *C. albicans* isolates worldwide has led to the fascinating observation of geographical specificity. Organisms can be divided into five different groups called clades, based on the arrangement of their DNA sequences. Clades I, II, and III predominate in the eastern and mid-western United States, clade SA is predominant in South Africa, clade E is the predominant clade in Europe, while clades I and III are the major clades in the southern United States and in South America[4]. The relationship between colonization with a particular *C. albicans* clade and the likelihood of development of a symptomatic infection or the effectiveness of a particular treatment regimen remains to be examined.

IMMUNOLOGY

The immune defense mechanisms that protect against the conversion of vaginal *Candida* colonization into a symptomatic infection have been largely inferred from studies on mice and rats. Innate immunity appears to be the first line of defense against a *C. albicans* infection in these animals, followed by development of acquired cell-mediated immunity. There is also evidence that local vaginal immunity, as opposed to systemic immunity, is paramount in defense against experimental vaginal candidiasis.

Recent advances in identification of components of the innate immune system have broadened the understanding of the immunological mechanisms important for protection against vulvovaginal candidiasis in women. Mannose is the most common monosaccharide present on the surface of *C. albicans*; it is rarely present on the mammalian cell membrane. Therefore, chains of mannose sugars (mannan) are immunogenic and anti-mannan antibodies have been identified in most individuals. These antibodies may function in the systemic immune defense against *Candida* by promoting opsonization and complement activation. However, since most women with vulvovaginal candidiasis are positive for these antibodies, their utility in preventing a vaginal infection by this organism in humans remains uncertain; a component of the innate immune system that also recognizes mannose residues appears to be important in anti-*Candida* immunity. Mannose-binding lectin (MBL) is a protein present in the circulation and other biological fluids that specifically recognizes mannose residues on microbial surfaces. Consequences of MBL binding to microorganisms are activation of the complement cascade on the microbial surface leading to cell lysis and opsonization by phagocytic cells with cell surface receptors for MBL or complement components. MBL binding to *C. albicans* has been demonstrated. Furthermore, MBL was identified in vaginal secretions and women with RVVC were shown to be deficient in vaginal MBL levels[5]. This indicates that MBL is an important component of the vaginal immune defense against *Candida*. The decreased vaginal MBL concentrations were shown to be associated with possession of a variant allele of the MBL gene, suggesting a genetic basis for RVVC in some women.

Toll-like receptors are also components of the innate immune system. They are molecules on the surface of phagocytic cells that react with specific molecular patterns that are unique to microorganisms. Microbe binding to toll-like receptors results in activation of pro-inflammatory cytokine production, stimulation of phagocytosis, and induction of cell-mediated immunity. Two of the toll-like receptors, TLR2 and TLR4, have been shown to recognize *C. albicans*.

Resistance to development of a *Candida* vulvovaginal infection in laboratory animals is dependent on phagocytic activity that is stimulated by production of pro-inflammatory cytokines that activate cell-mediated immunity (Th1 cytokines) and inhibited by production of anti-inflammatory cytokines (Th2 cytokines). Results of human investigations have paralleled these studies in that induction of local Th1 immunity appears to be protective against candidiasis, while a predominant Th2 immune response is associated with increased susceptibility to develop a clinical *Candida* infection[6]. Recent studies have demonstrated that vaginal epithelial cells also produce low levels of cytokines in response to *C. albicans* and may, therefore, also contribute to the immune defense against vulvovaginal candidiasis[7].

As mentioned above, an intact cell-mediated immune system is essential for prevention of a symptomatic vulvovaginal *Candida* infection. Several different areas of investigation have now provided mechanisms to explain this observation. One of these mechanisms appears to involve *Candida* mannan. T cell-derived antigen binding molecules (TABM) are components of T lymphocytes released during an immune response. They are antigen-specific and are associated with the immunosuppressive cytokine, transforming growth factor β (TGF-β). Women with RVVC were shown to have increased levels of TABM specific for *Candida* mannan, and binding of mannan to TABM resulted in the release of bioactive TGF-β and an inhibition of the cell-mediated immune response to *C. albicans*[8]. This suggests that a *Candida* vaginal infection and the release of mannan which binds to mannan-specific TABM may promote the release of the associated TGF-β. This, in turn, inhibits the local cell-mediated immune response and further permits *Candida* proliferation. Women with a genetic deficiency in MBL production would seem to be at greatest risk for TABM-mediated immunosuppression and RVVC due to a relative inability to bind up sufficient quantities of mannan to prevent this process.

Peripheral blood mononuclear cells from women with active RVVC are less responsive to *Candida* antigens *in vitro* than are samples from the same women when in remission or samples from control women. One mechanism to explain this observation is the elevated release of prostaglandin E_2 (PGE_2) from macrophages of RVVC patients in response to this microorganism[9]. PGE_2 is a potent suppressor of cell-mediated immunity and an enhancer of vascular permeability. In the presence of PGE_2 *Candida* present in the vagina can proliferate to higher concentrations. Furthermore, PGE_2 promotes the yeast to mycelium transition of *C. albicans*, thereby increasing its ability to invade mucosal tissues[10]. The capacity of *C. albicans* to promote its persistence by also producing PGE_2 has been demonstrated[11].

Thus, in those women that are harboring *C. albicans* in their vagina as a commensal microorganism, any mechanism that increases vaginal PGE_2 levels would promote *Candida* proliferation and germination, and increase susceptibility to a symptomatic infection. One mechanism that increases vaginal PGE_2 concentrations is a vaginal allergic response. An allergic reaction can be elicited in the vagina of sensitized women by *Candida*, other microbial products, intrinsic semen components or allergens ingested by the male sexual partner and present in his semen, components of vaginal medications or contraceptive products, or environmental allergens[12]. The local release of histamine stimulates high levels of PGE_2 production by macrophages and results in the local inhibition of cell-mediated immunity. It can easily be seen, therefore, that an underlying vaginal hypersensitivity reaction may be an underlying cause of vulvovaginal candidiasis. In these cases, treatment with an anti-fungal medication will bring only temporary relief of symptoms, but if the underlying allergic response is not addressed the woman will remain highly susceptible to recurrences.

Human semen contains the highest concentrations of PGE_2 of any body fluid. It is not surprising, therefore, that frequent sexual intercourse may also promote development of a symptomatic *Candida* infection in those women who are harboring this microbe as a commensal. In addition, in cases of a man with a genital tract allergy, the transfer of allergen plus the corresponding IgE antibodies to the female sexual partner may result in the induction of an allergy-related *Candida* vaginitis in a nonallergic woman[13].

The ability of *C. albicans* to inhibit the expression of genes involved in other immune defense mechanisms such as defensins production, neutrophil killing, and apoptosis has also been suggested based on experimental investigations. Thus, *C. albicans* has evolved numerous strategies to evade immune destruction and to persist within the vagina.

DIAGNOSIS

There are a number of myths about the diagnosis of *Candida* vulvovaginitis. The most common and overriding belief by doctors is that *Candida* vulvovaginitis is an easy diagnosis to make, either by a patient's phone description of symptoms, the gross appearance of a vaginal discharge at the time of the vaginal examination, or the quick perusal of a hanging drop preparation of vaginal secretions with an office microscope. One study of Obstetric-Gynecologic residents at a major medical center reported only half of the patients thought by these physicians to have a *Candida* vaginitis had the diagnosis confirmed by culture or PCR testing[14]. Physician overestimates of the frequency of vaginal infections are additionally fueled by the observations in gynecologic articles that women can have a *Candida* infection when yeast forms are not seen on the microscopic examination. The emphasis is always upon under-diagnosis, not over-diagnosis.

Patients also overestimate their ability to self-diagnose a vaginal *Candida* infection. The best study at a single investigation site showed only 37.4% of women who were sure they had a *Candida* vaginitis were actually culture positive[15].

The diagnosis of *Candida* vulvovaginitis begins with a history, searching for clues. The general questioning approach has been detailed in Chapter 3 with two categories, those patients with the initial episode and those with recurrent problems. In acute cases, the focus should be upon recent or current antibiotic use, while in recurrent situations, the physician should determine if the problem occurs with consistency in the premenstrual period, and does sexual activity initiate or increase the symptoms. Another historical aid is the patient's allergic tendencies, i.e. asthma, hay fever, eczema, or chronic sinusitis. This can identify a woman more at risk for an allergic vulvovaginitis who may be superinfected with yeast.

The physical examination is important, not to confirm the diagnosis of *Candida* vulvovaginitis, but to suggest alternative diagnoses and to focus upon anatomic sites for specimen collection. Three-quarters of the women with vulvar vestibulitis have an excessive discharge and have often been repeatedly treated by physicians for a nonexistent *Candida* vulvovaginitis that will not be confirmed by culture. When inspecting the vulva before the insertion of a speculum, pressure with a cotton-tipped applicator at vestibular gland sites will produce excruciating pain and confirm the diagnosis of vulvar vestibulitis (**30**). If the inspection of the vulva of a

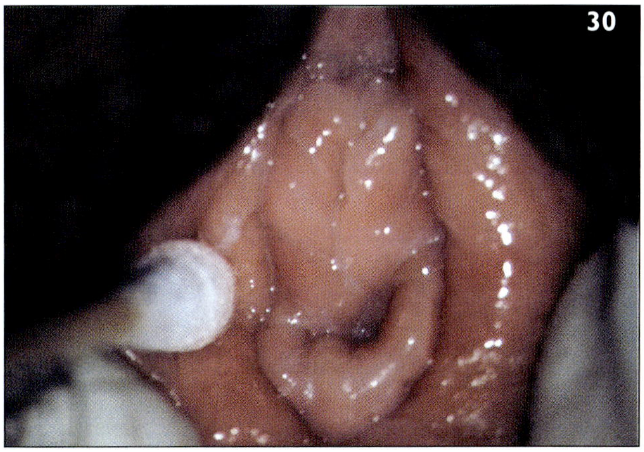

30 Inspection of the vulva before the insertion of a speculum. Pressure at the vestibular gland site results in severe pain and confirms the diagnosis of vulvar vestibulitis.

post-menopausal woman reveals inflamed tissue with adherent white plaques (**31**), the plastic spatula should be employed to scrape off a tissue sample to be placed upon a drop of 10% potassium hydroxide (KOH) to examine under the microscope. A more inflamed vulva with white plaques is shown in Figure **32**. In each case, the presence of hyphae on microscopic examination confirms the diagnosis (**33**). This quick diagnostic step is important, for some women have a similar vulvar picture not due to yeast (**34**).

The vaginal examination combines both inspection and specimen collection. Physicians in some cities should not use tap water to ease speculum insertion because at these sites the water is very alkaline, which can lead to an inaccurate determination of the vaginal pH. The care providers should follow a defined order of specimen collection. They should use a plastic spatula to collect a sample of vaginal secretions to place upon a drop of saline and then a drop of 10% KOH on slides. This reduces, but does not eliminate, all particulate matter on a slide that can be mistaken by inexperienced microscopists for a *Candida* form. In addition, it can be a helpful aid in the evaluation of the symptomatic woman who has started her menstrual period. Figure **35** shows the saline preparation of such a patient; Figure **36** shows how KOH eliminates the red cells from the microscopic field and hyphae can be seen. Figure **37** shows debris on the slide that a harried clinical microscopist can mistake for a *Candida* form; Figure **38** shows the cotton threads teased from a cotton-tipped applicator and added to a drop of saline on the slide, and Figure **39** shows a whirl of cotton fibers exfoliated from an applicator used to collect a specimen.

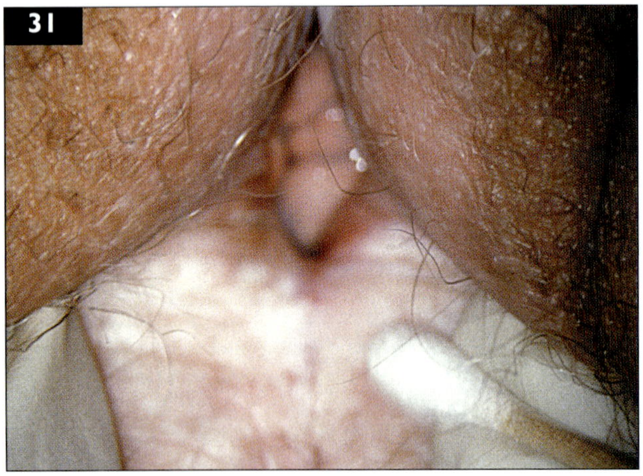

31 A menopausal woman with lichen sclerosis. A plastic spatula should be gently scraped over these plaques to secure tissue to be placed in a drop of 10% potassium hydroxide on a microscopic slide.

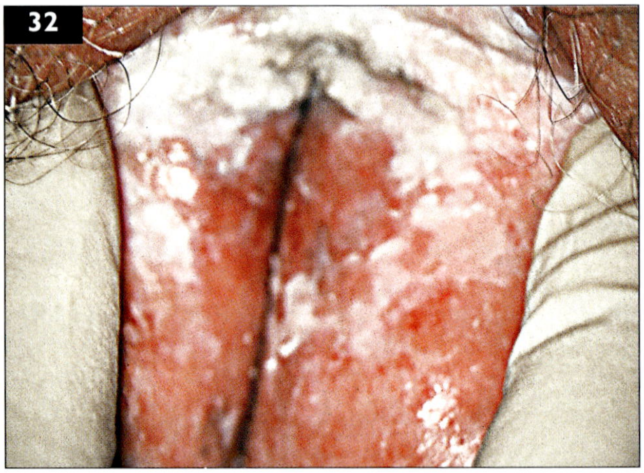

32 A more inflamed vulva with white plaques noted.

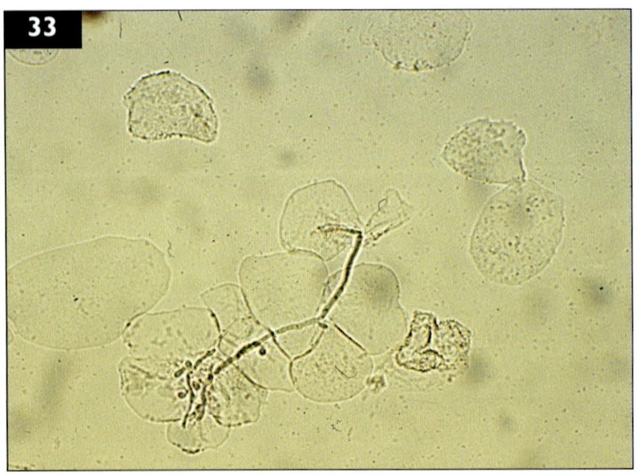

33 The microscopic examination of a vulvar scraping and potassium hydroxide suspension. The presence of hyphae confirms the diagnosis of *Candida* vulvitis.

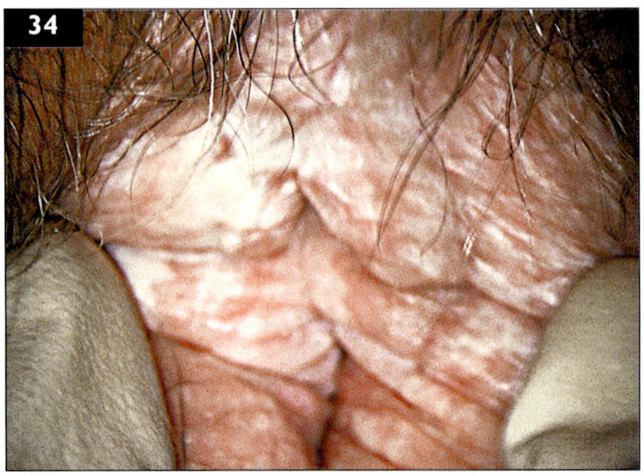

34 An inflamed vulva with white exudate. Microscopic examination of the potassium hydroxide preparation showed no hyphae, and culture had no growth of yeast.

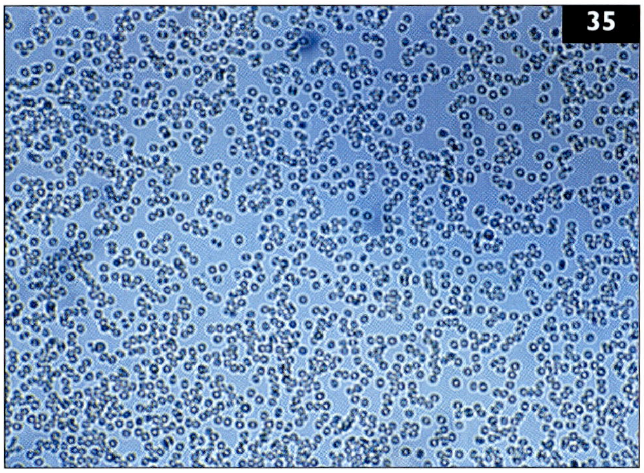

35 Microscopy of a saline preparation of a woman with symptoms, who has started her menses.

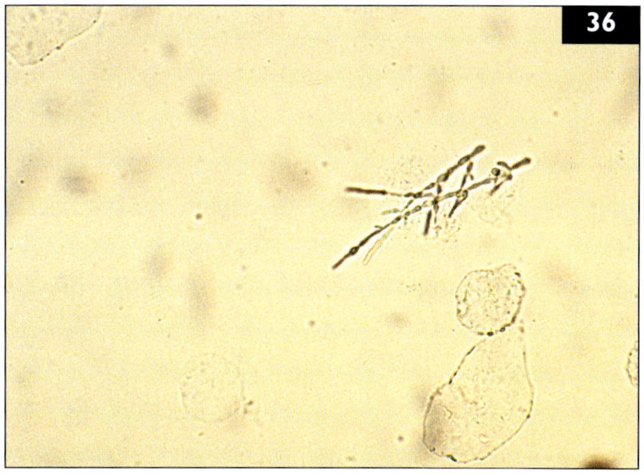

36 The same microscopic field as **35** in a potassium hydroxide preparation. The red blood cells have been lysed and hyphae are visible.

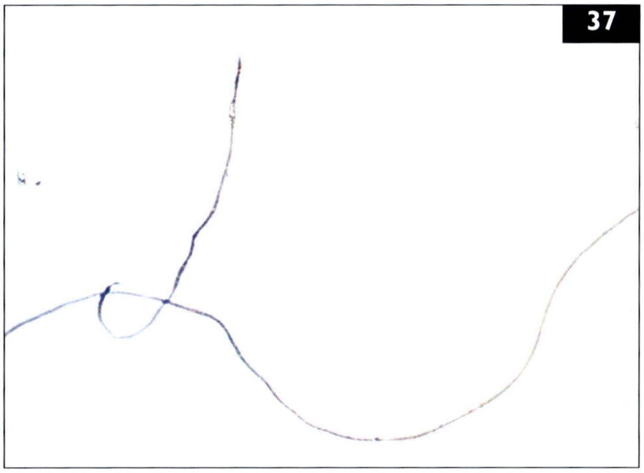

37 Debris on a slide, sometimes mistakenly assumed to be a *Candida* form.

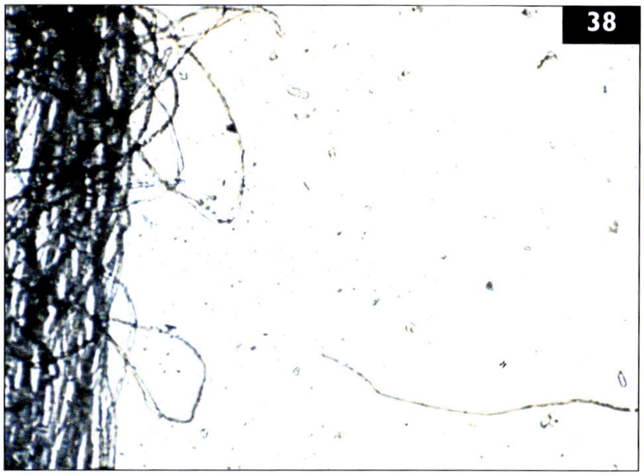

38 Large numbers of cotton threads extruded from a cotton-tipped applicator.

39 Large numbers of cotton threads found on microscopic examination when the cotton applicator was rubbed against the vulva to obtain a specimen.

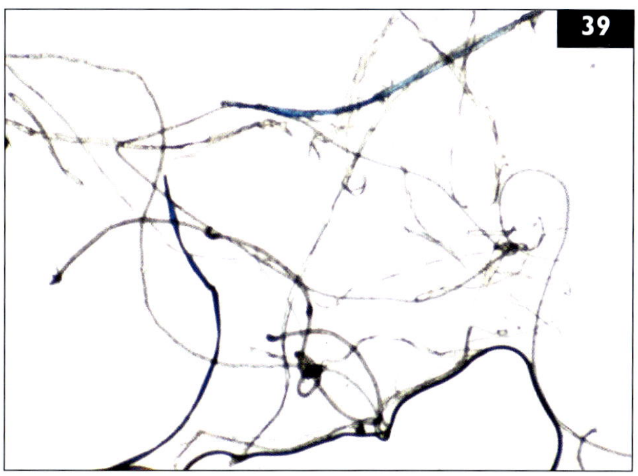

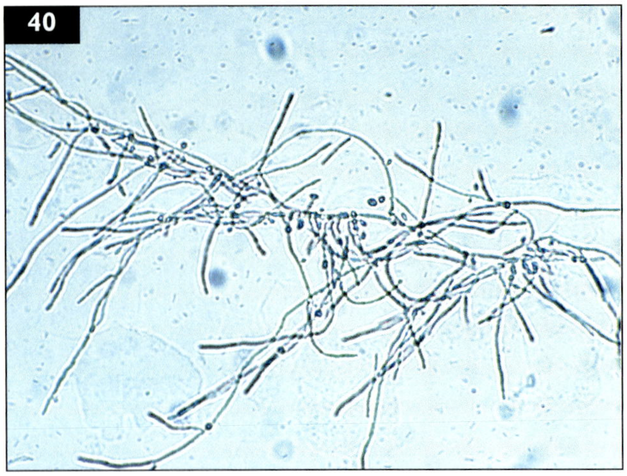

40 A complex mass of hyphae seen in a potassium hydroxide preparation of a vaginal sample of a woman with *Candida* vulvovaginitis. The contrast with **39** is obvious. The cotton threads are smooth without the rounded expansion sites, the buds seen on the yeast forms. (Being a child of the 1930s, it reminds the author of the depiction of Popeye's biceps!)

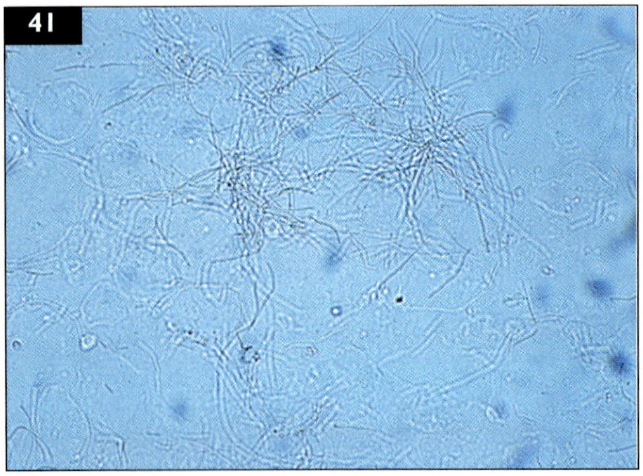

41 A tangled mass of long filamentous lactobacilli. The culture grew lactobacilli, no yeast.

Figure **40** shows a complex intertwined mass of hyphae, while Figure **41** shows a mass of long filamentous forms of lactobacilli. No buds are seen on these bacterial forms. The contrast between the evidence of a *Candida* infection (see **40**) and no *Candida* infection (**39, 41**) is striking.

Using the plastic applicator does not eliminate the possibility of finding cotton threads on the slide, it only reduces the numbers. Figure **42** shows a single strand of cotton found on a hanging drop microscopic examination when the plastic spatula was used to obtain the specimen. These strands can be found in vaginal pads and tampons as well, or be present after prior cleansing of the slides and will not be completely eliminated by the use of a plastic spatula. Figure **43** shows a solitary fungal form on microscopic examination. Again, the contrast with Figure **42** is obvious.

Most women with a *Candida* vaginitis will not have an inflammatory wet mount smear, but the hyphae can be hard to detect in the midst of squamous cells (**44**). There can be an inflammatory microscopic picture in a woman with a vaginal yeast infection that further obscures the presence of hyphae (**45, 46**). The diagnosis in these hard-to-determine cases can be confirmed by viewing the KOH preparation, which diminishes the backdrop of squamous cells and white cells, reducing them to ghost cells (**47**). The same problem with the saline preparation is seen in women with a *Candida* vaginitis with only spores present. These spores are not visible on the saline preparation (**48**). In another patient with fewer squamous cells present on the saline preparation, the spores are visible in the open area between the squamous cells (**49**). The spores are visible in the KOH

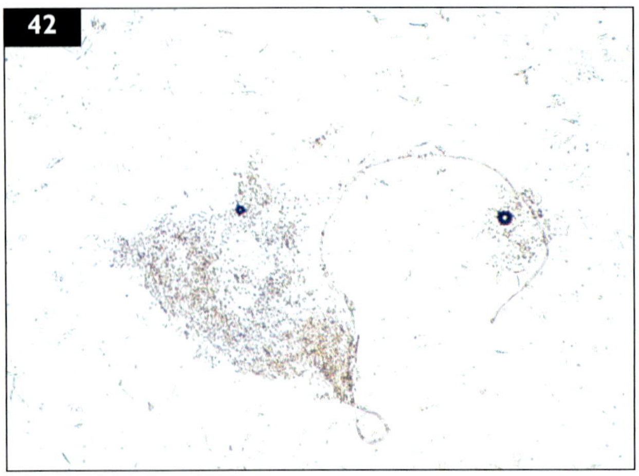

42 A single strand of cotton fiber found in a hanging drop suspension when a plastic spatula was used to obtain vaginal secretions.

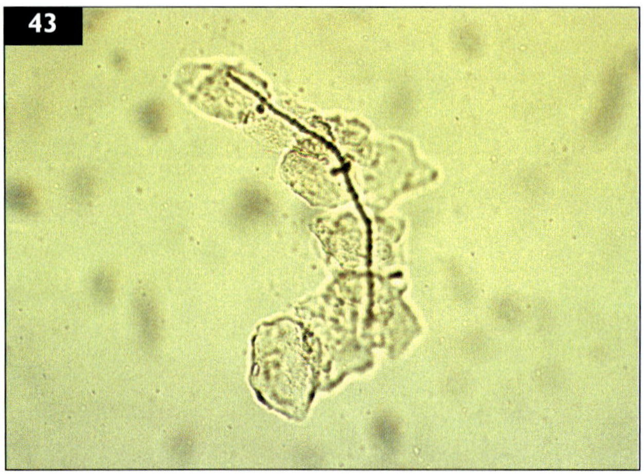

43 A single hyphal form. Buds are apparent and stand in marked contrast with the smooth surface form of the cotton thread.

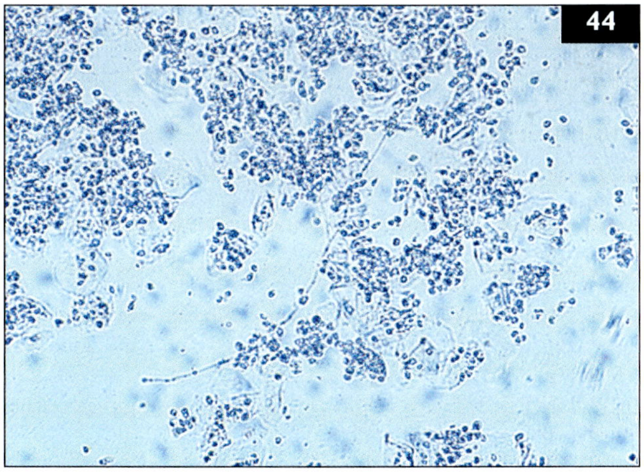

44 Hyphae are difficult to detect because of their attachment to vaginal squamous cells in a saline hanging drop suspension.

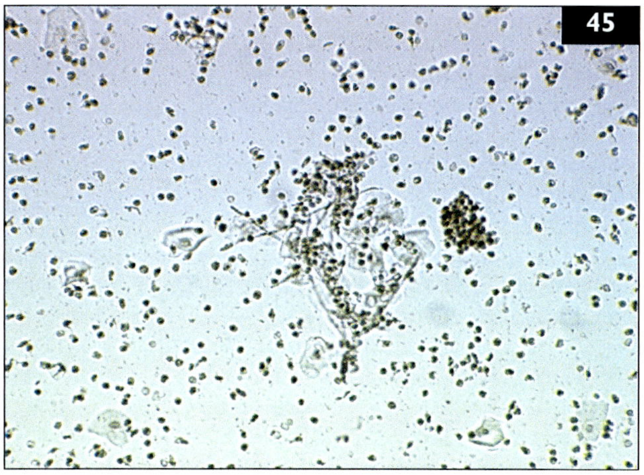

45 The saline preparation of an inflammatory vaginitis in which hyphae are seen with difficulty.

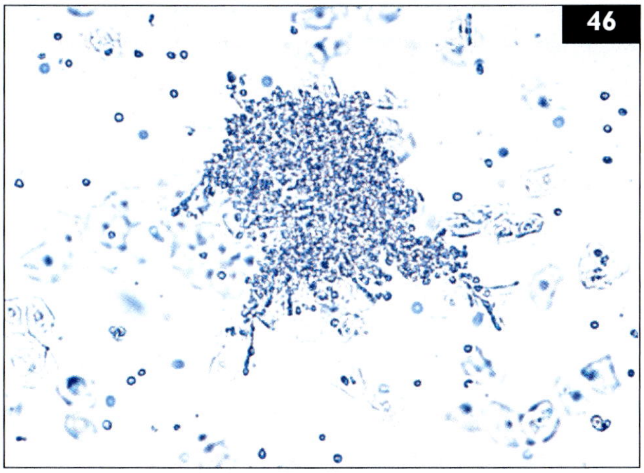

46 Another inflammatory saline preparation in which hyphae are seen with difficulty.

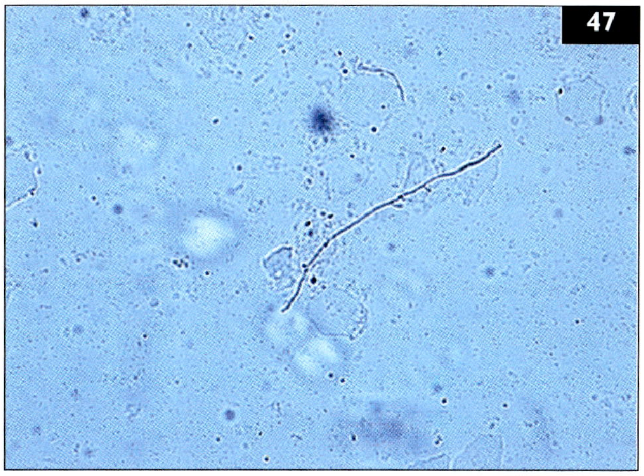

47 Hyphae easily seen in a potassium hydroxide preparation from the patient shown in **45**, in which the squamous cells become 'ghost' cells.

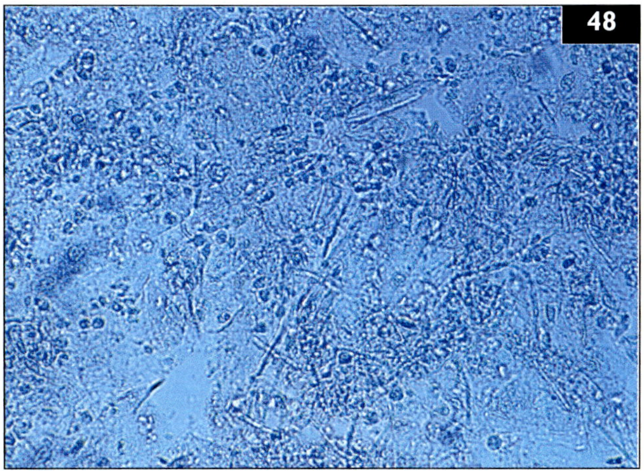

48 Microscopic examination of saline preparation. No spores are visible.

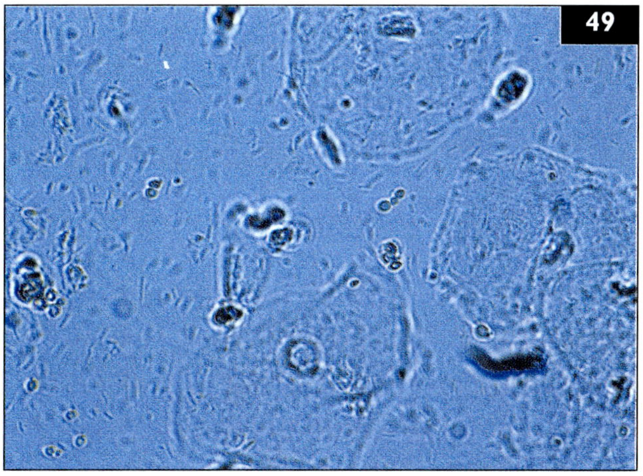

49 Microscopic examination of a saline preparation in which there are fewer squamous cells. Spores are visible. The culture grew *Candida glabrata*.

preparation (**50, 51**). In these women, a culture is particularly important to identify the possible presence of nonalbicans *Candida*.

Next, a cotton applicator should be used to sample secretions from the lateral vaginal wall and applied to the pH paper. Most patients with a *Candida* vulvovaginitis have an acid vaginal pH. A sample of vaginal fluid should then be obtained for a bacterial and *Candida* culture. The culture is important in acute cases, because it verifies the microscopic and clinical diagnosis. If positive, the patient will be empowered in the future to believe she has a vaginal yeast infection if a similar set of symptoms recurs. In women with chronic or recurrent vaginitis, the culture is of particular importance. For many women, the culture will be negative, indicating that an active *Candida* infection is not the cause of their symptomatology. In addition to confirming the diagnosis in culture-positive women, the isolates can be identified to determine the presence of nonalbicans *Candida*, particularly *Candida glabrata*.

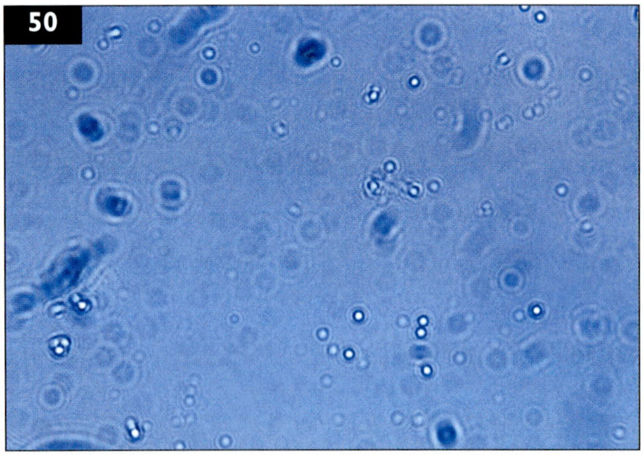

50 Spores become identifiable in a potassium hydroxide preparation.

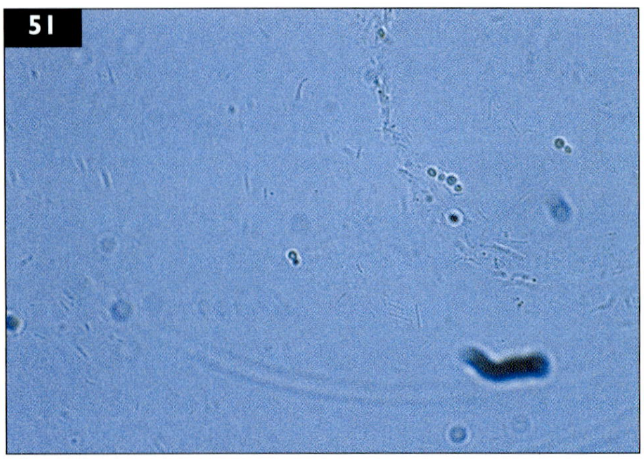

51 Easily identifiable spores in a potassium hydroxide preparation. The culture grew *Candida glabrata*.

TREATMENT

There is a number of 'reflex' therapeutic decisions by either physicians or members of the medical care team that can be disadvantageous to the patient. Some women, particularly those who have used anti-fungal creams repeatedly, can develop a vaginal allergic reaction, a contact dermatitis. They report intense vaginal burning with the application of the vaginal cream that can persist overnight. Sometimes, incorrect phone advice is given by a member of the medical care team. This vaginal burning is not a normal or an expected response that indicates the medicine is vigorously attacking the yeast. These women should never be counseled to continue using this vaginal product. Instead, they should be advised to immediately wash out as much of the vaginal medication as possible and not to use it again.

There is a wide range of local and oral medications available for use in a woman with an initial acute *Candida* vulvovaginitis. A partial listing of those available in the United States and the UK at the time of publication is presented in *Table 7*[16]. There is no evidence that any one of these regimens is superior to another. The choice for the physician should be based upon considerations of convenience of the selected therapeutic regimen for the patient.

There has been a number of predictable therapeutic trends with local vaginal anti-fungal medications over the past few decades. The azoles have almost entirely replaced the polyene preparation, nystatin, because of their increased activity against albicans, the most common isolate in women with *Candida* vulvovaginitis. This increased anti-fungal activity, plus the packaging of larger individual doses in creams, suppositories, and vaginal tablets has resulted in a reduction in the treatment regimen from 14 days to a 3-day or single dose in some instances. For albicans, resistance to the azoles is almost unheard of, with rare cases reported in HIV-positive patients. There is no convincing clinical evidence that any one local azole is superior to another. These facts should be kept in mind when evaluating patients that fail therapy. Larger doses of a different azole used for a longer period will probably not increase the treatment success rate. The physician must also keep in mind there are side-effects seen with these local medications.

The azoles used locally can be irritating to the vagina, particularly in the higher-dose single vaginal application regimens. A more common local vaginal irritant is propylene glycol, a chemical preservative used in most vaginal creams and suppositories. For the propylene glycol-sensitive patient, this local inflammatory reaction is a severe one with patients reporting debilitating vaginal burning. The patient and every member of the medical care team responsible for her care should be aware that this is an adverse reaction, not a normal response. If such patients need vaginal anti-fungal medications in the future, they should try a vaginal anti-fungal cream free of propylene glycol or one of the vaginal anti-fungal tablets. In addition, the oral azoles ketoconazole, fluconazole, and itraconzole are now available. They are popular choices with fastidious women who either do not relish placing foreign objects in the vagina or do not like the increased messiness of the vaginal cream or suppository. Fluconazole has largely replaced the original azole, ketoconazole, because only a single dose is needed. Studies have shown therapeutic levels of the fluconzaole in the vagina 3 days after oral administration. Liver toxicity can be seen with a prolonged daily dosing regimen, particularly in patients with underlying liver disease.

For the woman who remains symptomatic after treatment, or the woman with repeated vulvovaginal symptomatology, the treatment decisions are much more complicated.

The first step in the care of these patients is to determine the diagnosis. This point needs to be stressed, for over three-quarters of the symptomatic women referred to the vaginitis clinic at Cornell with a chronic yeast vulvovaginitis have no yeast present on vaginal culture. The basis for this determination is the culture. The physician should check that the clinical laboratory will be sure to plate the specimen on Sabouraud's media and that they can identify the species isolated. For the patient with negative cultures, the potential sources of problems and therapeutic approaches are detailed in Chapter 12: Allergic Vulvovaginitis.

Pregnant women with acute *C. albicans* vulvovaginitis place therapeutic restrictions upon the physician ordering medications. Fetal abnormalities have been documented in pregnant women receiving long-term fluconazole treatment. Although no newborn abnormalities have been noted in pregnant women who have received the single dose therapy prescribed for acute *C. albicans*, the noted teratogenic effects should put this drug off the list of acceptable drugs for pregnant women. Local azoles or nystatin can be prescribed.

There are several diagnostic steps to take in the patient with recurrent or chronic vulvovaginitis who is culture-positive for *C. albicans*. The physician should document the relationship to increased symptomatology and sexual activities, and determine whether or not the male is circumcised. Although circumcision is done in nearly all newborn males in the United States, there are many immigrant males from around the world who have not been circumcised. Circumcision is not routinely practiced in the UK. In chronic cases of vulvovaginitis, it is wise to have someone examine and culture the often symptomatic men. Even males who do not harbor *Candida* can contribute to a persistent chronic *C. albicans* vulvovaginitis. Some women are allergic to substances in the ejaculate and the vaginal reaction with an increase in local PGE_2 production creates an environment favorable to the growth of *Candida*. There are other factors associated with intercourse that can be deleterious. Some women are allergic to the latex in condoms or the nonoxynol nine that coats most commercial products, and this also can increase local PGE_2 production. These are clinical situations where modifications in sexual practices to avoid the woman's exposure to these allergens can be helpful. There is also evidence that oral sexual contact can be responsible for some cases of recurrent *Candida* vulvovaginitis. These matters must be explored in the history taking followed by an oral cavity examination and culture of the sexual partner, if indicated.

There should be caution and careful consideration given to the therapeutic regimen for women with a persistent and recurrent vulvovaginitis. Although treatment failures are not due to *C. albicans* resistance, those with recurrent infections seem to do better with more than one dose of fluconazole or 10–14 days of local vaginal treatment. Physicians shouldn't disregard the long half-life of fluconazole and the fact that therapeutic levels are present in vaginal fluids 3 days after the oral administration of this drug. The daily prescription of this drug for 15–30 days makes no sense. In addition to not adding any therapeutic advantage, this dosage regimen increases the possibility of an adverse liver reaction. The alternative choices of care for women with the supposed *Candida* hypersensitivity syndrome have not proven effective. The Spartan-like restrictive low carbohydrate diet combined with the concomitant use of nystatin popularized by the book, *The Yeast Connection*, was no better than placebo when evaluated in a careful clinical trial[17]. Attempts to promote a

Table 7 Therapy for vaginal candidiasis

Drug	Formulation	Dosage regimen
Topical agents		
Butoconazole*	2% cream	5 g × 3 days
Clotrimazole*	1% cream	5 g × 7–14 days
	100 mg vaginal tablet	1 tablet × 7 days
	100 mg vaginal tablet	2 tablets × 3 days
	500 mg vaginal tablet	1 tablet single dose
Miconazole*	2% cream	5 g × 7 days
	100 mg vaginal suppository	1 suppositary × 7 days
	200 mg vaginal suppositary	1 suppositary × 3 days
	1200 mg vaginal suppositary	1 suppositary single dose
Econazole	150 mg vaginal tablet	1 tablet × 3 days
Fenticonazole	2% cream	5 g × 7 days
Tioconazole*	2% cream	5 g × 3 days
	6.5% cream	5 g single dose
Terconazole	0.45 cream	5 g × 7 days
	0.8% cream	5 g × 3 days
	80 mg vaginal suppository	1 suppository × 3 days
Nystatin	100,000 U vaginal tablet	1 tablet × 14 days
Oral agents		
Ketoconazole	200 mg bid	400 mg × 5 days
Itraconazole	200 mg bid	400 mg × 1 day
	200 mg	200 mg × 3 days
Fluconazole	150 mg	150 mg single dose

*: over-the-counter.

more healthy vaginal flora have not been effective. Neither oral nor vaginal *Lactobacillus* was effective in preventing *Candida* vulvovaginitis after antibiotic treatment[18]. Some patients maintain their own dietary restrictions for symptom relief or are aware that certain foods bring on symptoms. This could be a placebo effect or their symptoms could be the result of a food allergy.

In those patients with culture-documented chronic or recurrent *C. albicans* vulvovaginitis, the therapeutic strategy will shift from a single course of therapy to protracted maintenance treatment schemes. This strategy is based upon two important observations: it works for many patients, and there is evidence that these women have increased levels of *C. albicans* in their vagina even when they are between episodes and asymptomatic. There is a wide range of treatment regimens available that should be employed for at least 6 months. If the patient prefers a local vaginal treatment, the weekly use of clotrimazole 500 mg can be prescribed[16]. The oral azoles have appeal, for they are effective and less messy. Ketoconazole, 100 mg given daily for 6 months was effective, as was itraconazole 50–100 mg daily[16]. Alternatively, weekly fluconzaole 150 mg is effective and has the benefit of once weekly rather than daily dosing. After 6 months of treatment, 90.8% remained well without a clinical recurrence as compared to 35.9% of patients receiving placebo. This benefit was not maintained after treatment stopped. Six months later, only 42.9% were clinically cured as compared to 21.9% in the placebo group[19]. For those patients in whom there is a concern about the long-term use of these azoles, one study indicated that 600 mg of boric acid given vaginally during the first 5 days of the menstrual cycle for 6 months was quite effective[20]. The problem of recurrence after the end of treatment remains a constant.

HIV-infected women pose special problems in the care of their *Candida* vulvovaginal infections. They are more likely to have azole-resistant *C. albicans* present, even in those women who are not on long-term oral azole prophylaxis. Those women on long-term azole prophylaxis also have a higher than expected recovery of *C. glabrata* species. The care of these women requires culture and the identification of nonalbicans species so that appropriate therapy can be planned. They are important patients to identify and treat, for symptomatic HIV-infected women with a *Candida* vaginitis are shedding increased numbers of copies of HIV-1 RNA in cervicovaginal secretions[1]. Untreated, they are at a greater risk for HIV transmission. Fortunately, Wang *et al.* (2001)[21] found that successful treatment of vulvovaginal candidiasis was associated with a three-fold reduction in the prevalence of HIV-1 DNA in cervicovaginal secretions.

Those patients with recurrent vulvovaginal infections can be saddled with immune shortcomings against vaginal *C. albicans* infections and not as the result of resistant albicans infections[5]. Currently, there are no specific therapies for these immune deficiencies, but it should be a focus for future therapeutic research.

Those patients with acute or recurrent nonalbicans pose a number of different diagnostic and therapeutic problems for physicians. For diagnosis, it is important that the laboratory can go beyond the characterization of these isolates as nonalbicans and identify the species recovered. The physicians should be most concerned about the identification of *C. krusei* and *C. glabrata*. *C. krusei* is most resistant to azoles, while *C. glabrata*, although it appears sensitive to the azoles in the laboratory, often does not respond clinically to azole therapy. When culture-positive for either of these strains, these alternative therapies should be planned. *C. krusei* is a rare isolate in patients with *Candida* vulvovaginitis. In these patients, topical boric acid resulted in a cure in the majority of cases[22]. If boric acid fails, prolonged treatment (6 weeks) with topical clotrimazole followed by maintenance treatment with topical nystatin should prove effective. A much more common nonalbicans isolate is *C. glabrata*. The preferred treatment is 600 mg boric acid in a gelatin capsule administered vaginally for 2 weeks. It should be noted that boric acid is poisonous and has been removed from commercial products because of its potential toxicity, especially for children. Three grams taken orally may be fatal to a child[23]. It is not well absorbed through the vagina, but cases of neurotoxicity (nausea, headaches, disorientation) have been reported with prolonged intravaginal use. For women who are treatment failures with such a regimen, Sobel *et al.* (2003)[24] have shown remarkably good results using a specially made flucytosine cream administered as a nightly 5 g intravaginal dose for 14 days.

Some physician interventions may not be appropriate in these patients. A diagnostic requirement for women with chronic vulvovaginitis repeated in every edition of gynecologic texts is that they should be screened to see if they have unsuspected diabetes mellitus. The yield is so low that this testing should be restricted to patients with risk factors for diabetes. With the increasing problem of obesity in the youth of the United States and Europe and the concomitant increase in diabetes mellitus, more screening may be done in the future. A popular therapeutic intervention in women with chronic vulvovaginitis is the physician-applied local vaginal treatment with the dye gentian violet. There are potential problems with this approach: it is often used in women who do not have a *Candida* vulvovaginitis, it usually does not work and, sometimes, women can have a severe reaction to the dye with excruciating vaginal burning that intensifies rather than relieves their symptoms. The most frequent mistake that physicians make in women with chronic or recurrent vulvovaginitis is always to attempt to make a diagnosis and treat the patient at the first clinical contact. There is no dishonor in holding off therapy when in doubt, until all culture results are available. This avoids mislabeling the patient's problem and utilizing treatment interventions that will not help or at times will worsen the problem.

Chapter 5

Bacterial Vaginosis

BACKGROUND

To paraphrase the title of Shakespeare's play, *Much Ado about Nothing*, the current Obstetric-Gynecologic literature overemphasis upon bacterial vaginosis (BV) as the cause of almost everything could be titled, *Much Ado about Something That Is Poorly Understood.* The 'much ado' is highlighted by repeated reiterations that this is the number one cause of vaginitis in the United States and western Europe, with the more concerning emphasis about its alleged role in the causation of premature labor, pre-term premature rupture of membranes, pelvic inflammatory disease, *Chlamydia trachomatis* infection, human immunodeficiency virus (HIV) infection, cervical cancer, post-operative pelvic infection after hysterectomy, post-operative pelvic infection after pregnancy termination, and post-partum endomyometritis. Women reading lay publications have been bombarded with the theme that BV is 'Public Health Enemy Number One'.

There are a number of reasons for reservations about these claims. Is BV the number one cause of vaginitis? This depends upon the patient population receiving care. The studies citing this fact have been done in young sexually active women, usually not in monogamous relationships. In these studies, frequent recurrences of this problem are noted. In contrast, in women in more stable sexual relationships, *Candida* vaginitis is more frequently perceived as a problem. In the Cornell vulvovaginal referral practice over the course of a year, dozens of women are seen with presumed chronic or recurrent *Candida* vaginitis as compared to the rare patient seen with a problem with recurrent BV. This is not due to the referring physician's failure to diagnose BV. In the majority of patients seen with supposed recurrent *Candida* vaginitis who are not culture-positive, BV is rarely found.

In addition, the overwhelming emphasis upon the importance of BV as a widespread public health problem is based upon epidemiologic studies. Epidemiologic studies can show relationships that are not necessarily cause-and-effect. A good illustration of this is contained in a whimsical story told by Michael Fitzpatrick: 'The Japanese eat very little fat and suffer fewer heart attacks than the British or Americans. The French eat a lot of fat and also suffer fewer heart attacks than the British or Americans. The Japanese drink very little red wine and suffer fewer heart attacks than the British or Americans. The Italians drink excessive amounts of red wine and suffer fewer heart attacks than the British or Americans. Conclusion: Eat or drink what you like. What kills you is speaking English'[1]. Associations do not equal causation. One prospective study of sexually active women in Pittsburgh, Pennsylvania showed no link between the presence of BV and an increased incidence of pelvic inflammatory disease[2].

The pathophysiology of BV seems to be straightforward. There is a marked reduction in the number of H_2O_2-producing lactobacilli in the vagina and an overgrowth with high concentrations of three groups of bacteria. These include *Mycoplasma hominis* and *Gardnerella vaginalis* and anaerobes which account for the foul odor often associated with this syndrome.

The etiology is unclear. There is evidence that it is related to sexual activity. It is much more common in sexually active women who have more than one sexual partner. In contrast, it has been reported in celibate women, and treatment of the male sexual partners with antibiotics has not improved the cure rates or eliminated the risk of recurrence.

There are many potential sources of confusion for the physician caring for the patient with BV. These women with similar microbiologic alterations in the vagina can have a wide variety of clinical presentations. They can be symptomatic, complaining of a vaginal discharge or vaginal malodor. In contrast, many women who meet the BV diagnostic criteria of an excess number of vaginal bacteria and an altered bacterial flora with few or no lactobacilli, have no symptoms. In addition, the vaginal alterations from normal can vary. The term 'bacterial vaginosis' was originally selected to label a vaginal condition in which inflammation was not a predominant aspect of the syndrome. Those patients with increased numbers of bacteria and the predominant presence of 'clue' cells, vaginal squamous cells whose surface is peppered with bacteria, have few or no white cells (WBCs) present (**52**); hence, the use of the term, 'vaginosis,' not 'vaginitis'. In contrast, there are patients with this increase in the number of bacteria and the shift in the bacterial flora, who also have an outpouring of WBCs on saline microscopic evaluation (**53**). This is an important sub-group for the physician to recognize and an important reason to favor office microscopy as the preferred diagnostic strategy, because it dictates more immediate testing in these women. This population, with a marked inflammatory response, can have another infectious problem in addition to BV, including *Trichomonas vaginalis*, *Neisseria gonorrhea*, or *Chlamydia trachomatis*. This presence of an excessive number of WBCs should be a wake-up call to the clinical care team to obtain the necessary tests to rule out these other sexually transmitted diseases. These clinical hints are only obtained at the time of the patient visit by the use of office microscopy evaluating the wet mount saline preparations. Confirmation of an increased number of WBCs on the Gram-stained smear is unfortunately only achieved after the patient has left the office. The opportunity to get important confirmatory tests has been lost. Finally, there are wide variations in individual responses to the alterations in the vaginal flora seen with this condition. Over time, some women have a spontaneous cure with the vaginal flora returning to normal, while others have recurrent or persistent problems despite local vaginal or oral antibiotic treatment. BV encompasses a wide range of clinical conditions.

Despite these inconsistencies about the diagnosis, at least one study has shown an increased magnitude of genital tract HIV shedding in women with a Nugent score diagnosis of BV[3]. This could be a factor increasing the risk of HIV transmission from the infected woman to her sexual partner or to the newborn at the time of delivery.

MICROBIOLOGY

Bacterial vaginosis is characterized by a profound change in the composition of the vaginal microbial flora. The concentration of lactobacilli, particularly hydrogen peroxide (H_2O_2)-producing lactobacilli, is greatly reduced while levels of *Gardnerella vaginalis*, *Mycoplasma hominis*, and anaerobic *Prevotella*, *Bacteroides*, *Porphyromonas*, and *Mobiluncus* species drastically increase. A recent study using nucleotide sequencing of polymerase chain reaction (PCR)-amplified 16S rRNA gene segments found a new bacterium, *Atopobium vaginae*, present in the majority of patients with BV and rarely present in normal women[4]. The net effect is a dramatic increase in the total number of bacteria seen when a wet mount or Gram stain of vaginal secretions is observed under light microscopy[5]. In addition, the adherence of large numbers of *G. vaginalis* to exfoliated vaginal mucosal epithelial cells (clue cells) is also readily observed in secretions from women with BV. These changes result in an elevation in the vaginal pH and, in some women, the presence of a malodorous discharge. Other women with a vaginal flora consistent with a diagnosis of BV have no clinical symptoms. Interest in BV has been greatly stimulated by reports of its association with HIV transmission[6], post-abortal and post-surgical pelvic infections[7], and preterm birth[7,8]. However, antibiotic treatment of BV in pregnant women to prevent pre-term birth has been largely, but not exclusively, unsuccessful[9–12]. In addition, a recent investigation demonstrated that metronidazole treatment has the potential to select for *Bacteroides* species with increased pathogenicity[13].

Several unanswered questions remain concerning microbiological aspects of BV. It remains unclear whether the decrease in lactobacilli is the primary event and precedes the overgrowth of the other microorganisms, or whether the proliferation of *G. vaginalis* and the anaerobes occurs first and causes the disappearance of the lactobacilli. Furthermore, it is completely unknown what triggers this massive alteration in the vaginal ecosystem.

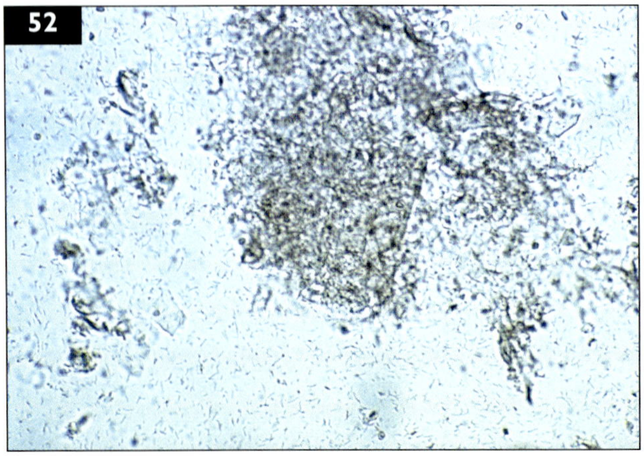

52 Microscopic examination of a saline hanging drop preparation. There is an increased number of clue cells, an increased number of bacterial forms, and no white blood cells.

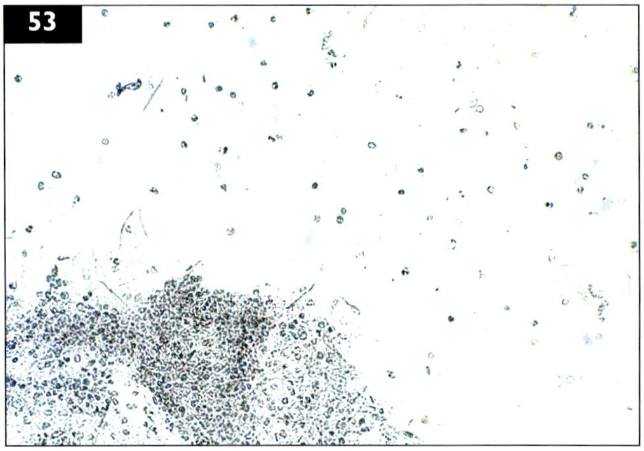

53 Microscopic examination of a saline preparation, with increased number of clue cells, increased number of bacterial forms, and an increased number of white blood cells.

Longitudinal studies have clearly demonstrated that the vaginal flora does not remain constant in most women, but is unstable and subject to almost daily fluctuations in the overall composition and concentration of the different microorganisms[14]. In addition, antibiotic treatment of BV results in only a temporary shift in the microbial flora in many cases. Greater than 30% of bacterial vaginosis patients will have a recurrence by 3 months. This implicates endogenous factors as being responsible for the alterations in the composition of vaginal flora. Alternatively, studies of women who have sex exclusively with women have demonstrated that when one partner has BV the other partner usually is also positive for the same microorganisms[15]. Similarly, having a greater number of heterosexual sex partners and not using a condom are also associated with acquisition of BV[14]. This suggests that BV may be a sexually transmitted disease involving the passage of an as yet unidentified etiologic agent. However, antibiotic treatment of male partners of women with BV does not reduce the rate of recurrence. It has also been postulated that acquisition of lactobacillus-specific bacteriophages, from a sexual partner or from consumption of phage-containing dairy products, may be responsible for the decrease in vaginal lactobacilli[16]. If H_2O_2 produced by lactobacilli inhibits proliferation of *G. vaginalis* and anaerobes in the vagina, than phage-mediated lysis of these organisms may remove a critical control factor. However, a recent study has demonstrated that in peri- and post-menopausal women the marked decrease in the concentration of vaginal lactobacilli is not followed by an increased growth of BV-associated microorganisms[17]. This is consistent with the decrease in lactobacilli being a secondary consequence, and not a primary cause, of anaerobic overgrowth in the vagina.

IMMUNOLOGY

BV is not called bacterial vaginitis due to the absence of clinical evidence of inflammation and the absence or scarcity of inflammatory cells in the vaginal discharge. However, there clearly are immunological alterations associated with acquisition of BV. The majority of these studies have been performed by Cauci, Guaschino, and colleagues in Italy[18–20]. Women with BV have an almost 20-fold increase in vaginal interleukin (IL)-1β concentrations in their vagina as compared to women with a lactobacilli-dominated microbial flora. Thus, there is in fact a strong host pro-inflammatory immune response to this altered microbiological flora. What is striking, however, is the absence of subsequent activity along the pro-inflammatory pathway. IL-1β typically induces production of IL-8 which promotes neutrophil migration to the site of pro-inflammatory activity. No increase in vaginal IL-8 concentration or neutrophil levels are apparent in vaginal secretions from women with BV. It appears that one or more of the BV-associated microorganisms is able to short-circuit the immune response by inhibiting IL-8 production or stability. Humoral immunity is also affected by BV-associated microorganisms. IgA antibodies to the *G. vaginalis* hemolysin have been identified in only 30% of women with BV. In the remainder, IgA-derived degradation products have been found.

Microbial proteolytic enzymes have been implicated in the inhibition of cell-mediated and humoral immunity in women with BV. Patients who lack IL-8 and IgA anti-hemolysin have high concentrations of the hydrolytic enzymes, sialidase and prolidase, in their vagina. These enzymes have been shown to inhibit IL-8 activity.

BV appears to be a heterogeneous disorder with two populations of women based on distinct immunological profiles. Vaginal levels of IL-8 and IgA anti-hemolysin are inversely correlated with local concentrations of sialidase and prolidase. Evidence is accumulating to suggest that it is only the sub-group of women with elevated proteolytic enzymes that suffer the sequela of BV. While there is no association between BV patients as a whole and pre-term birth and low birthweight, patients with elevated vaginal sialidase and prolidase levels and low concentrations of IgA anti-hemolysin have a strong association with adverse pregnancy outcome[20]. This suggests the inability of some women but not others to neutralize the negative effects of BV-related microorganisms or their products on vaginal cell-mediated and humoral immune responses. This may be responsible for the variability observed in the pathogenic potential of this syndrome, as well as the conflicting results of antibiotic treatment trials. It also appears that vaginal sialidase or prolidase activity may be better markers than clinically- or Gram stained-defined BV or an elevated vaginal pH for risk of adverse BV-related pathology.

DIAGNOSIS

Just as there are a variety of clinical presentations, the diagnosis of BV can be achieved in more than one way. In symptomatic patients who complain of either an excessive vaginal discharge, or an unpleasant vaginal odor, or both, a focused history can be helpful. In the patient with an acute first episode, whether there is a new sexual partner and if the patient has been exposed to the male ejaculate should be determined. In patients with a recurrent problem, there are three areas of concern in history-taking: (1) Is it related to intercourse?; (2) Has the patient been exposed to the male ejaculate?; and (3) What medicines has she used in the past for this problem and how have they worked for her?

For symptomatic women, an immediate office diagnosis can be made using an added assessment to the Amsel criteria of three of four findings being present, including a thin homogenous vaginal discharge, vaginal pH higher than 4.5, release of a fishy odor from the vaginal discharge placed in 10% potassium hydroxide (KOH), and vaginal epithelial cells heavily coated with microorganisms (clue cells)[5]. This approach is simple and easy to do, avoiding the delay associated with sending a vaginal smear to the laboratory to be Gram stained and evaluated under the microscope. Using a plastic spatula, a portion of the excessive vaginal discharge should be obtained and stirred on two slides, one holding a drop of normal saline and the other a drop of 10% KOH. Immediately after adding the vaginal secretions to the KOH solution, the physician should sniff above the slide, seeking a pungent fishy odor, a positive whiff test caused by the amines elaborated by the overgrowth of anaerobic bacteria. This is present in nearly all symptomatic patients. Then a cotton swab should be applied to the lateral wall of the vagina and touched to pH indicator paper. The pH is above 4.5 in nearly all of these women. Then, the saline preparation should be viewed under the microscope. The old criteria for the diagnosis focused upon the importance of clue cells, squamous epithelial cells covered with bacteria, with 20% or more of these epithelial cells meeting this criteria. Figures **52** and **54** show a microscopic view of a saline preparation with clue cells present, an obvious altered bacterial flora with low or no lactobacilli, and few or no WBCs. Figure **55** shows individual clue cells. Figure **56** shows a high-power view of a clue cell. Figure **53** shows a low-power view of clue cells with an abundance of WBCs. Figure **57** shows a high-power saline view with no lactobacilli.

There are other important microscopic clues that help cement the diagnosis. The microscopic examination of the KOH suspension is an important confirmatory test. It removes the confounding backdrop of epithelial cells and permits a direct view of an increased number of bacteria present with few or no lactobacilli in sight (**58–60**). Gilbert Donders from the European Union has also emphasized the fact that the characterization of the number of lactobacilli in the vaginal fluid is more accurate with the wet mount than with the Gram stain[21]. If the saline preparation has more than the expected numbers of WBCs (see **57**), tests should be obtained to rule out the presence of *Trichomonas vaginalis*, *Neisseria gonorrhea*, and *Chlamydia trachomatis*, although the yield is low. The standard vaginal culture plays

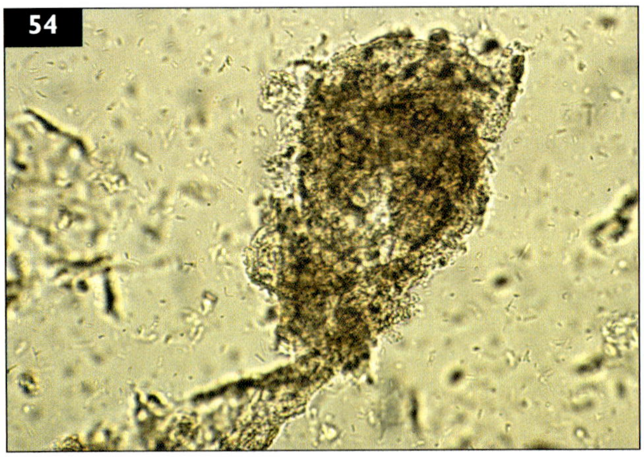

54 Microscopic examination of a saline preparation with clue cells, an altered flora, with a rare lactobacillus and a rare white blood cell.

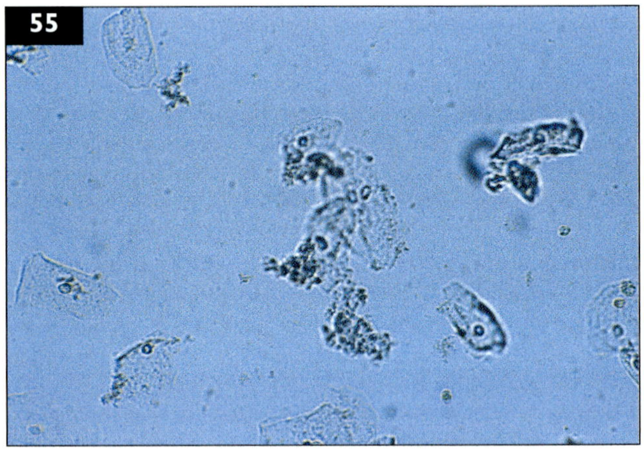

55 Individual clue cells seen on saline preparation.

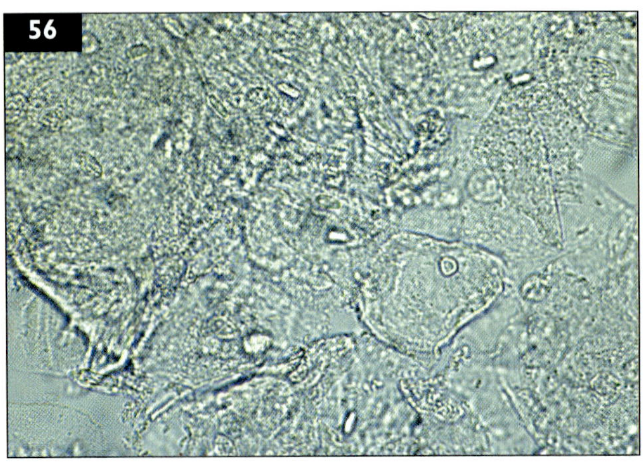

56 A high-power microscopic view of clue cells.

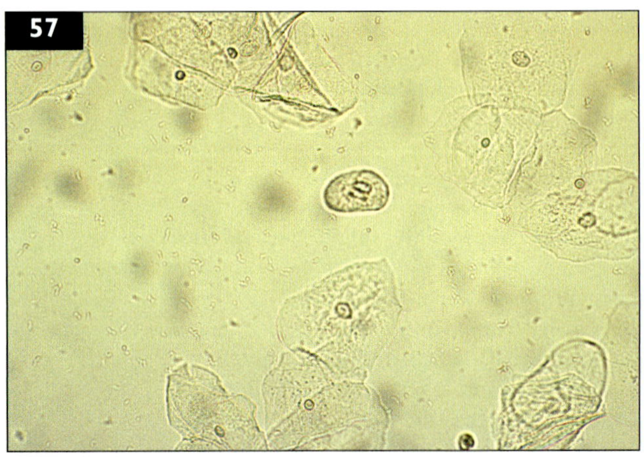

57 Microscopic examination of a saline preparation with no lactobacilli visible.

no role in the diagnosis of BV, because this syndrome is not characterized by a specific pathogen, but instead an overgrowth of bacteria normally found in the vagina. *Gardnerella vaginalis* can be recovered from the vagina of an asymptomatic woman without the major alterations in vaginal flora seen with BV. This microbiologic view of the nonspecific microbiologic nature of BV with no specific pathogen may be changed in the future as more sensitive microbiologic techniques are employed in the study of this syndrome. Using nucleotide sequencing of PCR-amplified 16S rRNA gene segments, a bacterium only recently identified, *Atopobium vaginae*, was present in 21 of 22 patients with BV and in only two of 24 normal patients[4].

The alternate diagnostic method is to obtain a vaginal smear and send it to the laboratory to be Gram stained and evaluated microscopically by laboratory personnel. This has the advantage of the utilization of more skilled microscopists, but has the disadvantage that a positive test result indicating BV is only available after the patient has left the examining room. This requires a subsequent contact with the patient to prescribe treatment. Also, the finding of an inflammatory response occurs after the patient visit. More troubling, some patients who fit the Nugent criteria for the diagnosis of BV with a score of 7–10, do not meet the immediate clinical criteria of an elevated vaginal pH, a positive whiff test, and the presence of more than 20% of the vaginal epithelial 'clue' cells. Although most patients overlap, i.e. they are positive by both Nugent and Amsel

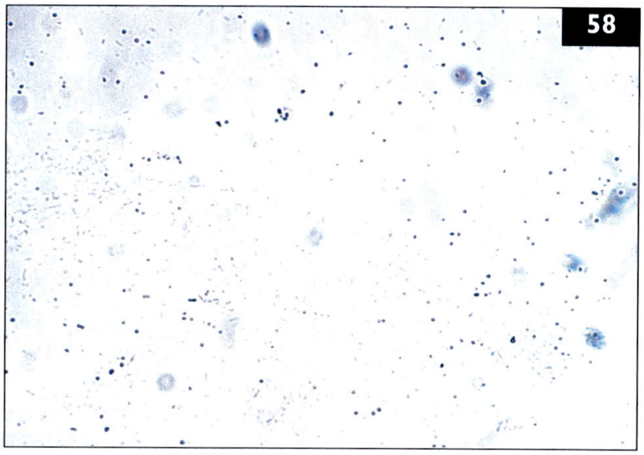

58 Microscopic examination of a potassium hydroxide preparation, with increased number of bacteria and a paucity of lactobacilli.

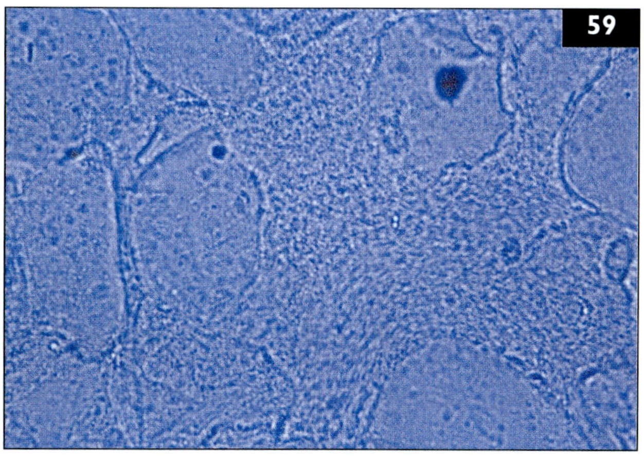

59 Microscopic examination of a potassium hydroxide preparation, with increased number of bacteria and no lactobacilli.

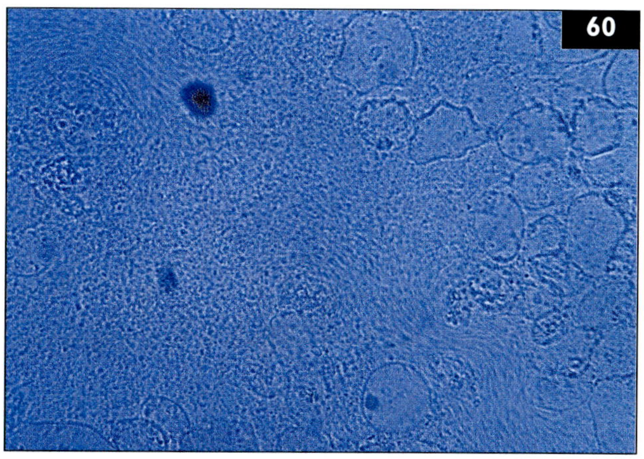

60 Microscopic examination of a potassium hydroxide preparation, with increased bacteria and no lactobacilli.

criteria, some patients are positive with only one testing regimen (*Table 8*). The Nugent test is more sensitive. A higher number of women surveyed by these two diagnostic schemes will have a diagnosis of BV using the Nugent method[22]. This is an important point to note. Epidemiologic and clinical studies of BV will have two different populations when one or the other of either Amsel or Nugent criteria are used. In one study, the more sensitive Nugent test showed a correlation between BV and increased genital tract shedding of HIV. In contrast, no increase in HIV shedding was noted in those women in whom BV was diagnosed by the Amsel criteria[3].

Other diagnostic options for clinicians who do not have a microscope available are test kits. The advantage of this approach is an immediate diagnosis for these doctors who are not likely to do pH paper testing as well. A number of systems are available: there is a DNA probe test for high concentrations of *Gardnerella vaginalis* (Affirm™); a card test for the detection of elevated pH and trimethylamine (Fem Exam®), and a card test for the detection of proline aminopeptidase (PipActivity Test Card™)[23]. The disadvantages are the different sensitivities and specificities in making the diagnosis when compared to either the Nugent or Amsel criteria. The medical care team's use of these kits must be coupled with an awareness that, again, different populations are identified than have been noted when Amsel or Nugent schemes are used. In addition, these tests do not detect those women with large numbers of WBCs present in their vaginal secretions.

Asymptomatic women with BV must by necessity be detected by screening tests. The burden on the physician is to determine what population to screen. What asymptomatic patients with BV will benefit from treatment? This is still an area of controversy. Pregnant patients with BV have been observed to have a higher than expected rate of pre-term labor and delivery and post-partum pelvic infection[23]. Although the treatment strategies are still not clear, this population at risk should be identified. One simple screening scheme obtains a vaginal pH and a whiff test with 10% KOH with every vaginal examination. If the pH is greater than 4.5 or the whiff test is positive, it can be followed with a microscopic examination of vaginal secretions in saline and 10% KOH preparations. Some gynecologic patients are screened as well. Similar tests can be done in every patient evaluated prior to a scheduled vaginal or abdominal hysterectomy, and in all those patients in whom it is planned to traverse the endocervical canal and enter the uterine cavity. These include pregnancy termination, endometrial biopsy, dilatation and curettage, hysterosalpingography, and intrauterine device insertion. This diagnostic screening technique is not the standard of care in the United States.

Most of the literature experience with screening has occurred in pregnant women, using Nugent criteria for the diagnosis with a score of 7–10 confirming the diagnosis. The Nugent screen can also be used in gynecologic patients if there will be a delay from the time of the office examination until the procedure is done. In addition, the Nugent screen can be used in HIV-infected women[3]. The aforementioned test kits could also be used in these populations. One interesting screening approach in asymptomatic pregnant women has been championed by Dr. Udo Hoyme in Germany[11]. At the time of their first pre-natal visit, the patients are given disposable plastic examining gloves with a strip of pH paper attached to the index finger. During the pregnancy, they examine themselves on Monday and Friday mornings and report to the medical care team if the pH paper tests alkaline so that they can be evaluated and treated. This scheme provides more frequent surveys of the vaginal flora than aforementioned testing tied to scheduled patient visits.

Table 8 Comparison of Amsel and Nugent criteria for bacterial vaginosis (BV)

	Amsel BV+	Amsel BV–	Total
Nugent BV+	150	93	243
Nugent BV–	13	361	374
Totals	163	454	617

TREATMENT

Since there is a wide variety of presentations in women with BV, each category will be discussed separately. Symptomatic patients with BV should receive treatment to relieve their discomfort. The therapeutic strategy for the patient with the first episode is straightforward: all of the options rely on the use of one of two antibiotics, metronidazole and clindamycin given orally or, alternatively, with the use of a vaginal preparation. Having more than one option available permits the tailoring of the therapeutic regimen to meet the needs of each individual patient. There is a number of factors that will influence the final health care provider's decision. The most effective therapeutic regimens seem to be oral metronidazole 500 mg bid for 7 days or metronidazole gel 0.75% (5 g) intravaginally, once a day for 5 days. Some women have problems with this antibiotic. There is an antabuse-like reaction when women on oral metronidazole are exposed to alcohol, and the long half-life of metronidazole means that in addition to avoiding liquor, wine, or beer while taking this antibiotic, they must continue to refrain for at least 24 hours after the last dose. The risk of this reaction with intravaginal metronidazole has not been quantified, but the same prohibition should be in place, for some of the vaginal metronidazole will be absorbed. Some women dislike the metallic taste after oral metronidazole ingestion or have abdominal discomfort when taking this medication for the prescribed 7 days.

Another alternative metronidazole regimen recommended by the Centers for Disease Control (CDC) is a large single dose of metronidazole (2 g)[23]. The advantage is that this avoids the 7 days of therapy that can be socially disruptive. The disadvantage is that this regimen is not as effective as the 7-day oral regimen or the 5-day vaginal treatment. Some women refuse metronidazole therapy because they are allergic to it, did not like how they felt when they previously took it, or have neurologic problems that make the risk of peripheral neuropathy from the use of metronidazole unacceptable.

Fortunately, there is the alternative of using a clindamycin product. None of the clindamycin alternatives is as effective as the 7-day oral or 5-day vaginal metronidazole regimen. Clindamycin vaginal cream 2% can be used with 5 g applied intravaginally for 7 days. If the patient is fastidious or dislikes the messiness of the 7-day treatment with the cream, clindamycin vaginal ovules (100 g) can be prescribed, to be inserted vaginally daily for 3 days. Occasionally, patients have a local reaction to the cream, usually due to propylene glycol, a preservative present in this formulation, and the subsequent vaginal burning and increased vaginal discharge is often worse than the original problem. Some of this vaginal clindamycin is absorbed, and rarely patients have developed pseudomembranous entercolitis after using one of the vaginal products. For the patient who does not want to use a vaginal clindamycin product, oral clindamycin can be prescribed 300 mg bid for 7 days. For the patient with an acute episode, most of the regimens work in the short term with an immediate resolution of symptoms. Other problems can occur. Patients given oral or vaginal antibiotics can develop a *Candida* vaginitis. This occurs more commonly with the clindamycin products. When it occurs, it represents another vaginal infection to be treated and is a setback for the patient.

The problem patient for the physician is the woman who presents with recurrent symptomatology, 1–6 months later. Both diagnostic tools and therapeutic options are limited, in part because of the narrow focus of most investigations of BV to date. There has been an inordinate amount of epidemiologic studies linking BV to a host of female problems, and the microbiologic focus has trained primarily on the absence of H_2O_2-producing lactobacilli in the vagina. The therapeutic options are limited. The approved antibiotic regimens, metronidazole and clindamycin, are highly effective against most anaerobic bacteria, but have minimal if any effectiveness against the other bacteria found in high numbers in many of the patients with BV, including *Gardnerella vaginalis*, *Mycoplasma hominis*, and the anaerobes, the *Mobiluncus* species. The newly discovered bacterium, *Atopobium vaginae*, is resistant to metronidazole[4]. Studies involving the introduction of H_2O_2-producing lactobacilli that attach to the epithelium have not proven effective.

This is the diagnostic and therapeutic void that faces the physician evaluating these patients. There are no readily available laboratory measures to determine the persistence of an overgrowth of *Gardnerella vaginalis*, *Mycoplasma hominis*, and the *Mobiluncus* species. There are no studied alternative antibiotic regimens to determine effectiveness in these women. The physician is left in the void of empirical antibiotic intervention with either metronidazole or clindamycin. A frequent scenario is to treat the first or sometimes the second recurrence with one of the CDC-approved antibiotic regimens, sometimes for a longer period of time or change the antibiotic used, substituting clindamycin for metronidazole or *vice versa*. If recurrence continues, Dr. Jack Sobel in Detroit has tried a vaginal metronidazole regimen twice weekly for up to 6 months[24]. Most patients are asymptomatic while on this regimen, but many have the recurrence of symptoms when the medication is stopped. Many women pinpoint the recurrence of symptoms after exposure to the ejaculate of a particular male partner. Is it reinfection? That doesn't seem likely in view of the failure of antibiotic treatment for the male to improve the rate of cure. However, perhaps the wrong antibiotic has been used. Alternatively, the male ejaculate is very alkaline, can cause an outpouring of vaginal secretions, and create a vaginal environment favorable for the overgrowth of bacteria if an allergen or an allergen and IgE are present in the ejaculate[25,26] and, finally, the ejaculate is immunosuppressive and may tip the balance in the vagina leading to an overgrowth of bacteria. Some of these patients have fewer recurrences when their male uses a condom. For this strategy to work presumes that the women are not allergic to latex and the nonoxynol nine, used to coat these products. Another possibility in these difficult-to-treat patients is the finding in a black population, using culture-independent methods, that normal flora for some is dominanted by anaerobes that produce amines; vaginal odor for these women is sometimes normal (Larry Forney, PhD, personal communication).

Guidelines for the treatment of asymptomatic patients are often tentative rather than fixed. There are many disagreements about strategies of detection and treatment. The ante-partum pregnant patient is a case in point. There is no dispute that some women detected with BV have a higher incidence of pre-term labor and delivery. What is in question is the appropriate strategy. The current wisdom in the United States is to screen pregnant women with a history of a prior premature labor at the time of the first pre-natal visit. The current treatment regimens proposed for this specific population with BV are either oral metronidazole 250 mg tid for 7 days or clindamycin 300 mg orally bid for 7 days[23]. One large National Insitutes for Health (NIH)-sponsored study showed no reduction in the prematurity rate with metronidazole treatment of asymptomatic women with BV. This was a flawed study, for the treatment was delayed from 1–8 or more weeks from the time the vaginal slide was collected to be sent to a central laboratory for Nugent score analysis[9]. In contrast, two European studies showed a reduction in the pre-term delivery rate when the diagnosis to treatment interval was started. The German study with bi-weekly screening and immediate evaluation showed a reduction in the prematurity rate when a variety of oral and vaginal treatments was employed[11]. In a study in Vienna, all treatment was begun within 7–10 days of the visit when slides were obtained for diagnosis and the pre-term delivery rate was reduced[27].

Leaving this controversy aside, the relationship between BV and an increased risk of post-partum endomyometritis should dictate a therapeutic intervention if BV is diagnosed. No data suggest that intervaginal treatment in this situation is any less effective than the oral route, so metronidazole gel (0.75%), 5 g intravaginally daily for 5 days can be employed. This avoids the more broad disruptions of the vaginal flora with clindamycin that favor the post-treatment overgrowth of enterococci, *Escherichia coli*, and *Candida*. For the patient allergic to metronidazole, clindamycin cream 2% (5 g) given intravaginally for 7 days is another option.

There is a host of pre-procedure asymptomatic patients in whom screening for BV and treatment can be beneficial. These include patients about to undergo a hysterectomy or a pregnancy termination. It also should include those patients who will have instrumentation in which instruments, devices, or radio-opaque materials will be introduced into the uterine cavity. Patients that are candidates for screening include those for endometrial biopsy, dilatation and curettage, insertion of an intrauterine device, and those for hysterosalpingography. The Nugent screening method can be employed if there will be a delay between the screen and the procedure. Otherwise, an immediate screen should be used, with a delay in the procedure until treatment has been accomplished. The treatment guidelines for these BV-positive women are the same as noted in the asymptomatic pregnant woman. One final group for BV screening and treatment is the ever-increasing population of women undergoing in vitro fertilization procedures. Vaginal invasive procedures are an integral part of this process. Ova retrieval is accomplished with transvaginal aspiration of ova and the insertion of embryos into the uterus is performed transvaginally. The Nugent technique can be employed to screen these women before such procedures are employed and intravaginal treatment as previously outlined should be appropriate.

Another population for Nugent screening is the HIV-infected patient. There is clinical evidence that they are more likely to transmit the infection to their sexual partners[6], and those that have a Nugent screen diagnosis of BV have higher HIV counts in cervical vaginal secretions[3]. This is an important population for surveillance and treatment, but the effectiveness of treatment in lowering the risk of HIV transmission is not known.

Chapter 6

Trichomonas vaginalis Vaginitis

BACKGROUND

There has been a great change in American physicians' attitudes about *Trichomonas vaginitis* since the introduction of metronidazole into clinical practice in 1963. Before that, there was no effective treatment regimen, and practicing physicians faced the daunting task of ministering to a large number of women with an uncomfortable, persistent, and annoying vaginal discharge in which medications might temporarily relieve symptoms, but would not eradicate the problem. Although some women were able to eliminate the organism with local vaginal defense mechanisms, the majority had a persistent chronic infection. For these women, the mantra was similar to the one applied to genital herpes today: *Trichomonas* was forever. Metronidazole changed all that. The effectiveness of this treatment has remarkably reduced the incidence of the infection, and this has been seen in all Western industrialized countries. Currently, in the Cornell referral vulvovaginitis clinic, there is rarely more than one patient a year seen with a symptomatic *T. vaginalis* vaginitis. This probably relects the upper middle-class social status of this referral patient population. In contrast, using polymerase chain reaction (PCR) testing of low-income pregnant women, *T. vaginalis* was detected in 22 of 219 patients (10%)[1]. Similarly, a PCR *T. vaginalis* detection study of sexually active low- or middle-income adolescent women in Indiana, USA, identified infection initially in 16 of 268 (6%) of the participants; 57 of 245 (23.2%) of the study population with at least 3 months of follow-up had at least one infection[2]. In addition, this is a common sexually transmitted disease (STD) in third world countries that have a parallel high incidence of human immunodeficiency virus (HIV) infections. One study of men attending STD and dermatology clinics in Malawi found an incidence of 17%[3]. Physician awareness of this infection will be dependent upon the composition of their patient population.

For many private practitioners, just as the frequency of *T. vaginalis* vaginitis has dropped in upper middle-class practices, some long-held opinions about these infections have had to be modified. The old view was that this infection was readily recognized by clinicians. These patients were symptomatic and desperate with a chronic, frothy, malodorous discharge with vulvar and vaginal inflammation. The diagnosis was easy to make, for motile trichomonads could easily be detected on microscopic examination of vaginal secretions mixed with a drop of saline. The reality is far from this. Many infected women have no symptoms or symptoms too mild to call to the attention of the health care provider. The sensitivity of the wet mount microscopic examination is closer to 50% rather than 100%.

The impact of this infection upon the pregnant woman remains unclear. The Vaginal Infection in Pregnancy (VIP) study showed an association between a positive vaginal culture for *T. vaginalis* and an increased rate of pre-term labor and delivery[4]. In the United States, the pre-term delivery rate for African-Americans is twice the general rate, and in the VIP study, one-third of these pre-term births were apparently associated with a *Trichomonas* infection[4]. Inexplicably, treatment of these infected women with metronidazole was shown to increase further the prematurity rate, rather than lower it[5,6].

HIV-infected women with a *Trichomonas* vaginitis should be a special focus for the physician. The inflammatory vaginal response to this infection probably increases the HIV viral load in the cervical vaginal secretions of these women, and increases the risk of transmission of the HIV infection. At least one study has suggested that a *T. vaginalis* vaginitis doubles the rate of HIV transmission[7].

There are some observable trends in treatment. Concomitant treatment of the male lowers the risk of re-infection and more resistant strains of *T. vaginalis* have been recognized that require larger doses of metronidazole and, if this fails, treatment with tinidazole.

MICROBIOLOGY

T. vaginalis vaginitis is the number one nonviral sexually transmitted infection worldwide with an annual incidence of 3×10^8 cases. It is a sexually transmitted protozoan and a common cause of mucopurulent cervicitis and vaginitis[8]. However, in many women, infection may be asymptomatic. The number of asymptomatic infected women appears to increase during pregnancy. There is no relation between the number of organisms present in the vagina and clinical signs and symptoms. This indicates that individual host immune and genetic factors influence the consequences of a *T. vaginalis* infection.

The organism is haploid and has six chromosomes. A unique attribute of *T. vaginalis* DNA is that one-quarter of the genome is repetitive and apparently does not code for any proteins. The protozoan is motile due to the presence of four anterior flagella and a single flagellum attached to an undulating membrane. Upon entry into the vagina, *T. vaginalis* coats itself with a multitude of host proteins, plasminogen, fibrinogen, IgG, transferrin, albumin, lactoferrin and, by so doing, evades recognition by the immune system. In addition, *T. vaginalis* releases an array of cysteine proteases that effectively degrade all immunoglobulin isotypes[9]. Thus, in most infected women *T. vaginalis* is not spontaneously cleared and persists for long periods of time.

T. vaginalis adheres to and degrades mucin glycoprotein in the vagina. Four different adhesion proteins are then synthesized which allow the organism to attach to the vaginal epithelia. Eventually, *T. vaginalis* reaches the basement membrane where it binds to laminin and fibronectin. *T. vaginalis* binding sites in the epithelium are estrogen-dependent. This could explain why men are often asymptomatic *T. vaginalis* carriers, and why nearly every case of *Trichomonas* vaginitis is detected in women after puberty and prior to menopause. Men can become symptomatic, and one study implicated *T. vaginalis* in as many as 17% of nonchlamydial, nongonococcal urethral cases[10].

T. vaginalis utilizes exogenous cells to satisfy many of its nutritional requirements. It rapidly lyses erthyrocytes and incorporates the red cell membrane to obtain iron. This accounts for increased pathogenicity of this organism in the vagina during menstruation. *T. vaginalis* also effectively ingests lactobacilli, which may account for its association with bacterial vaginosis. Sexually transmitted microorganisms such as *Neisseria gonorrheoeae* and *Chlamydia trachomatis* are also ingested by *T. vaginalis*, and it has been hypothesized that this may facilitate the sexual transmission of these organisms. It has been suggested that a *T. vaginalis* infection may increase the rate of HIV transmission twofold[7]. Both HIV-shedding and the number of target cells may be increased in the vagina of *T. vaginalis*-positive women.

Some strains of *T. vaginalis* are infected by a double-stranded RNA virus[11]. The two types of *T. vaginalis*, type I with no virus and type II with viral particles in its cytoplasm, differ. The virus influences expression of *T. vaginalis* proteins and enables the organism to undergo phenotypic variation, a property absent from type I isolates. Identification of the specific types present in an individual may eventually prove to have implications for pathogenicity and treatment.

IMMUNOLOGY

The role of humoral and cell-mediated immunity in inhibiting *T. vaginalis* growth in the vagina had not been fully determined. The ability of the organism to evade recognition by different immune system components by coating its surface with host proteins, as well as by its capacity to undergo phenotypic variation and to release an array of strong proteolytic enzymes all combine to make for a poorly detectable immune response to vaginal infection. A comparison of *T. vaginalis* isolates from women who were asymptomatic with strains from women with clinical symptoms revealed that, following inoculation into a mouse model, IgA antibody production, CD4 T lymphocyte responses and interleukin-2 and interferon gamma production were significantly higher with the former organisms[12]. This further highlights the variability of *T. vaginalis* isolates.

Detection of *T. vaginalis* by microscopic examination of a wet mount of vaginal secretions is only about 50% effective. Inoculation of secretions into Diamond's medium increases sensitivity but takes several days for analysis. The use of gene amplification techniques allows rapid and accurate detection of this microorganism[1,13]. About 12% of *T. vaginalis* isolates appear to be clinically resistant to standard doses of metronidazole. A new antibiotic, tinidazole, appears to be able to overcome this resistance[14].

DIAGNOSIS

The work-up of the patient with an acute symptomatic *T. vaginalis* infection varies from that for the patient who is asymptomatic. The symptomatic woman presents with a complaint. She is uncomfortable because of an irritating, excessive vaginal discharge. In these acute onset cases, there are points in the history that will aid the diagnostic and therapeutic focus. Physicians need to determine if the patient has had a recent sexual encounter with a new male partner and if she has been exposed to that male's ejaculate. These patients also should be queried about self-medication, for many will have used over-the-counter vaginal anti-fungal medications or have douched, with very short-term relief followed by the resumption of symptomatology. In these women, it is important to try to make a proper diagnosis while the patient is still in the office. The physician should not depend upon gross physical findings, although there is often an excessive purulent vaginal discharge with bubbles present and vulvar and vaginal inflammation in these patients. Gross findings can be misleading. Figure **61** shows a frothy vaginal discharge of a patient who had bacterial vaginosis (BV), not *Trichomonas* vaginitis. The often-cited pathognomonic signs of a frothy vaginal discharge and strawberry spots on the cervix (colpitis macularis) are infrequently present and are not specific to *T. vaginalis* patients. The same pattern of vaginal sample collection mentioned previously is followed. A plastic spatula is used to place a portion of the vaginal fluid in a drop of saline and on a drop of 10% potassium hydroxide (KOH) on microscopic slides. A whiff test of the KOH preparation is done before putting a cover slip over the drops. A cotton

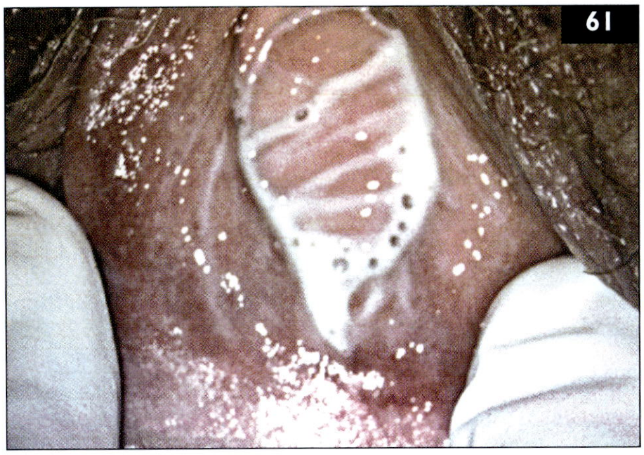

61 Frothy vaginal discharge. The patient had bacterial vaginosis, not *Trichomonas* vaginitis.

swab should then be stroked against the side wall of the vagina to obtain a pH measurement and to obtain a sample of the vaginal fluid for bacterial, fungal, and *Trichomonas* culture, using either modified Diamond's media or the InPouch *T. vaginalis* test for the latter. For the symptomatic women seen with this problem, the pH is nearly always alkaline and the whiff test is usually positive, as the *T. vaginalis* infection is often accompanied by an overgrowth of anaerobic bacteria. At this point, the parallels with BV are obvious. The physician then moves to the microscopic examination of the saline and KOH suspensions. An early sign signaling the possibility of a *Trichomonas* infection is the presence of a wide array of white blood cells (WBCs) on the initial microscopic examination (**62**). On higher power, Figures **63** and **64** show the microscopic examination discovery of trichomonads in the saline preparation. There are some caveats to be followed when doing this test that will

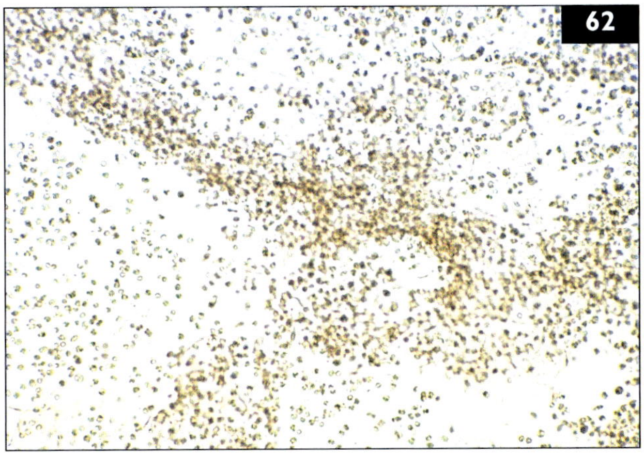

62 Low-power microscopic view of a patient subsequently found to have *Trichomonas* vaginitis. The field is covered with white blood cells.

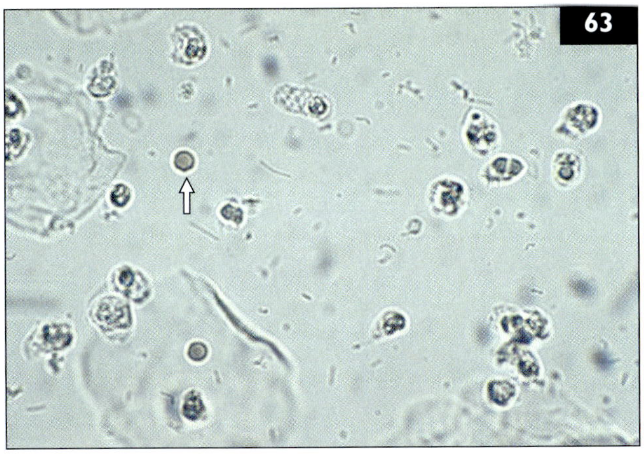

63 A motile trichomonad (arrow) seen in a higher-power microscopic examination of a saline preparation.

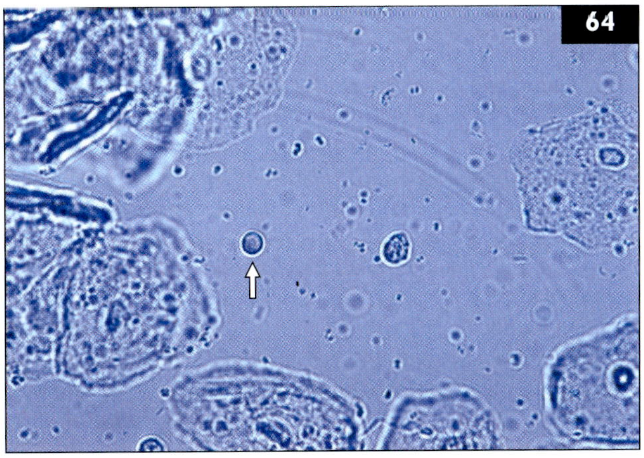

64 A motile trichomonad (arrow) seen in a high-power microscopic examination of a saline preparation. The flagella were not visualized with this frame.

increase the probability of seeing the motile trichomonads on the saline preparation. These flagellated protozoa are not hardy survivors outside of the vaginal environment. For the best results, the saline slide must be examined as soon as possible but, unfortunately, some clinics store their saline sources in a refrigerator overnight. Cold saline is a sure means of eliminating the flagellated movements of the trichomonads. If there are no motile trichomonads, it is understandable that an inexperienced microscopist doing a hurried examination might mistake a WBC for a trichomonad. The sizes are similar, but the WBC has a more distinct nucleus (**65**, **66**). For this population of medical care providers, confirmatory tests are good quality control to measure the adequacy of the microscopist's performance. A positive test confirms the microscopic diagnosis, especially when there are no motile trichomonads. There is a number of confirmatory testing techniques commercially available. These include modified Diamond's media, the InPouch *Trichomonas vaginalis* test (Biomed Diagnostics), and a *Trichomonas vaginalis* polymerase chain reaction (PCR) test. The PCR test is the most sensitive of the available tests, but has not yet been approved by the Food and Drug Administration (FDA)[15]. In addition to being used as confirmation, these tests should also be considered in the evaluation of patients with an inflammatory vaginitis with an elevated pH, in whom motile trichomonads are not seen on microscopic examination. Physicians should not depend solely upon the microscopic examination to make the diagnosis. In a recent study, only 52% of the women who had culture or PCR evidence of a *Trichomonas* infection were diagnosed by the wet mount examination[16]. For the physician without a microscope, these other culture or PCR tests should be used in patients with an inflammatory vulvovaginitis in whom there is a clinical suspicion of a *Trichomonas* infection. The problem with this approach is that there will be a delay in days from the time the patient is seen until the report is available for the heath care team.

The next category of patients that requires diagnostic consideration is those women with a *T. vaginalis* infection who are asymptomatic. There is a variety of patients that will require some physician interventions. The largest group is the patient whose Pap smear report returns days later with the notation that trichomonads are present. These patients require a return visit for evaluation, because these Pap smear findings are not specific; false-positives occur and, in a patient with a validated *T. vaginalis* infection, treatment of the woman and her male sexual partner is mandated. To confirm or deny the Pap smear report of a *Trichomonas* infection, these patients should be called back for the previously noted office tests with culture or PCR utilized if motile trichomonads are not seen on microscopic examination.

There are two other groups of asymptomatic women that should be screened for the presence of trichomonads. The first are those same patients that were screened for BV in whom the physician plans to do a vaginal or abdominal hysterectomy, a pregnancy termination, endometrial biopsy, dilation and curettage, hysterosalpingography, or intrauterine device insertion. Specifically, the medical care provider should get a culture or a PCR for trichomonads when a patient with an elevated pH, a positive whiff test, also has an inflammatory vaginal smear in which the clinic microscopist cannot see any motile trichomonads. The same regimen should be followed in pregnancy whenever a vaginal examination is done and the physician finds either an alkaline pH or a positive whiff test. If there is an inflammatory picture found on saline microscopy with no motile trichomonads, further tests for the presence of *T. vaginalis* should be performed.

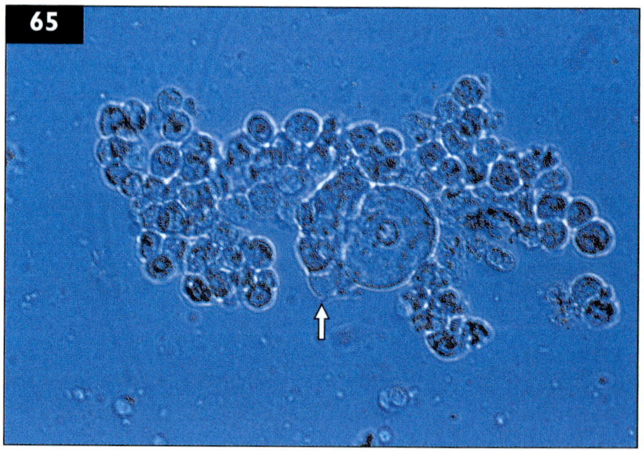

65 A trichomonad (arrow) in a saline preparation of the vaginal secretions of a post-menopausal woman. It is next to an immature squamous cell and the same size as the many nearby white cells.

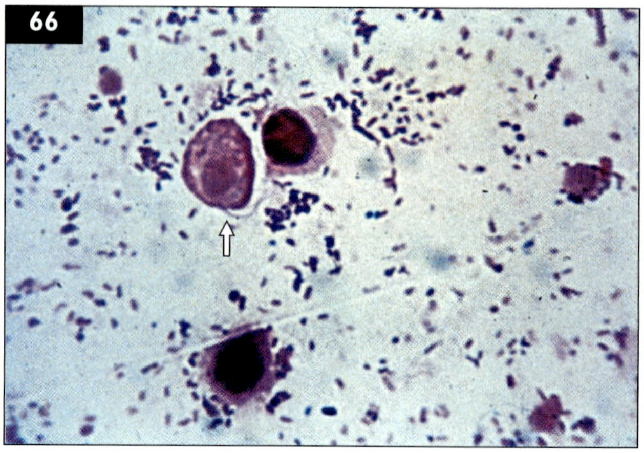

66 A trichomonad (arrow) noted in a Pap smear taken from an asymptomatic woman. To the right of the trichomonad is a white cell.

TREATMENT

The treatment for the symptomatic gynecologic patient with *T. vaginalis* vaginitis is well established and not controversial. The sex partners should be treated as well before these women become sexually active with them again. The current treatment recommended by the CDC is metronidazole (2 g) orally in a single dose[15]. There is less disruption in lifestyles with a single dose of metronidazole than treatment spread over several days, and the asymptomatic male is more likely to be compliant with a single dose of metronidazole than with the alternative regimen of metronidazole 500 mg bid for 7 days. This is especially important in the HIV-infected patient where compliance is important to achieve a cure and lower the risk of HIV transmission. These patients should be advised of the possibility of an antabuse-like reaction to alcohol with severe nausea and vomiting and they need to be aware that metronidazole has a long half-life. No alcoholic beverages should be ingested in the first 24 hours after the last dose of metronidazole.

There can be other setbacks in the care of these patients. Vaginal metronidazole should not be considered, as the tissue levels of the medication are not high enough to ensure acceptable cure rates and result in less than 50% of those achieved by the oral medication options[17]. Since it was approved by the FDA in May 2004, an alternate treatment regimen is tinidazole (2 g) orally. As tinidazole has a much longer half-life than metronidazole, no alcoholic beverages should be ingested for 3 days after the drug has been taken. Some women fail treatment with either of these regimens. The advice from the CDC in the metronidazole failure cases is straightforward. They should be re-treated with 7 days of metronidazole 500 mg bid and, if that fails, a 2-g dose of metronidazole once a day for 3–5 days. If that fails, consultation with the CDC is recommended[15]. In one study evaluating treatment failures with this dosage regimen, 87% of these patients were ultimately cured with a mean dose of 2.6 g of metronidazole given over a mean period of 9 days[18].

Some physicians have a jaundiced view of these CDC proposals for initial treatment failure. Over the years, in the authors' vulvovaginitis clinic, there has been a number of patients who have remained infected despite this approach. These infrequent patients seen in consultation have been a very interesting group for study. Usually, their infection symptoms have begun after a single unprotected sexual encounter with a partner they have not seen again. Also of interest, in those women who remain sexually active with the same male, there has not been a positive test for trichomonads from the male ejaculate. Admittedly, the numbers of these women are small. The common problem of metronidazole treatment failure for these women is that they cannot tolerate the daily 2-g dose of metronidazole. One strategy that can be employed in these women is to admit them to the hospital and treat them with intravenous metronidazole 4 g a day. The availability of outpatient intravenous medical services in the United States offers the option of treating these women as outpatients. In addition to this strategy, success has been reported using another member of the nitromidazole group, tinidazole[19]. Two regimens have been used with success: oral tinidazole 500 mg qid for 14 days, along with intravaginal use of tinidazole 500 mg bid for 14 days. Alternatively, a higher dose has been used: oral tinidazole 1 g tid for 14 days and vaginal tinidazole 500 mg tid for 14 days. In the patients failing this therapy, topical paromomycin can be tried. This has to be made up in a local pharmacy[20].

Patients who cannot take metronidazole present another difficult and not yet resolved therapeutic problem for clinicians. They have a variety of reasons to be in this category. Usually, the problem is one of metronidazole allergy. Desensitization can be tried, but this is an uncommon medical problem, and physicians have little experience with the desensitization regimen. Some patients with neurologic problems are not candidates for metronidazole treatment. In the authors' vulvovaginitis clinic one patient developed a peripheral neuropathy after high-dose intravenous metronidazole therapy. Fortunately, this resolved, but took several months. Also, there was one patient with symptomatic multiple sclerosis who had a more resistant *T. vaginalis* vaginitis. After failing with local therapy with an alternative vaginal medication, she was found free of infection 2 years later, probably related to her own immune response.

In those women who are not able to take metronidazole, local medications can be used. The use of a local anti-fungal preparation fenticonazole has been evaluated in Europe and has been associated with the elimination of trichomonads in some of the women studied[21]. The success rate with this approach is too low to have a place in primary therapy, but there could be a role when metronidazole is not an option for an individual patient. Alternatively, paromomycin can be prepared in a local cream and used locally, 250 mg per 4-g application to be used nightly for 14 days[20]. The problem with this approach is that some women can have a serious local reaction to this preparation and have to cease its use before the vaginal trichomonads are eliminated[19].

The treatment of asymptomatic women with a proven *T. vaginalis* vaginitis requires the physician's judgment with a careful balancing of the projected benefits and risks. These can vary with the population under scrutiny. For the nonpregnant woman noted to have trichomonads on a Pap smear and confirmed by subsequent evaluation, treatment of the patient and her sexual partner with a single dose of 2 g of metronidazole seems appropriate. The rationale for treatment is that these patients can subsequently become symptomatic with an inflammatory vulvovaginitis if not treated. The basis for any therapy of patients with asymptomatic *Trichomonas* vaginitis prior to hysterectomy or procedures involving instrumentation of the endocervical canal and the introduction of instruments, intrauterine devices, or radio-opaque dyes into the uterine cavity has not been established by prospective study. The lower genital tract tissue inflammation associated with most *Trichomonas* infections is probably not conducive to the best results with invasive procedures, for there is a concern about an increased rate of post-treatment infection. In these situations, the 2 g metronidazole treatment of the patient and her sexual partner can be employed before the intervention is done.

Pregnancy raises a series of still unresolved questions for the physician who discovers a *Trichomonas* infection in an asymptomatic patient. On the one hand, there are associations with this infection that are of concern. These women have an increased incidence of pre-term labor and delivery[4]. There also is the possibility of an increased rate of post-partum infection. On the other hand, treatment of these women with metronidazole seems to increase the rate of pre-term labor and delivery[5,6]. There are concerns about the study designs of each of these reports that call into question their conclusions. In the first study, an inordinately high dosage of metronidazole was given. These pregnant women were given 2 g of metronidazole in two separate doses 48 hours apart, and this 4-g regimen in divided doses was given again 4–8 weeks later. In the second study, the numbers of patients studied were small and metronidazole was one of three antibiotics given to these women. The problem of pre-term delivery was only found in patients who received first-trimester administration of metronidazole. In infected asymptomatic pregnant women, physicians should be concerned about the potential development of an inflammatory vulvovaginitis, as well as the association with an increased risk of post-partum infection. Because of this, one option would be to treat these women and their sexual partners with a single 2-g dose any time the infection is discovered after the first trimester of pregnancy. This is not currently recommended by the CDC, because of the failure of the metronidazole intervention study to prevent pre-term labor and the higher incidence of pre-term delivery in treated patients.

Chapter 7

Desquamative Inflammatory Vaginitis

BACKGROUND

Desquamative inflammatory vaginitis (DIV) is a clinical malady that is usually not recognized by doctors responsible for the care of these symptomatic, distressed patients. There are many reasons for this. It is an uncommon condition even for savvy infectious disease experts who have a referral practice filled with patients who have chronic vulvovaginal problems that have not responded to the care of their primary physicians. In this referral practice setting, Sobel found 51 patients with DIV among 7,000 (0.73%) patients seen over a 7-year period[1]. This disease mimics other inflammatory vulvovaginal infections that are much more commonly seen. These patients have gross and microscopic vaginal inflammation that is associated in the minds of most practitioners with *Trichomonas* vaginitis. DIV can also be confused with menopausal vulvovaginitis for it is more commonly seen in older women who have a paucity of mature vaginal squamous cells seen on microscopic examination of the saline preparation. This is a condition that Donders, an esteemed European investigator of vaginitis, would characterize as distinct from bacterial vaginosis (BV) and that he has named aerobic vaginitis[2].

Although the first clinical description of this infectious entity was published nearly 50 years ago[3], it remains today in the 21st century a poorly understood malady for women. Over the ensuing years since that first publication, a number of clinical observations have provided insight into the underlying etiology of DIV. This is an infection encountered primarily in older women. In Sobel's series[1], the mean age was 41.8 years (range 21–66 years) and 19 of the 51 patients (37.2%) were menopausal. In the majority of the women seen, they are of an age, either perimenopausal or menopausal, where they are witnessing a decline in their endogenous production of estrogen. Many of the women with this condition at Cornell are menopausal and, in common with the experience cited by Sobel[1], were not taking hormone replacement therapy when the symptoms began. This syndrome is almost entirely encountered in Caucasian women. In Sobel's series, 48 of the 51 (94.1%) were Causasian. At Cornell in New York City, all of these patients have been white and nearly all were Jewish and of Ashkenazi origin. This target population suggests there could be a genetic link to this disorder. Finally, the nearly uniform therapeutic success of vaginal clindamycin, the typical lack of lactobacilli on microscopic examination, and the frequency of cocci suggest an alteration in the vaginal bacterial flora. This shift results in increased numbers of bacteria susceptible to clindamycin, and this is a factor in the vaginal inflammatory response. The most frequent isolate on culture is the Group B streptococcus, but in Sobel's series this was recovered in only 44% of the cases[1]. Sobel has also noted that clindamycin's success may also be related to its anti-inflammatory activity by inhibiting pro-inflammatory cytokines[4]. The presence of large numbers of immature squamous cells has been the basis for the theory of accelerated desquamation of vaginal cells and the name applied to this syndrome[5]. More than this cannot be surmised from the available data. The paucity of women with this inflammatory syndrome is a major factor in our lack of scientific progress that would increase our understanding of this syndrome

MICROBIOLOGY

DIV is primarily a diagnosis of exclusion. It is defined as a clinical syndrome consisting of an exudative inflammatory vaginitis with a nonodorous purulent vaginal discharge in which diagnoses of trichomoniasis, endometritis, cervicitis, and an infection of the upper genital tract have been excluded. When viewed under a microscope, the vaginal secretions contain a large number of polymorphonuclear leukocytes, parabasal cells and naked nuclei[1]. The vaginal flora of women with a diagnosis of DIV is characterized by a large number of Gram-positive nongroup A cocci, and the absence of lactobacilli. The vaginal pH is markedly elevated. Distinct from BV, clue cells are absent and there is an absence of a vaginal odor.

It remains unclear whether DIV is due to a microbial infection, or whether the observed microbial colonization is merely a secondary effect of a dermatologic disorder such as erosive lichen planus[1,6,7]. The alleviation of symptoms following treatment with intravaginal clindamycin[1,7] is consistent with an infectious etiology. If antibiotic therapy fails, an alternative diagnosis is vulvovaginal erosive lichen planus. This can be diagnosed by biopsy with the specimen subjected to special staining by a dermatopathologist. Women with erosive lichen planus often have concurrent oral lesions, including erythema around the base of the teeth, or chronic recurrent painful buccal or gingival erosions. Oral surgeons call this condition the oral–genital syndrome. Group B streptococci, a predominant microorganism cultured from women with DIV, is not considered to be a vaginal pathogen. It remains to be determined using gene amplification technology whether a nonculturable microorganism may be involved in the pathology of DIV.

IMMUNOLOGY

One of the defining characteristics of DIV is a large influx of polymorphonuclear leukocytes into the vagina. This observation plus the inflammatory state of the vagina strongly suggests that there is marked cell-mediated immune activation associated with this syndrome. Estrogen treatment is ineffective for DIV, suggesting that the inflammation is not due to the withdrawal of this hormone. Studies have yet to be conducted to characterize the cytokines and other soluble inflammatory mediators associated with DIV.

DIAGNOSIS

It is not easy to make the diagnosis of DIV. It is an uncommon clinical problem, and the clinical, microscopic, and culture findings are not unique to this condition. Often, it is confused with other, more common entities. These women present with the symptoms of an inflammatory vulvovaginitis. The patients referred to the Cornell Vulvovaginitis Clinic have seen many physicians with no clinical response to vaginal and local anti-fungal preparations, local and oral metronidazole, local and oral estrogens, and local clindamycin given with the standard duration of therapy. Upon inspection, they have evidence of a copious vaginal discharge and, upon insertion of the speculum, an excessive purulent discharge is present, which when wiped away reveals inflamed vaginal mucosa (**67**). This inflamed mucosa had been incorrectly judged by a referring physician as the strawberry hemorrhages of *Trichomonas*. This is a distinctive clinical finding and varies from cervicitis in which the inflammation and discharge is restricted to the cervix. Examination of the vaginal discharge reveals an alkaline pH. When added to a drop of the 10% potassium hydroxide (KOH) on a slide, no amine odors are present, and the microscopic examination is striking, although not distinctive. Under low-power microscopy, there are many epithelial cells and white blood cells (WBCs) (**68**). There is an outpouring of WBCs (**69–71**), and this should set off a warning bell to the examining physician that this woman might have a sexually transmitted disease. The microscopic field should be scanned thoroughly for trichomonads and another portion of the specimen sent for polymerase chain reaction (PCR) test for *Trichomonas vaginalis*, *Neisseria gonorrhea*, and *Chlamydia trachomatis*. In patients with desquamative inflammatory vaginitis, all will be negative. On continued microscopic perusal of the saline preparation in this menopausal woman, there are few mature vaginal squamous cells (**71**). This is similar to the saline preparation of a breast-feeding post-partum patient with a persistent irritating vaginal discharge (**72**).

Diminished estrogen must play a role. The saline microscopic preparation from women with DIV shows no lactobacilli and an increased number of bacilli (**73**). The KOH preparation in another patient showed no lactobacilli and many cocci (**74**). The vaginal culture has no distinctive

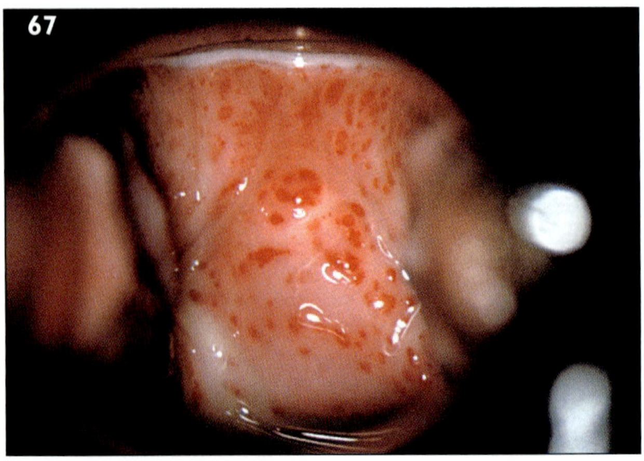

67 The gross vaginal findings of a patient with desquamative inflammatory vaginitis after copious amounts of purulent material had been removed from the vagina.

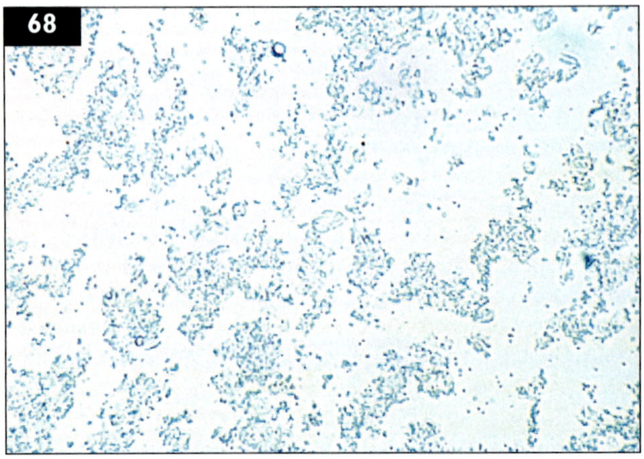

68 A low-power view of a patient with desquamative inflammatory vaginitis. Many squamous cells and white blood cells are present.

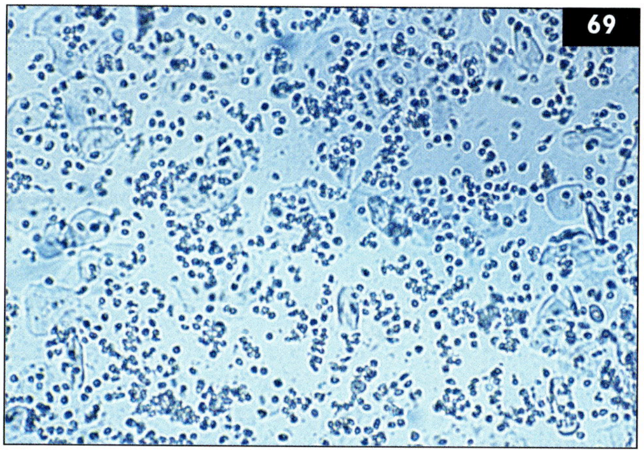

69 An overabundance of white blood cells on microscopic examination of the saline preparation of a symptomatic premenopausal woman with desquamative inflammatory vaginitis.

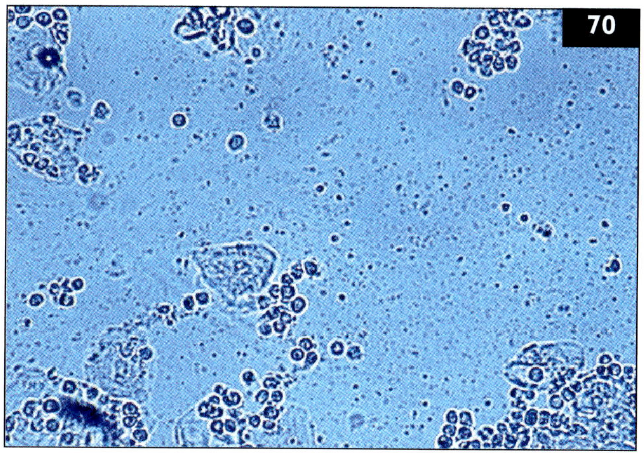

70 Microscopic scan on the edge of a saline specimen from a patient with desquamative inflammatory vaginitis, showing increased white cells and no lactobacilli.

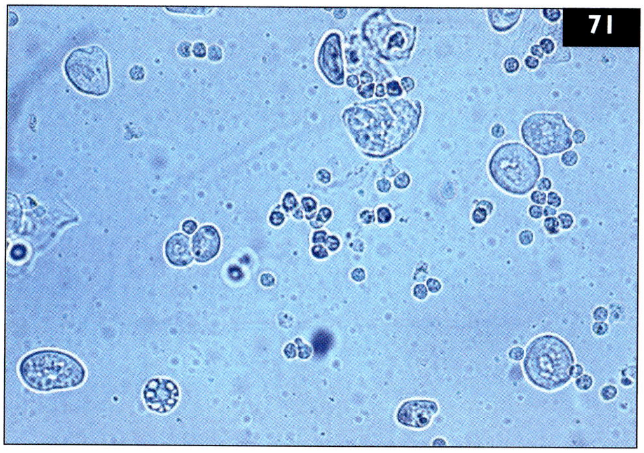

71 A menopausal woman with desquamative inflammatory vaginitis; there is a paucity of mature squamous cells seen on microscopic examination of a saline preparation.

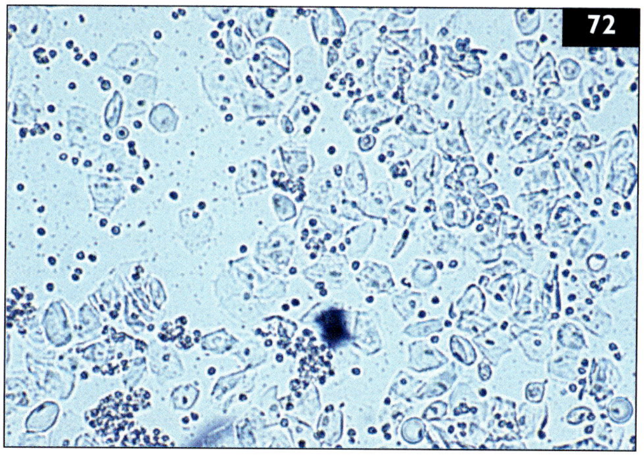

72 A breast-feeding post-partum patient with desquamative inflammatory vaginitis, with many white cells and few mature squamous cells on microscopic examination of a saline preparation.

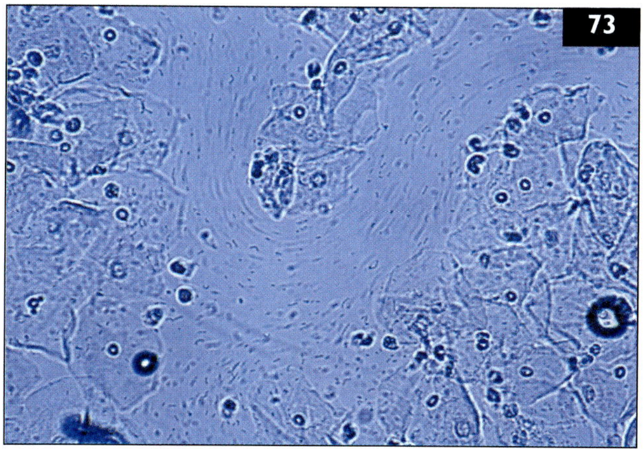

73 High-power view of a potassium hydroxide preparation from a patient with desquamative inflammatory vaginitis. In areas free of cells, swirling numbers of bacteria are present.

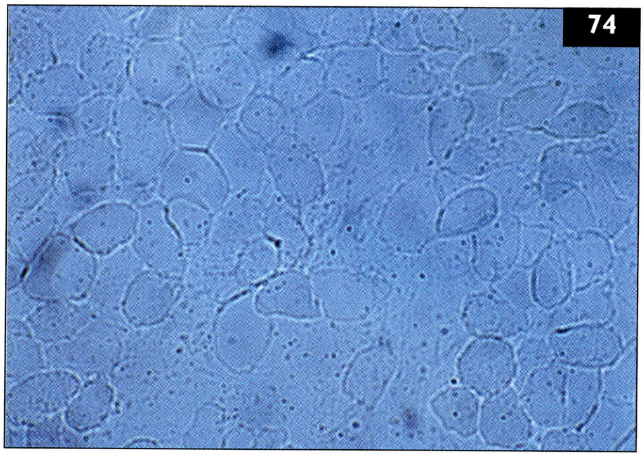

74 Potassium hydroxide microscopic evaluation from a patient with desquamative inflammatory vaginitis. No lactobacilli are present, only cocci.

pathogen, although the Group B streptococcus is frequently isolated. For most physicians, the diagnosis finally becomes apparent as they ponder the total picture. This may be at the first visit or when the laboratory reports are available. These patients have a remarkable degree of vaginal inflammation as seen by the gross appearance of the vagina, the huge volume of purulent discharge, the total field coverage by WBCs on microscopic examination, and negative cultures and PCR testing for *Candida*, *Trichomonas vaginalis*, *Neisseria gonorrhea*, and *Chlamydia trachomatis*. By this time everything clicks in place and the diagnosis of DIV can be made.

TREATMENT

There is no more satisfying group of patients to treat than these women with DIV. They are desperate, for they have this profuse, disgusting (to them) discharge that has been unsuccessfully treated by one physician after another. Physicians have to be aware of this uncommon condition. The beauty of this awareness is that the treatment is straightforward and so successful. Clindamycin vaginal cream 2% should be prescribed, and the patient should insert 5 g intravaginally at bedtime for 14 days. Sobel has reported a dramatic reduction in signs and symptoms with this treatment regimen[1]. After time passes, about 30% will relapse with a similar clinical and laboratory picture. When this occurs, a similar 2-week course of intravaginal clindamycin can be prescribed, followed by the periodic use of intravaginal estradiol in cream twice a week, or the vaginal estrogen tablet weekly. The rationale for the additional vaginal estrogen treatment is that it will create a vaginal environment more favorable to the growth of lactobacilli[8]. This is done with an awareness that estrogen alone has not been successful in the treatment of these women when they are at the height of symptomatology. There are women who will not use any exogenous estrogen. In these patients, an acid vaginal gel can be used once a week in conjunction with an intravaginal 600 mg boric acid capsule also once a week. These patients can insert one medication on Sunday night and the other on Wednesday night. The hope here is that these medications will restore the vaginal pH to a normal level for a period of time and create an environment more favorable to the growth of lactobacilli. Successes have also been seen with the periodic use of an intravaginal corticosteroid. Sobel reported success with 10% hydrocortisone (5 g) used daily for 2 weeks; after initial response, there needs to be slow titration of the steroid therapy[4]. There have been no studies to determine the effectiveness of either estrogen or substances to lower vaginal pH on the frequency of recurrences in these women.

Despite the current success of clindamycin intravaginal therapy, more needs to be known about this condition so that better directed treatments can be devised. There are clouds on the horizon; the Group B streptococcus, which is a predominant member of the bacterial flora in nearly half of these women[1], shows an increasing level of resistance to clindamycin[9]. The distinctive characteristics of this patient population suggest that a genetic factor is involved. It is known that a significant number of women with vulvar vestibulitis[10] and recurrent *Candida* vaginitis[11] have a specific gene polymorphism that is the underlying cause of the malady. This population of women with DIV should be the target for future genetic evaluations.

In contrast, the treatment of erosive lichen planus can be discouraging. This syndrome typically causes a vaginal discharge identical to DIV, with many inflammatory cells, increased parabasal cells, and the absence of lactobacilli. Women with biopsy proven ulcerative vulvovaginal lichen planus have only a transient response to antibiotic therapy and may require chronic use of potent systemic anti-inflammatory agents, more commonly used to prevent rejection of transplanted organs. Severe cases of erosive lichen planus may result in disabling degrees of inflammatory stenosis or agglutination of the upper portion of the vagina. In some cases, the syndrome can lead to the development of squamous carcinoma. Awareness of this possibility and the repeated use of the Pap smear are important in these women.

CHAPTER 8

GENITAL HERPES

BACKGROUND

There are two separate story lines that describe genital herpes (HSV-1 and HSV-2) infections in women. The first is the focus upon the symptomatic patient that was the vogue of medical attention in the 1970s and early 1980s. This was the pre-heterosexual human immunodeficiency virus (HIV)-era, where oral contraceptives prevented an unwanted pregnancy and pre-marital sexual activity with more than one partner was the rule, not the exception. The great fear was the acquisition of genital herpes, and physicians' knowledge of this infection was too sharply focused. Over time, it has been discovered that this narrow emphasis overlooked the largest portion of women with genital herpes. The medical dogma of the early 1980s was that women with this condition became very ill with their first outbreak, with perineal pain, fever, and voiding difficulties so severe in some instances that they had to be catheterized. The first infection was a sentinel event, easily recognized by the patient and the physician. Afterwards, these patients were instructed to be alert to the perineal tingling that occurred prior to the visible outbreak of perineal vesicles. These women were instructed that this was a time frame in which they could transmit the virus to a sexual partner and they should avoid intimate contact. At the onset of labor, these patients could inform their doctor of the possibility of a herpes eruption.

The theme was for the patient's personal responsibility that would avoid transmission of the virus to a sexual partner. It was a nicely constructed theory. Unfortunately, it has become apparent in the last two decades that this view applies to a minority of the patients who have a genital infection with HSV-1 or HSV-2. The breakthrough in this new understanding of the wide range of clinical presentations with genital herpes has come from the use of HSV-1 and HSV-2 antibody testing in the adult American population. Study after study showed that many more women and men were antibody-positive for HSV-2 than those with a history of genital herpes. One study of a general population group in the United States led to the estimation that 20% of adult Americans are infected with HSV-2, an increase of 30% since the late 1970s[1]. The incidence of HSV-2 infection is even higher in high-risk populations. In a survey of HSV-2 antibody testing in five sexually transmitted disease clinics, HSV-2 antibody presence was higher in women than men, 52% vs. 32.4%, $P < 0.0001$, and higher in blacks than nonblacks, 48.1% vs. 29.6%, $P < 0.0001$. In this study, the majority of HSV-2 seropositive persons (84.7%) had never received a diagnosis of genital herpes[2]. The take-home message of these studies for the physician is that this high rate of undiagnosed HSV-2 infection contributes to the continued transmission of the disease. These studies imply that the majority of patients with genital herpes are asymptomatic. This view has been put into question by a study in 2000[3]: when patients were identified as seropositive by serologic testing and educated about their HSV-2 infection, 62% reported having typical herpetic lesions. In addition, there are many modifiers that can influence the clinical presentation of these women. Prior exposure to HSV-1 and the development of HSV-1 antibodies can lessen the severity of the HSV-2 infection. It is also apparent that the first recognized episode of genital herpes might be the first symptomatic recurrence of an earlier, unrecognized primary infection. For the practicing physician today, this should translate into a higher suspicion of the possibility of herpes, with viral culture of any vulvar lesions plus wider use of testing for HSV-1 and HSV-2 antibodies.

There are trends in the pathophysiology of genital herpes infection that are important for the physician responsible for the care of women. The differences in positive HSV-2 antibody status between the sexes suggest that men transmit the virus to susceptible women more efficiently than women transmitting the virus to susceptible men[2]. The frequency of genital herpes caused by HSV-1 is increasing in the United States. Better living conditions and better personal hygiene have reduced the number of small children who have HSV-1 oral infection with the subsequent development of antibodies. As a result, there are more adult men and women susceptible to HSV-1 infection. For the physicians viewing the initial outbreak of genital herpes, there are no clinical signs or symptoms to distinguish a genital tract infection caused by HSV-1 from one in which the infectious agent is HSV-2. In this clinical situation, the infectious agent should be determined by culture and confirmed by accurate antibody testing. This is important information, for in the nonpregnant patient, the rate of both symptomatic and asymptomatic subsequent recurrences is much less with HSV-1 infections than HSV-2 infections[4]. For the pregnant patient, the risk of transmission of HSV-1 to the fetus is greater than with HSV-2[5], and the risk of transmission to the fetus is much greater with a primary infection than the first symptomatic recurrence of an earlier unrecognized primary infection.

There are two populations of women in whom genital herpes infection poses additional therapeutic concerns for the physician. The untreated HIV-positive patient is much more likely to be shedding HSV-1 or HSV-2. If she has an outbreak, she is more likely to transmit the HIV to a susceptible sexual partner. The pregnant patient must be assessed carefully in the ante-partum period and again when she is admitted in labor, for she runs the risk of transmitting the infection to the newborn. Fortunately, the incidence is low and it varies by country. It is more common in the United States, one in 1,800[6] to one in 8,700[7]. In contrast, the number of recognized cases of neonatal herpes in the United Kingdom is much smaller, only one in 60,000 births[8]. This difference in incidence will influence any suggested screening and treatment guidelines for pregnant women.

MICROBIOLOGY

Genital herpes is caused by a double-stranded DNA virus, herpes simplex virus (HSV). The two closely related members of this family responsible for genital infections are HSV type 1 (HSV-1) and HSV type 2 (HSV-2). HSV-2 is a genital pathogen and sexually transmitted while HSV-1 infects both genital and nongenital tissues. Antibodies to HSV-2 are first identified in individuals during the teenage years and peak by age 40. In contrast, HSV-1 antibodies are present in children below the age of 5 years and the incidence continues to rise until age 70. HSV is a neurotropic virus and, following infection and replication in epithelial cells in the genital mucosa, peripheral nerves become infected. HSV establishes a latent infection in neurons where it is inaccessible to the host immune system. A recurrent infection occurs when HSV replicates in the neuronal cells, is transported through axons to the original infectious site, and new epithelial cells become infected fostering new cycles of viral replication.

Genital herpes is one of the most prevalent sexually transmitted diseases in the United States and worldwide, both in developed and underdeveloped countries. The percentage of adults in the United States infected with HSV-2, as determined by the presence of type specific antibodies, approaches 25%. Interestingly, there has been a recent large increase in the percentage of genital HSV infections due to HSV-1, especially in women. In one study of women at a mid-western American university, the proportion of newly diagnosed genital herpes due to an HSV-1 infection increased from 31% in 1993 to 78% in 2001[9].

Only about 10–25% of seropositive individuals claim to have had an observable manifestation of the infection, i.e. a genital lesion. This nonrecognition of being HSV infected is a major problem for viral control and transmission, since most new HSV infections are acquired from individuals who were not aware of their viral status[3]. Contrary to commonly held beliefs, asymptomatic shedding of HSV-2 from the genital tract occurs at a similar rate in men as in women[3]. Therefore, in discordant couples where only the male partner is seropositive, seroconversion of the female partner can eventually occur even if no lesions develop in the male. The intermittent and unrecognized emergence of virus at genital sites can explain the apparent sudden appearance of genital herpes in women involved in long-term, mutually monogamous relationships. The possible long interval between virus acquisition and development of a clinically apparent genital lesion also explains the development of genital herpes in women who have been sexually inactive for varying periods of time.

The most serious consequence of genital herpes is neonatal herpes. In women who are seronegative for HSV-1 and HSV-2 during their pregnancy, initial seroconversion near the time of labor is associated with neonatal acquisition of herpes and a significant rate of peri-natal morbidity and mortality. Conversely, maternal seroconversion during the first or second trimester is not associated with an increased rate of adverse pregnancy outcome[5]. The rate of neonatal herpes can be reduced by cesarean delivery and limiting the use of invasive fetal monitoring in those women with positive cultures during the time of labor. Most importantly, neonatal herpes can be prevented by instituting measures to stop the acquisition of HSV-1 and HSV-2 during the third trimester in seronegative female partners of discordant couples[10]. Since most adults who are infected with herpes are not cognizant of this fact, it is imperative that both male and female partners receive serological screening for HSV-1 and HSV-2 during the first pre-natal visit.

IMMUNOLOGY

Immune responses to genital herpes virus infection do occur as evidenced by the accuracy of serological tests to determine exposure to HSV-1 and HSV-2. The induced immune reactivity does not prevent initial viral acquisition or the sporadic reactivations of viral proliferation and infectivity. However, the duration, severity, and frequency of HSV reactivation appear to be related to the functional capacity of the individual's anti-viral immune defenses.

Herpesviruses appear to have evolved mechanisms to blunt the effectiveness of anti-viral immune defense mechanisms. Infection of genital mucosal epithelial cells by viruses triggers the production of type 1 αβ interferon. The interferon up-regulates a multitude of genes in infected cells as well as in adjacent uninfected cells to prevent viral replication. However, HSV-1 and HSV-2 are more resistant than most other viruses to the action of αβ interferon, suggesting that these viruses encode an interferon inhibitor. There is only a relatively small decrease in viral titer following exposure to this interferon. Similarly, although complement-mediated lysis of free viruses or virus-infected cells is another anti-viral immune mechanism, an HSV surface protein binds complement component C3b and, thereby, diminishes complement activity. Later manifestations of anti-viral immune defense mechanisms, such as neutrophils and macrophage chemotaxis and phagocytosis, natural killer cell lysis of virus-infected cells, and stimulation of dendritic cell activation and differentiation, are also inhibited to varying degrees by HSV[11].

There have been attempts to develop a therapeutic vaccine against HSV-2 or to limit the extent of reactivation with immune modulators. The most effective immune-based methods to prevent genital herpes acquisition or its reactivation, an anti-HSV vaccine, immune adjuvants to boost selected aspects of anti-viral immunity, or development of inhibitors of HSV-anti-immune molecules, remain to be determined.

DIAGNOSIS

Diagnosis requires a physician alert to the possibility of a genital herpes infection. When the patient is asked what is their problem, the response that they have a vulvar or perineal irritation should bring immediately this possible diagnosis to the fore. The patient should be asked if they have ever had this problem before. If the answer is no, information should be obtained about a new sexual partner and what contraception the patient is using, for condom use lowers, but does not eliminate, the risk of infection. Queries about the male sexual partner's symptoms should be raised, although there rarely will be a positive response. The physical examination should check for the presence of an elevated temperature and the presence of tender inquinal lymph nodes. When initially viewing the perineum, the physician should ask the patient to point to the irritated site, for often these genital lesions are small and might be missed by a nondirected scan of the perineum.

Using a colposcope to magnify the area in question is a great help, and it is important to do a viral culture of any lesions, even when these patients are tender and in much pain. Figures **75** and **76** show the perineal lesions of a patient early in the course of a symptomatic first outbreak. These women are in acute distress, and the lesions are easily recognized. Figure **77** shows early healing perineal lesions of a patient with a primary outbreak 5 days after the onset of symptoms. Figure **78** shows the lesions of another patient with an HSV-2 infection 5 days after lesions first appeared. The lesions are obviously secondarily infected.

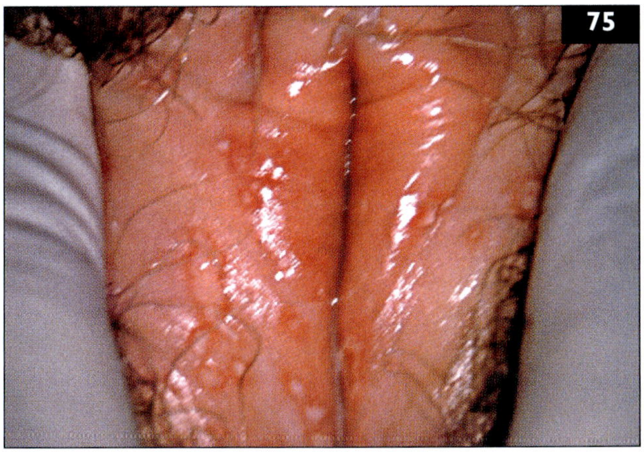

75 Perineal lesions of a patient seen early with symptomatic primary herpes infection.

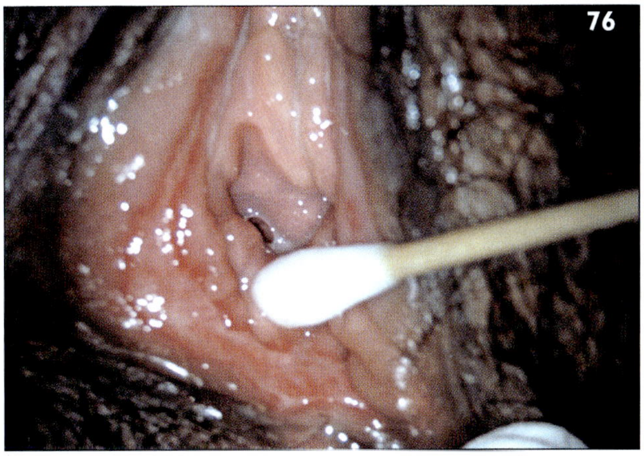

76 Perineal lesions of a patient early in the course of a symptomatic primary outbreak. Culture was positive for HSV-2.

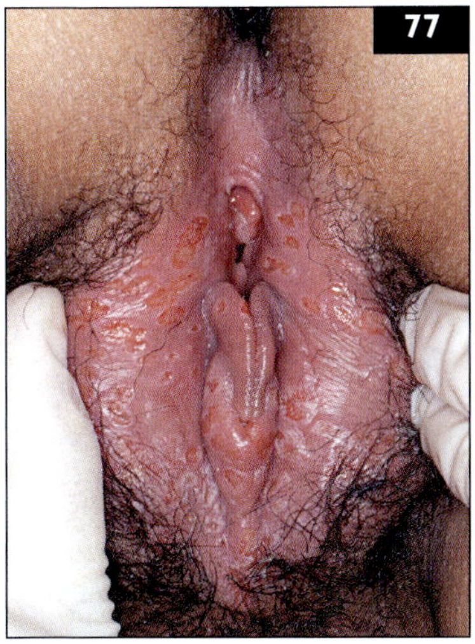

77 Perineal lesions of a patient with a debilitating primary outbreak 5 days after the onset of symptoms. Culture was positive for HSV-1.

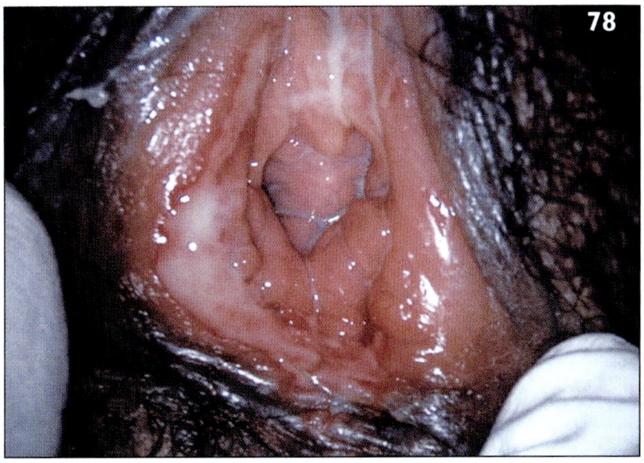

78 The appearance of genital herpes lesions 5 days after the initial outbreak. They are secondarily infected and very painful.

Not every woman with painful vulvar ulceration has herpes (**79**). This patient had negative herpes cultures and no herpes antibodies. In view of concomitant oral lesions, a tentative diagnosis of Behçet's disease was made. Patients are often unaware that they have genital herpes. Figure **80** is the picture of a patient who had a history of recurrent vulvar irritations near the rectum, which she attributed to recurrent yeast infections. She had no awareness that she had genital herpes. This was culture-positive for HSV-2. Figure **81** shows another patient with unsuspected genital herpes. In these cases (**80, 81**), the diagnosis was confirmed by the culture of small lesions that did not have a classic appearance of herpes. Patients seen late in the course of the disease will have crusted-over, healing lesions (**82**). These lesions were in same location that previous HSV-2 outbreaks had been noted.

It is important to culture the lesions and do HSV-1 and HSV-2 antibody testing in every patient seen with vulvar lesions. Without these two tiers of tests, culture and antibody screening, it is impossible to determine whether this is a primary or recurrent outbreak if the diagnosis is based solely upon the patient's history and the clinical findings. Tests other than culture are available to screen for herpes. Polymerase chain reaction (PCR) for HSV-1 and HSV-2 is a much more sensitive screen for herpes shedding[12], but the clinical significance of a positive PCR test for herpes as a marker for passing the virus to either a sexual partner or to the fetus is not known. The low numbers of virus detected by PCR possibly may not impose a risk of transmission. However, PCR is a more sensitive test than culture to evaluate whether the patient has an initial outbreak. This is also the time to perform serological studies

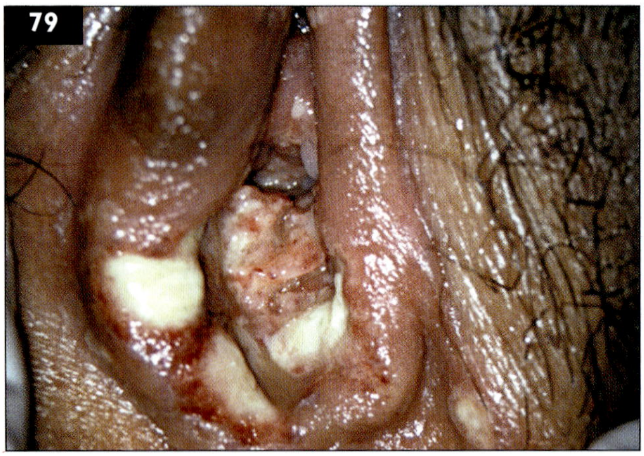

79 A patient with ulcerative disease of the vulva. Culture was negative for herpes and no blood antibodies were present to HSV-1 or HSV-2.

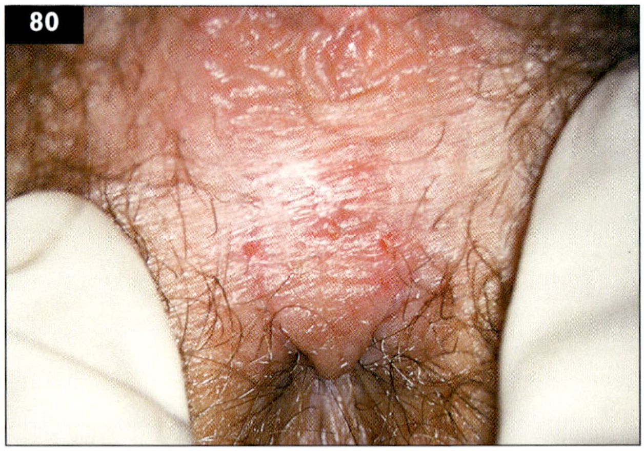

80 Patient with symptoms of vulvar irritation. She had small vulvar lesions culture-positive for HSV-2.

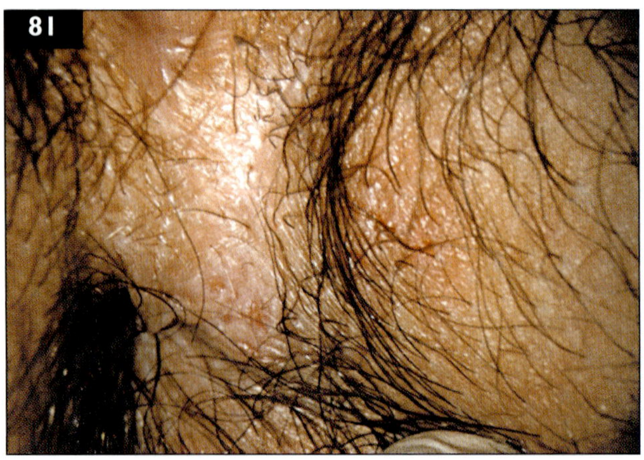

81 Patient with a history of recurrent vulvar irritation, which she attributed to *Candida*. Culture of these small lesions was positive for HSV-2.

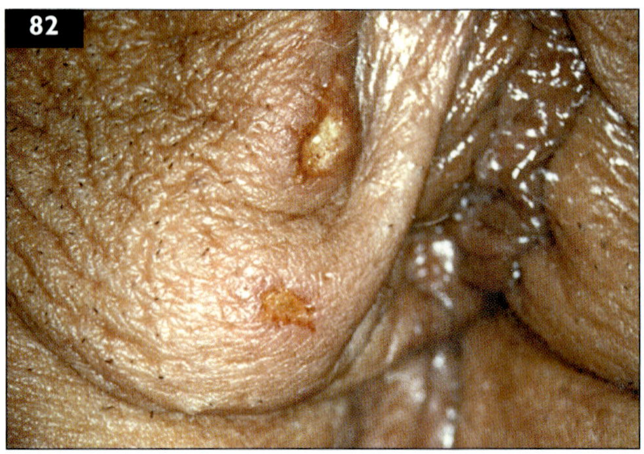

82 Patient with recurrent genital herpes, late in the clinical course with crusted healing lesions.

for HSV-1 and HSV-2 antibodies. If the culture is positive and no antibodies are present, this is suggestive of a primary infection. If the antibody tests are negative, they should be repeated in 4–6 weeks to confirm this diagnosis. If antibody tests are positive in a patient with an initial clinical outbreak, this indicates that she has a reactivation of genital herpes subsequent to an unrecognized first infection. In this case, the risk of transmission of the virus to the fetus is much less than if there were a primary genital herpes infection. Providing accurate information to the patient requires utilization of a laboratory where the most discriminating tests are available. Accurate type-specific assays for HSV-1 and HSV-2 antibodies must be based upon HSV-specific glycoprotein, a test commercially available since 1999[13]. Unfortunately, older assays that do not accurately distinguish between HSV-1 and HSV-2 antibodies are still on the market and are still being used in many commercial and hospital laboratories. The physician should be aware of the testing procedures used in the laboratory to which the specimens are being sent.

There are asymptomatic patients in whom the physician may be obliged to do herpes antibody testing. Since this is a sexually transmitted disease, testing of the woman should be paralleled by testing of the male sexual partner. There are three groups of women in whom this testing can be performed. The first is the nonpregnant woman who is about to begin a new sexual relationship and expresses a desire to avoid the acquisition of herpes. An antibody screen for HSV-1 and HSV-2 antibodies should be done for both partners. If the tests are discordant, i.e. one partner has antibodies and the other is susceptible, there is a risk of transmission of the virus to the susceptible partner. This is a particular problem if the woman is susceptible, for males are more likely to transmit the virus to a susceptible female than is the HSV-2-positive female to infect the susceptible male. The second area of optional testing is pregnancy. If the pregnant patient is HSV-1 or HSV-2 antibody-positive, the physician should advise her to alert the medical care team whenever any vulvar irritation or discomfort occurs so it can be evaluated and viral cultures obtained. This total concentration upon the HSV antibody-positive pregnant woman has dramatically switched. The physician can also detect the susceptible pregnant woman and obtain antibody testing of the male. Those men who are HSV-1 and/or HSV-2 antibody-positive can transmit the virus to susceptible pregnant mates. This population is important to identify, for one-half to two-thirds of the cases of neonatal herpes result from the mother acquiring a new infection in the third trimester of pregnancy and subsequently shedding virus in the lower genital tract while in labor. Overall, one study showed that 2% of susceptible women acquired HSV infection during pregnancy[5], but if the focus is placed on those at higher risk, i.e. discordant couples with a susceptible woman and an HSV-1 and/or HSV-2 antibody-positive male, the conversion is much higher (13%)[14]. The most jarring aspect of these observations is that for two-thirds to three-quarters of the women who acquired a herpes infection during pregnancy, neither they nor their medical providers were aware of the infection. Despite these concerns, screening for maternal type-specific HSV antibodies to prevent neonatal herpes was not recommended in one appraisal, because of concerns about costs, prenatal care delivery, and social duress[15]. In the British Isles with a reported incidence of neonatal herpes as one in 60,000 births, the costs of such a universal screening policy would be excessive[8]. One very good British analysis found no evidence for a public or individual health benefit for routine HSV-2 specific serology screening in antenatal patients[16]. The third group to focus upon is that of asymptomatic HIV-positive women. They should be screened for HSV-1 and HSV-2 antibodies, because they are much more likely to shed virus, and if they develop herpetic lesions, they are more likely to transmit HIV to a susceptible sexual partner.

TREATMENT

Treatment of the patient with a first clinical episode of clinical herpes requires an unhurried, nonjudgmental approach. After obtaining a history and identifying genital lesions suspicious of a herpes infection, cultures or PCR testing of the lesion should be performed, and herpes antibody tests should be obtained. It is sometimes difficult for a physician to make a definitive diagnosis at this initial visit, but if herpes is suspected, treatment should be begun immediately to lessen the severity and length of the symptoms. The physician should not be dogmatic about the diagnosis, and should emphasize that the diagnosis depends upon the laboratory findings. This is important. Too many women have been unnecessarily traumatized emotionally by a physician's hurried and incorrect diagnosis of genital herpes for a vulvar irritation. These women too often accept this wrong information as gospel for months or years. There is a variety of treatment regimens recommended by the Centers for Disease Control (CDC) in the United States[13] (*Table 9*).

Table 9 Treatment regimens recommended by the CDC

- Acyclovir 400 mg orally 3 times a day for 7–10 days

  Or

- Acyclovir 200 mg orally 5 times a day for 7–10 days

  Or

- Famciclovir 250 mg orally 3 times a day for 7–10 days

  Or

- Valacylovir 1 g orally twice a day for 7–10 days

An effective strategy is one in which the dosage is given two or three times a day, because this is an easier regimen for the patient to follow. When talking to the patient, the physician must remember that, for the woman involved, this is a highly charged emotional issue. A physician's disapproving attitude only adds to the patient's distress. The physician should state that the diagnosis is probably herpes, and that the medication should decrease their symptoms. This is not the end of their sexual lives and does not rule out the possibility of their becoming a mother in the future if they are of childbearing age. This emphasis upon age is important for this is not a disease limited to the young. Genital herpes can be diagnosed in menopausal women who have new sexual partners. In every patient, it is important to stress the fact that the prognosis and treatment options will be related to the results of the cultures and antibody studies. Another patient session should be scheduled in 1 week to 10 days to go over the laboratory findings, check their response to the medication, and offer some future guidance.

Armed with the culture reports and the blood HSV-1 and HSV-2 antibody studies, the stage is set for the follow-up visit. The physician must be prepared to deal with all of the variations in laboratory results. There are many combinations. The patient could have a negative herpes culture and no antibodies against herpes, in which case the symptoms were most likely not due to herpes; however, it is possible that the patient was seen when viral shedding had diminished to the point that the culture was not positive and it was too early in the infection cycle for antibodies to appear. This is the situation where the increased sensitivity of the PCR test is more helpful than culture. If culture is the test used, these women should be advised to have the antibody tests repeated in 4–6 weeks, and if no antibodies are then present, they can be reassured they do not have herpes. This is important, for there are patients who have been given the wrong diagnosis of genital herpes when they have never had a positive antibody test.

The next category is the patient with a positive culture for either HSV-1 or HSV-2 with no demonstrable serum antibodies. This indicates a primary infection and different advice should be given depending upon the herpes isolate. If it is HSV-1, the risk for recurrent eruptions is low, and this finding should be emphasized. They should be alerted to inform the physician if they have any symptoms suggestive of a recurrence so they can be re-evaluated. If the isolate is HSV-2, the patient needs to be counseled that recurrences can occur. The patient can be advised to keep a calendar to document the frequency of recurrences so that judgments can be made about either intermittent or prolonged treatment. They also should have a prescription for an anti-viral medication to be begun if they have prodromal symptoms. These women have questions that need to be addressed. Is their most recent sexual partner the source of the infection? Probably, but these partners could be asymptomatic shedders of the virus and not be aware that they have genital herpes. Contracting herpes is a medical event that terminates many relationships. Sexually active women, not in a monogamous relationship, have an important question. What is their sexual future? They should be aware that they do have the risk of spreading the virus to a susceptible male. The risk is greater if they have an outbreak, but these patients can have asymptomatic shedding of the virus. Although the numbers of virus recovered with asymptomatic shedding are much lower than when the women have lesions, infection can still occur. These women can be advised to inform any potential sexual partners that they have genital herpes. Too often, this ends the relationship. If the sexual partner is committed to the relationship, they should have HSV antibody testing to see whether they are susceptible. If susceptible, there are options available to reduce the risk. Obviously, the couple should avoid any intimate contact if there are either prodromal symptoms or genital vesicles or any genital lesions present. In addition, placing the woman on once daily valacyclovir reduces, but does not eliminate, the risk of transmission[17]. The most important long-term life question for many of these women is whether or not they can have a healthy baby. They should be advised that they will need to be monitored carefully and a cesarean section might be indicated at the time they go into labor if they have a genital outbreak, but with close observation they should look forward to having a healthy newborn.

The next group of women to counsel consists of those with a positive culture for HSV-2 and who have HSV-2 antibodies present. This is a patient having a nonprimary first symptomatic episode[3]. They have had a much less reactive first episode and must be instructed to learn to recognize the symptomatology associated with these episodes so they will be alert to them as warning signs. Again, in these women the frequency of outbreaks will determine the future therapeutic strategy.

In this patient who has been diagnosed with genital herpes, the strategy of how to deal with recurrent episodes should be in place before the next episode occurs. Effective episodic treatment must be given within a day of the appearance of lesions or ideally with prodromal symptoms. The patient should have an anti-viral agent on hand so that they are not requiring emergency prescriptions for the drugs. There is a wide range of treatment regimens available[13] (*Table 10*). Any of these regimens is acceptable.

Some women have frequent recurring episodes of genital herpes, six or more times a year. This disrupts their work and social lives and an appropriate option is to place these women on suppressive therapy. They should be counseled that such medication will reduce, but probably not eliminate the number of outbreaks. To date, this has been a highly effective strategy. These anti-viral medications are well tolerated for long periods of time, and the development of resistance of herpesviruses to these anti-viral agents has not yet been a problem. The many treatment regimens recommended by the CDC are noted in *Table 11*[13]. Patients should be advised that these regimens will also reduce, but not eliminate, the transmission of the virus to a susceptible sexual partner. They also should be aware that susceptible men are at lower risk than susceptible women in acquiring the virus. In one study comparing the use of valacyclovir 500 mg once a day to placebo in which condoms were used in varying degrees by the study population over an 8-month interval, the total HSV-2 infection rate in susceptible males was 6 of 499 (1.2%) valacyclovir partners compared to 9 of 497 (1.8%) who received placebo[17]. This was not statistically significant. Significance was achieved when the data on susceptible females were combined with that of susceptible males. This regimen for susceptible females shows an acquisition rate of 8 in 244 (3.3%) in the valacyclovir arm as compared to 18 of 244 (7.4%) in the placebo arm.

Patients who are HIV-positive present specific new problems for the physician. These immunocompromised women can have severe episodes of genital herpes that can be prolonged and painful. The episodic treatment regimens suggested by the CDC are shown in *Table 12*. If there is frequent recurrence, these women should be candidates for daily suppressive therapy (*Table 13*). HIV-infected women with genital ulcers are more likely to transmit HIV. In addition, this is the one population of patients in whom there should be concern about the possibility of the appearance of resistance to these anti-viral agents by herpes. If recurrences continue or persist, viral isolates should be obtained for a resistance screen and an infectious disease consult should be obtained after the sensitivity results are available, to help select the most appropriate anti-viral therapy.

Genital herpes in pregnancy carries with it the risk of transmission of the virus to the fetus. Fortunately, this is an uncommon event, noted in 1 in 1,800 to 1 in 60,000 deliveries[6,8]. In the past, the obstetrical focus has been upon the patient with a history of genital herpes. These women were under careful scrutiny with many mandates. The use of scalp electrodes or fetal scalp blood sampling would be avoided in the event that they were asymptomatically shedding the virus at the time of labor. If they had prodromal symptoms or a recent genital eruption when labor began, a cesarean section would be performed as soon as possible. A number of studies have also reported using suppressive anti-viral therapy for the last 4 weeks of gestation. This reduces the number of genital herpes outbreaks and reduces the frequency of asymptomatic shedding of the herpes virus, but the impact on the numbers of newborn infections due to herpes is not known[12].

Table 10 Treatment regimens for recurrent genital herpes

- Acyclovir 400 mg orally 3 times a day for 5 days

Or

- Acyclovir 200 mg orally 5 times a day for 5 days

Or

- Acyclovir 800 mg orally twice a day for 5 days

Or

- Famciclovir 125 mg orally twice a day for 5 days

Or

- Valacylovir 500 mg orally twice a day for 3–5 days

Or

- Valacylovir 1 g orally once a day for 5 days

Table 11 Recommended suppressive therapy for recurrent genital herpes

- Acyclovir 400 mg orally twice a day

Or

- Famciclovir 250 mg orally twice a day

Or

- Valacylovir 500 mg orally once a day

Or

- Valacylovir 1 g orally once a day

Table 12 Recommended suppressive regimens for recurrent genital herpes in HIV-positive women

- Acyclovir 400 mg 3 times a day for 5–10 days

Or

- Acyclovir 200 mg orally 5 times a day for 5–10 days

Or

- Famciclovir 500 mg orally twice a day for 5–10 days

Or

- Valacylovir 1 gram orally twice a day for 5–10 days

Table 13 Episodic therapy for genital herpes in HIV-positive women

- Acyclovir 400–800 mg orally 2–3 times a day

Or

- Famciclovir 500 mg orally twice a day

Or

- Valacylovir 500 mg orally twice a day

This narrowly focused strategy ignores the majority of newborns who are at risk for acquiring herpes from their mother at the time of labor and delivery. One option is HSV-1 and HSV-2 antibody screening on all pregnant women at the time of their first pre-natal visit. The population that is HSV-1 and HSV-2 antibody-positive with no history of genital herpes should be advised to report every incident of a vaginitis or vulvar irritation during pregnancy, so they can be examined and cultured to see if this an instance in which they have lesions and are shedding the virus. If they are, they should be instructed to recognize these reactivations and alert the physicians if they occur just prior to or at the onset of labor. The patients who require close follow-up are those susceptible to HSV-1 and HSV-2 infections. A primary maternal infection with either virus in the third trimester remarkably increases the risk of newborn infection. The value of screening and counseling has not yet been established, and the question of cost and effectiveness in view of the infrequency of neonatal herpes needs to be addressed before any screening program is established[15,16]. If a decision is made to screen routinely for HSV-1 and HSV-2 antibodies, there are three groups of susceptible women. The first has HSV-1 antibodies and none to HSV-2. Their sexual partner should be screened and, if HSV-2 antibody-positive, these mothers-to-be are at risk of acquiring an HSV-2 infection during pregnancy. To decrease this risk, the couple can perhaps use sexual abstinence, the male can use condoms during pregnancy, and the male could take a daily suppressive dose of valacyclovir. The next group consists of those with no HSV-1 antibodies and antibodies present to HSV-2. The sexual partner should be tested and, if HSV-1 antibody-positive, alerted that they have the risk of infecting the pregnant woman. An HSV-1 primary infection in a pregnant woman carries a higher risk of transmission to the newborn than a primary HSV-2 infection. This HSV-1 antibody-positive male could be advised to avoid oral–genital contact and, since HSV-1 can be recovered from genital infections, condoms could be used during pregnancy. Anti-viral suppression has not been studied in HSV-1 discordant couples, but it could provide added protection. Finally, HSV-1 and HSV-2 antibody-negative woman could have her sexual partner screened and, if HSV-1 and HSV-2 antibody-positive, the same advice could be given to the couple.

The future treatment of HSV-1 and HSV-2 infections will look beyond the current anti-viral regimens. Vaccine studies are underway and, if effective, they would be a tremendous preventive measure. In one study reported to date, a glycoprotein D-adjuvant vaccine was effective in women seronegative to HSV-1 and HSV-2. It was not effective in women who were HSV-1-seropositive and HSV-2-seronegative. It had no efficacy in men, no matter what their HSV-serologic status[18]. Immuno-enhancers, variations of the drug imiquimod, have been under study. They are applied directly to recurrent genital herpes lesions. Animal trials of this drug have been promising, for they have lowered the frequency of virus shedding. To date, the human trials have not proven effective.

Chapter 9

Human Papillomavirus Infections

BACKGROUND

There are two faces to the reality of human papilloma virus (HPV) infections in women. The overwhelming majority of patients with this most common sexually transmitted disease (STD) have no symptoms or cytologic signs of infection, and they rid themselves of the virus with no residual evidence of ever being infected. This is the silent majority of this widespread STD. A major component of physician opposition to universal HPV testing is that positive high-risk HPV tests will unnecessarily raise patients' anxieties over a disagreeable subject, an STD that has been linked to cervical cancer. There is strong support among physicians to the strategy of 'don't test, don't tell'.

A small minority of the patients infected with low-risk HPV strains will develop new growths, condyloma acuminata ('warts'), on the perineum, the rectum, or in the lower genital tract, the vagina or the cervix. These new growths are initiated by the presence of low-risk HPV types, so-called 'low-risk' for they are not associated with abnormal cervical, vaginal, or vulvar cytologic changes. With the current Food and Drug Administration (FDA) approved Hybrid Capture II testing, HPV types 6, 11, 42, 43, and 44 can be identified that are associated with this new tissue growth. Anyone testing asymptomatic women will find more positive low-risk HPV tests than women with visible lesions. The development of these visible lesions is a sentinel event for most women. It is a visible and palpable confirmation of the acquisition of an STD, to them a modern-day Scarlet Letter. Most want immediate treatment to rid themselves of these lesions, and they want to be assured that their removal will end their concerns about transmitting these viruses to any new sexual partner in the future.

There are other clinical situations in which these new lesions will be discovered. In the physical examination of a sexually active patient who complains of recent onset dyspareunia, warts can sometimes be discovered on inspection of the introitus. In a woman with a new vaginal discharge, vaginal or cervical warts can occasionally be identified at the time of the speculum examination. These women are usually appalled when informed of these discoveries. They feel violated, unclean and, again, want immediate treatment to eliminate the growths.

A similar scenario exists with high-risk HPV types. Most patients infected with high-risk HPV types are unaware of the infection and eliminate the virus without ever knowing they were infected. This immune response seems specific to the strain encountered so that elimination of one high-risk HPV type confirmed by negative Digene HPV testing can be followed by an infection with another high-risk HPV type. When these patients are Digene HPV-tested again, they will be positive. This is not the re-emergence of a prior infection that supports the widely held false assumption that these are lifelong infections, but instead is a new acquisition of a different high-risk HPV type. In a small percentage of women infected with high-risk HPV types, cellular changes occur that are reflected in cytologic reports as atypical squamous cells of undetermined significant (ASCUS), atypical glandular cells of undetermined significant (AGUS), low-grade or high-grade intraepithelial lesion (LSIL or HSIL), low-grade or high-grade glandular intraepithelial lesion (LGIL or HGIL), or frank squamous or glandular carcinoma. Depending upon the extent of the cellular changes, these abnormal Pap smears can lead to repeated tests at more frequent intervals or require biopsy confirmation, with subsequent treatment depending upon the tissue biopsy results.

Too many doctors and patients have misconceptions about the natural history of HPV infections. The patient's misinformed assumptions about HPV infection have been reinforced by the unfiltered data available on a variety of Internet Web sites, parts of which are wrong. HPV infections are not like varicella and herpes, in which the viruses persist in the human host for a lifetime. Instead, they are eliminated by the woman's own inherent host defense mechanisms. One careful study of sexually active female college undergraduates who had repeated polymerase chain reaction (PCR) testing for HPV showed that 70% of patients originally infected with HPV had eliminated the virus within 12 months and 91% in two years[1]. This immune response is very specific to the strain involved for, in a subsequent study of these same women after elimination of one high-risk HPV type, 70% had become infected with a new high-risk HPV type[2]. Obviously, there is a large number of asymptomatic women and men infected with various strains of HPV. They are the reservoir that continues the spread of HPV infection to other susceptible sexual partners. Most women eliminate these viruses remaining symptom-free, with no awareness they had ever been infected.

Physician awareness of the frequency of HPV infections has been increased in the last few years by the use of Hybrid Capture II testing, approved by the FDA and commercially available, applied in conjunction with the thin-prep Pap smear. Current HPV testing in the United States, Germany, and Britain has been population focused. It has been employed in parallel with the Pap test in women with a test result with the confusing nomenclature, 'atypical squamous cells of undetermined significance' (ASCUS). In the current strategy for care of these women, HPV screening confirming the presence of a high-risk HPV type dictates immediate physician intervention. This takes the form of colposcopic examination and biopsy of any abnormal appearing tissue, to be sure that more advanced cervical tissue changes are not present than appeared on the cytology report. Patients with an ASCUS smear and a negative high-risk HPV test do not require immediate colposcopy and instead can have a repeat Pap smear and HPV testing in 6 months. Since a Pap smear report of LSIL or HSIL dictates colposcopy and biopsy, HPV testing is currently not recommended to select patients who need biopsies in women with these Pap smears.

If cervical cancer is believed to be an infectious disease, this strategy with a focus upon established disease, i.e. an abnormal Pap smear, seems misdirected. With an infectious disease focus, a logical first step in a new paradigm of care would be to screen all sexually active women for the presence of the STD, high-risk HPV. Rather than wait for the progression of the infection to abnormal cervical cellular changes, these at-risk women would be identified early while they still had a normal Pap smear. Although this seems logical, a strategy of universal HPV testing is not currently justified. This most common STD yields many multiples of women infected with high-risk HPV types compared to the smaller number of these infected women who develop abnormal cervical cellular changes. Younger women, i.e. those under the age of 30 years with a high incidence of HPV infection, are particularly efficient in clearing HPV and eliminating early abnormal cervical changes without treatment. In contrast, women over 30 with a much lower frequency of HPV infection are less efficient in clearing HPV and more often require interventions to avoid progression of the abnormal cervical cellular changes. Universal testing today would require informing large numbers of asymptomatic women that they have a STD that has been associated with cervical cancer. This anxiety-producing information would then be followed by the physician's lame statement that no treatment is currently available to speed up the process of HPV elimination. Instead, these newly anxious women would be told to live with the infection and wait 4–6 months to have a repeat Pap smear and HPV test done. This is not a practical strategy.

The current alternative to universal screening in the United States has been to do HPV testing in sexually active women over the age of 30 who have had normal Pap smears in the past. This has also been suggested in the British Isles[3]. There is some logic to this guideline. These older women are not as efficient in the elimination of HPV as are sexually active teenagers and women in their early 20s. Because of this, they seem more likely to develop abnormal cervical cytology. Also, age 30 is an identifiable breakpoint in population studies when the frequency of invasive cervical cancer begins to increase. These women who are high-risk HPV-positive with a normal Pap smear are targeted for more frequent evaluations until they either develop abnormal cytology which will invoke some type of operative intervention or maintain normal Pap smears and become HPV-negative when they can be returned to a normal population category.

There is another high-risk population, HIV-positive women, in whom high-risk HPV screening has been recommended. A positive HPV test should dictate frequent follow-up visits with repeat Pap and HPV testing. A positive HPV test and abnormal Pap dictate operative intervention. All of these strategies invoke the use of HPV testing to enhance the cytologic screen. The focus remains on cytology, as it has been since the first reports of the potential benefits of cytologic screening in the 1940s.

The use of HPV testing may be expanded in the future if we change our focus from abnormal cytology to the asymptomatic viral infections that are the basis of subsequent cellular abnormalities. There soon will be two new strategies available to physicians. One will focus upon medical treatments to enhance the human host's process of virus elimination. This can take the form of immunomodulators, whose local application induces an increased production of interferon and pro-inflammatory cytokines to speed up the process of the woman's ridding herself of the virus. Alternatively, local injections or topical applications of interferon can be used to enhance the elimination of the virus. As a preventive measure, the most promising strategy will be the development of type-specific HPV vaccines that will prevent the acquisition of these viruses.

MICROBIOLOGY

HPV is a double-stranded DNA virus with a tropism for epithelial cells. Currently, more than 100 different HPV types have been identified, 40 of which infect cells in the ano-genital area. Approximately 18 different human HPV viruses have been shown to be potentially oncogenic and a necessary factor for the development of cervical cancer. These HPV types are classified as 'high-risk' HPV. Among the oncogenic HPV types, HPV 16 is present in about 50% and HPV 18 has been identified in 20% of cervical cancers detected worldwide. The other human HPV types that are responsible for only benign lesions are known as 'low-risk' HPV types. HPV is acquired chiefly through sexual intercourse, as indicated by the strong relationship between HPV acquisition and number of lifetime sexual partners, and is the most common sexually transmitted microorganism. Pre-natal HPV transmission as well as transmission by HPV present on fingers has also been documented. In the female, HPV can infect the vaginal introitus and vagina as well as the cervix. Anal intercourse can lead to anal HPV infections. Sexual activities between two women can also result in HPV transmission. In men, HPV infects the penile epithelium and the risk of infection is reduced in men who have undergone a circumcision[4]. Sexually active teenagers and women in their 20s frequently test positive for HPV, although in the vast majority of cases no clinical signs or symptoms of infection are evident. Utilization of a condom has been shown to be ineffective in preventing HPV sexual transmission. Immunity to HPV is type specific and, therefore, exposure to one HPV type does not prevent subsequent infection by other HPV types. Concomitant infections with more than one HPV type are common, especially in immunocompromised patients. In most women, cervical infections with HPV remain asymptomatic and are transient, becoming undetectable even by the most sensitive gene amplification assays after 1–2 years. This is also true for high-risk HPV types, leading to the conclusion that most high-risk HPV infections are, in reality, not a high risk for development of cervical cancer.

While the prevalence of HPV infection in women decreases markedly at about the age of 30, there is an increased likelihood of HPV persistence at this age. Furthermore, those HPV types associated with development of cervical cancer are more likely to persist than are low-risk HPV types[5]. It is the persistence of high-risk HPV types in some women, i.e. an inability of the immune system to spontaneously clear these viruses, that is strongly associated with development of pre-cancerous cervical lesions.

The physical state of HPV DNA within the epithelial cell greatly influences the malignant potential of the infection. In low-risk HPV infections, the viral DNA exists as a circular episome and is not integrated into the host cell's DNA. In cervical cancers, HPV DNA is found integrated into the cell's chromosomes. This integration disrupts the function of the HPV E2 gene, which is responsible for regulating the transcription of other viral genes. In the absence of a functional E2 gene, two other HPV genes, E6 and E7, are over-expressed and lead to uncontrolled cell growth and malignant transformation[6]. Both E6 and E7 inactivate the host proteins that restrict cell proliferation.

Although still not conclusive, evidence is accumulating that *Chlamydia trachomatis* might be a co-factor for HPV progression to malignancy[7]. A combination of several mechanisms might be involved. In women persistently infected with *C. trachomatis*, oxidative stress might result in alterations to the cellular DNA. Genetic alterations might increase the likelihood of HPV infection or activation of pro-oncogenic genes in cervical epithelia. Since apoptosis (programmed cell death) is inhibited by both *C. trachomatis* and HPV, survival of cells with altered DNA would be maximized in the presence of both infections.

IMMUNOLOGY

The abilities of HPV to persist in the genital tract for various periods of time, to be effectively transmitted to sexual partners, and to occasionally result in malignant transformation are consequences of the virus' properties of immune evasion[8]. The replication of HPV exclusively in epithelial cells and the absence of a blood-borne infection greatly limits contact between the virus and antigen-presenting cells. In addition, potentially immunogenic HPV capsid proteins are produced at low levels within epithelial cells, a property which also greatly reduces the potential for an effective immune response. The genes coding for HPV capsid proteins contain codons that are rarely utilized by mammalian cells. This assures that the availability of the appropriate transfer RNAs, and formation of the resultant proteins, will be limited. Other mechanisms of immune evasion involve the inhibition of anti-viral interferon alpha activity and interferon beta production by the HPV E6 and E7 proteins.

Approximately 30–60% of sexually active men and women are infected with HPV. In the great majority of cases virally infected cells are eventually eliminated by the immune system. Cervical cancer occurs in less than 1% of women with a cervical HPV infection. The ability of the host immune system to combat effectively an HPV infection, over a variable time period, strongly suggests that boosting the immune response through vaccination would be a successful approach in more rapidly eliminating this virus and, thereby, further reduce the incidence of cervical cancer. *In vitro* expression of the HPV L1 capsid protein leads to the formation of virus-like particles (VLPs) with high immunogenicity. Several groups, at Merck, Glaxo-SmithKline and the National Institutes of Health and centers in the British Isles and Europe, have taken advantage of this property and have initiated vaccine clinical trials using VLPs of various HPV types. The Merck HPV type 16 vaccine has shown excellent protection against HPV 16 infection and persistence[9].

DIAGNOSIS

The options for confirming the diagnosis of a visible new growth as condyloma acuminata or a wart are limited. Currently, the diagnosis is made by the physician's direct observation of new growth on the patient's perineum or vulva, a diagnosis often highlighted on mucosal lesions by the direct application of 10% potassium hydroxide (KOH) solution. Figure **83** shows the massive presence of warts on the mucous membrane of the vulva at the entrance to the

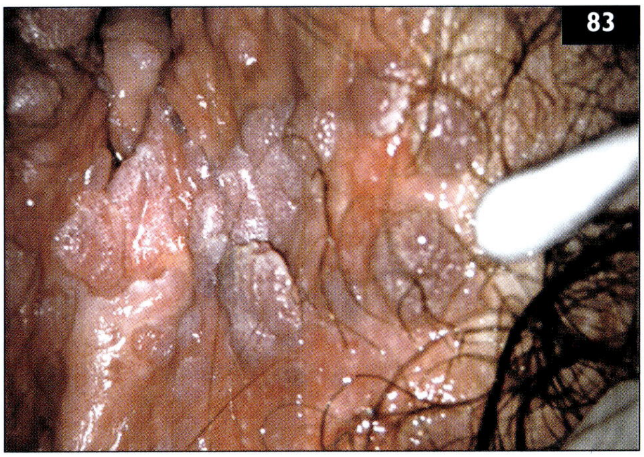

83 Multiple condyloma present on the mucous membranes of the vulva.

vagina. This is the type of illustration shown in most gynecologic textbooks. Fortunately, for physicians in practice it is a rare finding. Figures **84–89** show the more common presentations seen by the physician in an office gynecologic setting. Figure **84** shows a single small wart on the cornified squamous epithelium of the perineum. Figure **85** shows multiple small warts at the vaginal introitus. Figure **86** shows another patient with warts on the vulvar vestibule, a source of pain when intercourse was attempted. Figure **87** shows two warts near the clitoris, and Figure **88** shows a larger mucosal wart next to the hymenal ring. Figure **89** shows vaginal warts. Figure **90** shows a delicate, feathery wart growth on the cervix, highlighted by the application of KOH. Figure **91** shows a large condyloma on the cervix. There are no noninvasive techniques currently available to support this diagnostic suspicion by the detection of low-risk HPV types. The Digene Hybrid Capture II test is only approved for use in conjunction with cervical cytologic testing. PCR testing for HPV is not FDA-approved, and DNA probe testing for the presence of HPV requires tissue removed by biopsy. The result is that in most cases, the diagnosis is a visual one made at the time of the first visit, when a decision on the type of local therapy is made. For the patients who respond to therapy and the growths disappear, these limited diagnostic options are not a problem.

There is a large number of patients in whom this simple approach is not adequate. Most sexually active patients who come for the evaluation of new growths on the perineum or vulva are sure they have 'warts' and they are angry and upset with their sexual partners for giving them this visible problem. In many cases, their concerns are real and the growths are warts that can confirmed by biopsy (**84–88**). In other cases, these new growths do not have the distinctive look of a wart. Many of these patients will seek help after patient self-application treatment has failed. When these women are seen, a biopsy is an appropriate first diagnostic step to determine the nature of the lesion and DNA probe testing for HPV of the biopsied tissue can be done if the histologic picture does not confirm the diagnosis of condyloma. In many cases, the biopsy pathology report shows that the original diagnosis was in error. Figure **92**

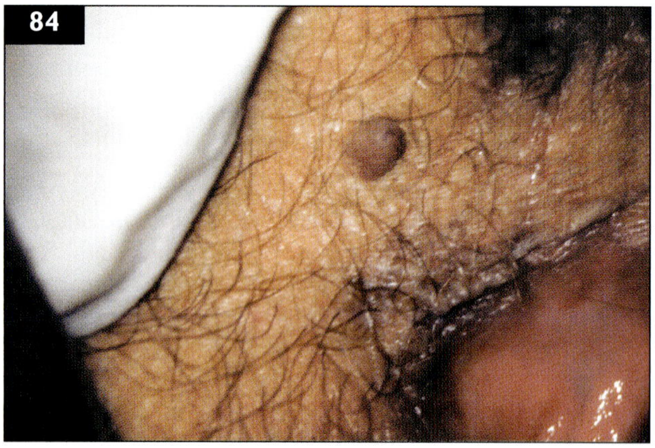

84 A single small wart on the perineum.

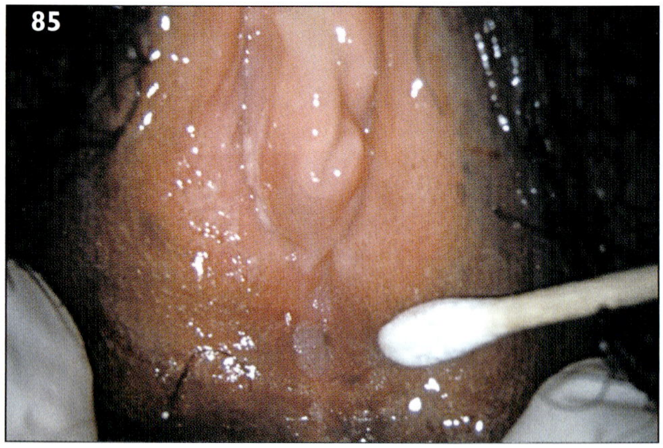

85 Multiple small warts at the vaginal introitus after acetic acid was applied.

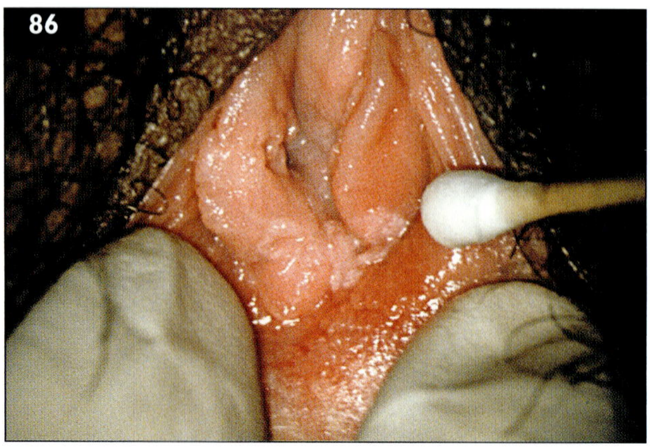

86 Small warts on the vulvar vestibule of a sexually active young woman.

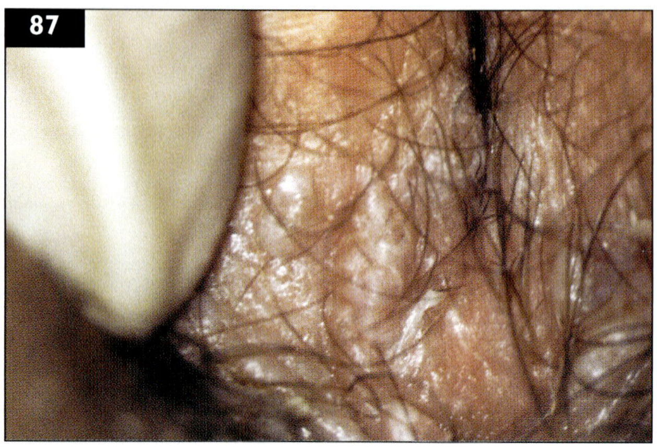

87 Two condyloma close to the clitoris.

illustrates the lesions of a woman unsuccessfully treated for warts who on biopsy had a hemangioma. Figure **93** shows the vulvar lesion of an upset patient who was angry with her significant other for giving her warts that had not responded to 5% imiquimod cream. The lesions were removed under local anesthesia with the pathologic diagnosis of an

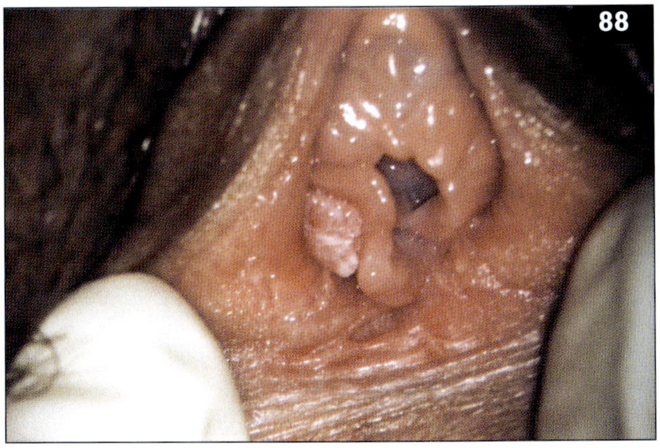

88 A large condyloma on mucous membranes next to the hymenal ring.

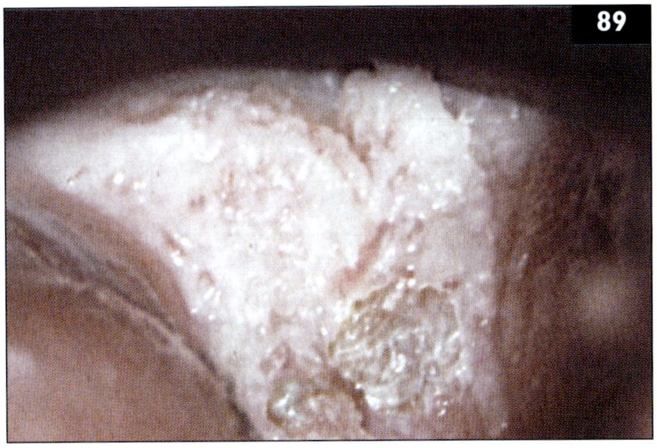

89 Extensive condyloma acuminata in the vagina.

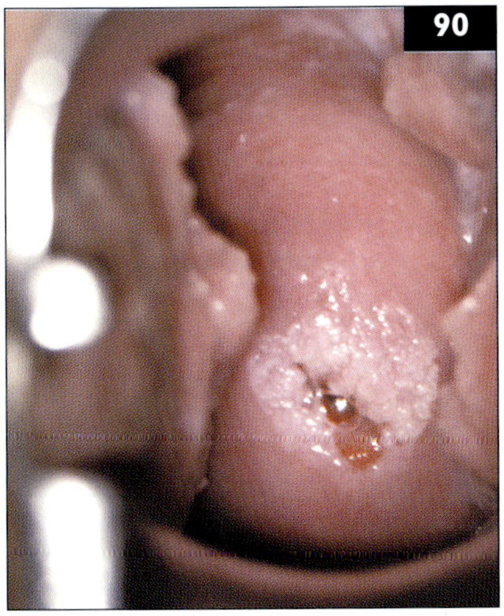

90 Fine condyloma acuminata on the cervix after application of 10% acetic acid.

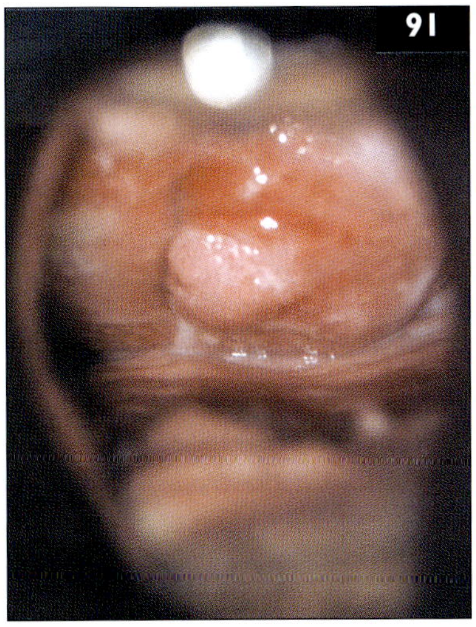

91 A large condyloma acuminata on the cervix after application of 10% acetic acid.

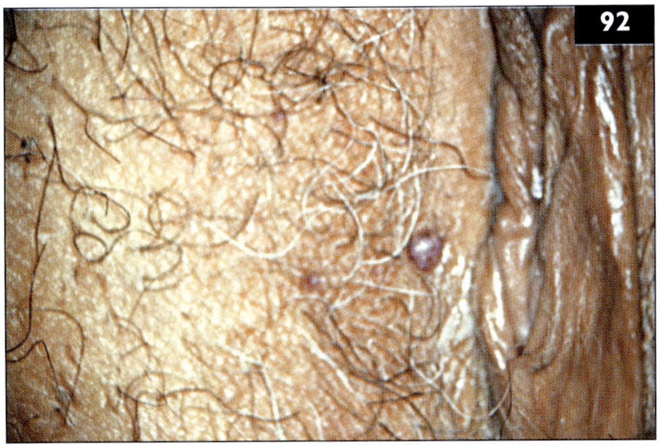

92 Suspected wart, unresponsive to imiquimod. Biopsy diagnosed a hemangioma.

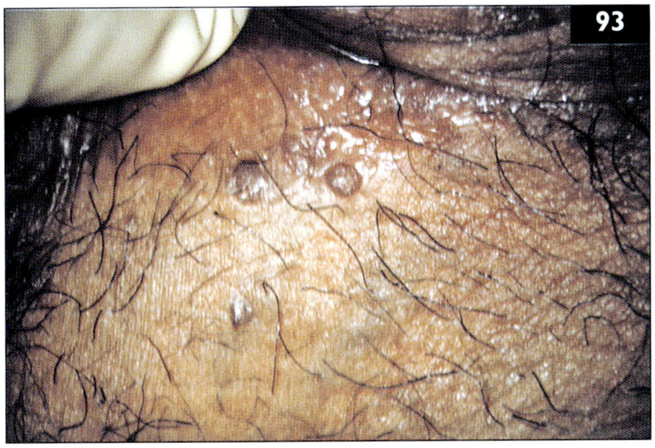

93 Assumed condyloma. Biopsy diagnosed an angiokeratoma.

angiokeratoma. Figure **94** shows another wart-like structure with the pathology diagnosis of acrochordon. Patients with micropapillomatosis labialis are often assumed to have genital warts (**95**). A gross inspection clue to the diagnosis is the symmetrical bilateral presentation of the lesions, which are confirmed by biopsy. Figure **96** shows the bilateral appearance of another patient with the lesions of micropapillomatosis labialis. It is easy to see that first inspection might confuse this condition with vulvar warts. A somewhat similar gross appearance on inspection of the vulva on biopsy proved to be low-grade squamous vulvar intraepithelial neoplasm 1 (VIN 1) (**97**). This illustrates the importance of biopsy in the care of these patients. Figure **98** shows the vulvar lesion, removed in its entirety, that proved to be a high-grade squamous VIN 111. A PCR test of a swab rubbed against this vulvar tissue was HPV 16-positive.

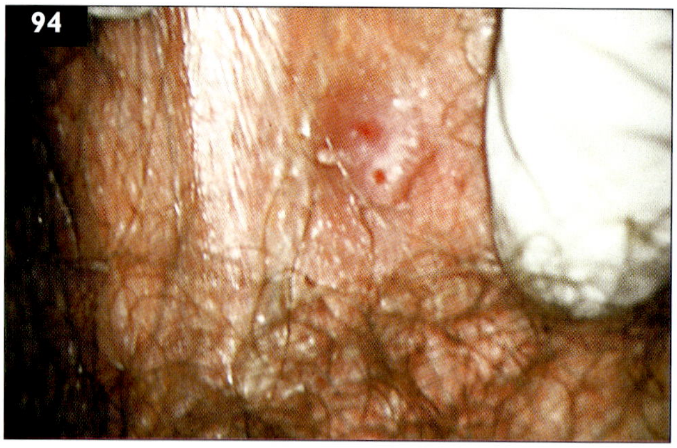

94 Assumed condyloma. Biopsy diagnosed an acrochordon.

Diagnostic testing for the presence of high-risk HPV types has become more widely used in the United States since FDA approval of the Hybrid Capture II test. The original Hybrid Capture I test was a nonradioactive, relatively rapid, liquid hybridization assay designed to detect five low-risk and nine high-risk HPV types. The Hybrid Capture II uses microtiter plates instead of tubes. It gave more reliable results with a lower detection limit and added four additional high-risk HPV types. This Hybrid Capture II test has many advantages. It is simple for the laboratory to perform and is done in conjunction with the collection of the Pap smear. There are no extra visits for the patient and no prolongation of the pelvic examination time. It is very sensitive and identifies 13 high-risk HPV types: 16, 18, 31, 33, 35, 39, 45, 51, 52, 56, 58, 59, and 68. The test has shortcomings that can make interpretation of the results difficult for the physician. It is a qualitative not a quantitative test, with the result either Yes, the virus is present, or No, it is not. Early in the course of infection when the patient is first tested, the patient can be shedding large quantities of virus. As the patient's immune system responds, the number of shed viral particles diminishes until they are eliminated. When a follow-up Hybrid Capture test is obtained later in the course of infection, when the number of shed viral particles may be much smaller, the result is still a Yes. The positive report gives the physicians no hint as to whether the numbers of shed viral particles are decreasing. The test also can be confusing to the patient and the physician in the event that a patient who originally tested positive and then found to be negative, subsequently tests positive again. This is not a re-exacerbation of the original HPV infection, but infection with a different high-risk strain. A positive high-risk HPV test only means that the patient is infected with at least one of the 13 high-risk HPV types. Finally, these are very sensitive tests and cross-well contamination of samples during processing can occur, resulting in a report of marginally positive HPV tests. One study found the proportion of cases at risk for these false-positive tests to be less than 3%[10].

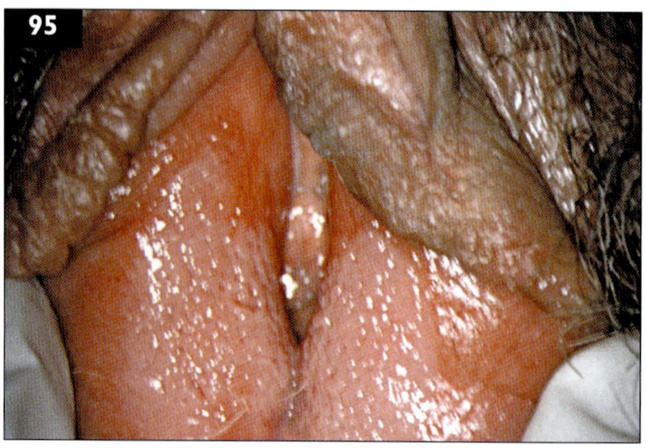

95 A patient with micropapillomatosis labialis. Each side of the vulva is a mirror-image of the other.

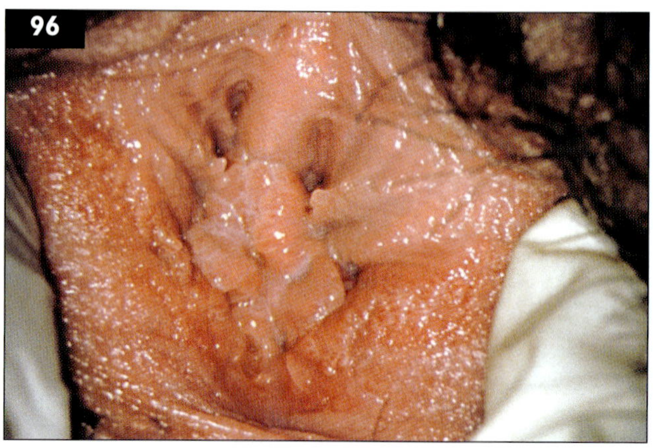

96 Another patient with micropapillomatosis labialis. The bilateral nature of the lesions is apparent.

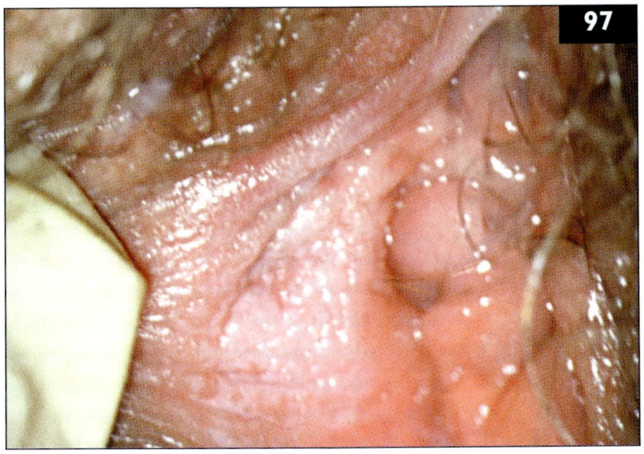

97 Vulvar lesion with different staining with the application of acetic acid to the field. Biopsy showed vulvar intraepithelial neoplasm I.

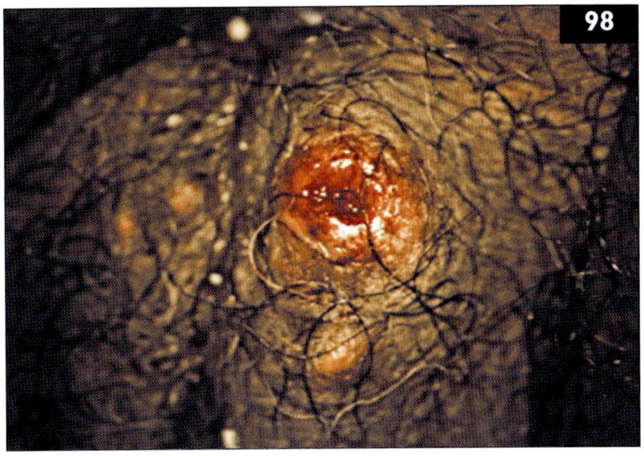

98 Raised vulvar lesion. Pathologic diagnosis was vulvar intraepithelial neoplasm III.

TREATMENT

The decisions about the mode of treatment of visible warts are influenced by their location. A wide range of therapeutic choices exists when these new growths are found on the cornified squamous epthelium of the perineum. The normal tissue adjacent to these 'warts' is more tolerant of any destructive therapy that extends to normal tissue edges beyond the wart than are lesions on the mucous membranes.

For rapid removal of these new unwanted tissue growths, a number of options is available. One approach is operative removal with the use of a local anesthetic, for it provides tissue to be sent to the pathology laboratory for a confirmatory microscopic diagnosis and DNA probe testing for HPV, if the tissue diagnosis remains in doubt. Care should be taken to avoid a too-deep incision into the normal dermis, and Monsel's solution (ferric subsulphate solution) can be applied locally to achieve hemostasis. Alternatively, freezing, heat, or laser can be used to destroy these lesions. Freezing the lesions with liquid nitrogen or a cryoprobe requires training with the use of this modality, and frequent employment of this intervention to maintain competence. Unless this is done, the result can be sub-optimal treatment that doesn't completely destroy the warts and which requires future office visits for re-evaluating the residual warty tissue. Of more concern is overtreatment, which can result in ugly scarring because of damage to adjoining normal tissue. Burning by cautery can also destroy the lesions. A potential problem is the occasional inability of the practitioner to measure the depth of the burn at the time of treatment, resulting in damage to the underlying tissue and subsequent scar formation. Finally, laser has the appeal of a high-technology approach with better control of the depth of the burn. There are concerns about the safety for the operator and helpers because the plume of smoke from the tissue treatment of these visible warts can contain HPV particles. And, of great importance in the United States at least, the laser equipment is an expensive capital investment and there is the temptation by some physicians to overuse this mode of therapy.

There are medical treatments for these visible lesions that can be used by the physicians. A big disadvantage of all of them is that they require repeated patient visits. This may not be a viable choice for many patients and physicians. If this approach is selected, podophyllin resin in tincture of benzoin can be applied directly to each wart and allowed to dry. There are legitimate concerns about (a) the increasing concentration of these tissue-toxic resins over time, and (b) the tissue reaction if any medication runs off the wart to normal skin. All patients receiving this treatment should be advised to wash it off 1–4 hours later. Another alternative is trichloracetic acid (TCA) or bichloracetic acid (BCA) applied directly to the warts. Again, the concern is spillage of the acid onto normal integument with subsequent burning and scarring.

There are two relatively new strategies that have been tried. One is the intralesional injection of 5% 5-fluorouracil (5FU). Another is the intralesional injection of one million units of interferon αβ, because successful treatment results in elimination of the warts without residual scarring. There is a number of drawbacks to the latter approach: it requires many office visits and several weeks after the last injection must elapse to determine if the treatment has been effective. More important, this is an uncomfortable mode of therapy for the patient. Every woman will have systemic symptoms after the first injection, such as general body aches and fever. Some have had repeated, though less severe, responses to subsequent injections. In addition, even though the amount of medication to be injected is small, it hurts when injected in this sensitive perineal area.

A convenient choice for treatment of small perineal condyloma acuminata is patient-applied therapy. Patients can apply local therapy repeatedly without visit after visit to the physician. There are two treatment choices available in the

United States. Podofilox 0.5% solution or gel is a purified lower concentration of the active agent in the podophyllin resin. These women are counseled to follow a unique treatment regimen. They apply the medication directly to the warts twice a day for 3 days to be followed by 4 days of no treatment. This cycle of care can be repeated for up to a total of 4 weeks. Again, this treatment can be irritating to the adjacent normal skin and the appearance of tissue ulcers during treatment is common, and subsequent scarring can occur. An alternative is the local application of 5% imiquimod cream directly to the warts on Monday, Wednesday, and Friday evenings for 4 consecutive weeks. Imiquimod is an immune-response modifier that increases the local production of multiple interferon messenger RNAs (mRNAs) and shows a reduction in virus load as measured by decreases in HPV DNA and mRNA for early HPV proteins[11]. It can be irritating to the underlying normal skin and must be washed off with soap and water 8 hours after application. The beauty of this treatment is that when successful, the warts disappear and there are no residual scars.

There are two groups of patients with visible warts who require special care: those who are pregnant and those who are HIV-positive. Pregnancy adds several dimensions to the care of women with condyloma acuminata. In some women, the warts proliferate to the extent that the vaginal introitus is a mass of friable tissue, an unfavorable site for any attempt at vaginal delivery. These large friable exophytic lesions should not be treated with either podophyllin resin or podofilox, because their large area of absorption permits systemic toxicity for both the mother and the fetus. Because of the size of these growths, any local medical therapy such as imiquimod, TCA and BCA can cause too much tissue inflammation when applied to large exophytic growths. Observation is not an option, for the other concern is that pregnant women with genital warts have 231.4 times the risk of delivering a newborn who will subsequently develop juvenile-onset recurrent respiratory papillomatosis than those free of warts[12]. Although this was a highly significant increase in risk the actual number of cases, 57 newborns with respiratory papillomatosis from 3,033 births (1.8%), in women with genital warts during pregnancy illustrate the low frequency of disease when visible warts are present. There is an even lower risk of HPV infection in the newborn in the face of HPV shedding in women using sensitive HPV DNA testing. In one study of 151 pregnant women, 54% had a positive test for HPV from cervical or vulvovaginals specimen at 34 weeks gestation. Despite this, none of the 151 infants developed clinical evidence of respiratory HPV disease[13]. Although there is a low risk of infants developing respiratory papillomatosis when delivered from women with visible condyloma acuminata, these lesions should be removed by operative excision or hot wire loop excision under local anesthesia prior to labor and delivery. In these cases the vulva should be re-examined at each subsequent pre-natal visit, for recurrences are not uncommon.

HIV patients who develop genital warts present two problems for the physician. They have more frequent recurrences following therapy and squamous cell carcinoma arising in or resembling genital warts may occur[14]. Because of this, local medical treatment is not an option. These growths should be removed either by scalpel or hot wire loop excision under local anesthesia with the tissue sent to pathology for microscopic evaluation and diagnosis.

Patients with lesions on the mucosa of the labia minora, vagina, or cervix pose a different set of treatment problems for the physician. Tissue fulguration therapy, (successfully used with the more resilient cervical tissue) when applied to the more sensitive mucosal membranes of the vagina and vulva, can cause scarring with subsequent problem, because of dyspareunia. The treatment of a patient with cervical warts (**90, 91**) should be straightforward. The lesions are biopsied to be sure that there is no more extensive pathology and, following this, the lesion can be removed in its entirety by excision, loop electrodiathermy excision procedure (LEEP), or ablated with freezing, cautery, or laser. The patient needs to be followed to check for recurrences but, usually, the cervix heals and the patient is free of problems. Applying the same regimen to the mucosa of the labia minora or vagina can result in tissue injury and scarring. The same concerns apply with most of the medical therapy options. On the labia minora, locally applied therapy to the wart by the physician (podophyllin, TCA or BCA) or by the patient (podofilox or imiquimod) all can extend to the surrounding normal mucous membranes, causing excruciating pain from tissue injury with subsequent scar formation. These reactions are seen to an even greater extent in the vagina where the removal of the speculum after treatment allows transfer of these irritating medications to normal vaginal mucosa with a potential for a mucosal burn. A popular therapy for vaginal warts in the 1970s was the intravaginal use of 5FU cream. The long-term problems seen in patients who had this treatment are the result of prolonged sequestration of this irritant in the posterior vaginal cul de sac, with ulceration and subsequent scar formation. For this reason, this treatment should be abandoned. What are the therapeutic options? A small biopsy under local anesthesia should be done to confirm the diagnosis of condyloma acuminata. Once this diagnosis is confirmed, the use of intralesional injection of interferon speeds up the process of wart elimination by the human host and avoids the problem of residual scar formation, but it has all the difficulties previously noted with this method of therapy, including frequent office visits and patient discomfort.

The next category of patients with HPV infection that requires therapy consists of those women with abnormal Pap smears. There is consensus about the use of HPV testing in patients with a Pap smear diagnosis of ASCUS. A positive test for a high-risk HPV type is a marker for the possibility of a lesion more advanced than noted by cytology. The current pathway of care is colposcopy with biopsy of any abnormal areas noted by acetic acid and iodine staining. HPV testing is currently not recommended in the United States and the British Isles for women with a Pap report of LSIL or HSIL, because this cytology report requires colposcopy no matter what the HPV tests show. One report using PCR testing for HPV cast additional doubt on the validity of the HPV screen, because high-grade lesions were confirmed by biopsy in women with these abnormal Pap smear reports who were PCR HPV-negative[15]. There may be value in doing HPV testing in women with LSIL or HSIL Pap smear reports. In one United States study, women with LSIL cytology and an initially HPV-positive report who subsequently become HPV-negative were unlikely to have problems with repeated abnormal Pap smears[16]. In another study in Holland, all 33 women to whose cervical changes progressed to CIN3 were persistently infected with high-risk HPV[17]. These interventions, colposcopy, biopsy, and the local use of astringents to control biopsy site bleeding probably enhance the local immune response and accelerate the process of HPV clearance and the return of cervical tissue to a normal state. This is especially obvious when looking at the results after cold knife conization or LEEP, where more cervical tissue is removed. The results with pre-invasive cancer, CIN1 or CIN2 break all the rules of cancer treatment. More than 70% of the women whose margins were not free of tissue abnormalities reverted to normal over time with no further therapy. There is justifiable concern about high-risk HPV infection in HIV-positive women. They have been noted to have high rates of recurrent and persistent cervical intraepithelial neoplasia[18]. Although logic suggests that the introduction of highly active anti-retroviral therapy would lower this risk, one study showed that no beneficial effects of highly active anti-retroviral therapy were seen[19]. These HIV-positive women should be followed closely with intervention dictated by cervical cytology abnormalities.

The final category of patients for care is those asymptomatic women with a normal Pap smear who are high-risk HPV-positive. Currently in the United States, the British Isles, and some countries in Europe, screening is an option in women over the age of 30. Those who are HPV-negative can be relegated to a less frequent Pap smear screening group and those who are high-risk HPV-positive can be followed with at least yearly Pap and HPV screens to see if they eliminate the virus and maintain a normal Pap smear or develop cellular cytologic abnormalities. This group was selected because of the low rate of HPV infection and the increased risk of abnormal cervical cellular changes. In contrast, the high frequency of high-risk HPV infection and the rapid clearance of these viruses in women under the age of 30 years with infrequent persistent cervical problems have eliminated them from HPV screening. If safe, effective immunomodulating agents were available that would accelerate the process of ridding women of these viruses, it would add support to the idea of a focus upon the etiologic agent, HPV, rather than more advanced stages of HPV infection when cytologic abnormalities are noted. Imiquimod, agents similar to imiquimod, and the local injection of interferon have the potential to accelerate the elimination of these viruses. They may be part of the new therapeutic strategy, targeting the pathogen, not the Pap smear. Obviously, prospective studies will be necessary to detect the efficacy of such an approach. Finally, prevention is the mainstay of care in any infectious disease. The effectiveness of an HPV 16 vaccine trial is an indication that this is feasible[9], and a quadravalent HPV vaccine trial is underway currently in the United States with two low-risk VLPs associated with warts HPV 6 and HPV 11, plus two high-risk VLPs associated with cervical cellular abnormalities and cervical cancer HPV 16 and HPV 18. Other trials are also underway in the United States and Europe. If these are successful, use of a vaccine in the future should reduce the frequency of HPV infections and the subsequent development of abnormal cervical cytology in sexually active women. In 2006, the quadrivalent vaccine Gardasil® was approved by the FDA in the United States, and by the European Union as well.

Chapter 10

Other Sexually Transmitted Diseases of the Vulva and Vagina

BACKGROUND

This is a grouping of clinical infections that is not part of the daily, weekly, or monthly outpatient office routine of most gynecologists. Physicians in clinics, emergency rooms, or sexually transmitted disease (STD) clinics that service the urban poor around the world, more commonly encounter STDs of the vulva and vagina. For the physician in private practice, these vulvovaginal conditions are rarely seen, and because of this, most physicians are unfamiliar with both the clinical manifestations and the available laboratory tests that can help confirm the diagnosis. Because these infections are uncommon, there can be problems with any diagnostic work-up. For an exercise in frustration, try to arrange for a dark field microscopic examination of the exudate of a suspicious vulvar lesion to rule out syphilis in a patient seen in an office, separate from a hospital! The equipment is rarely available and there are few physicians both competent and available to acquire the specimen properly and to evaluate the microscopic findings accurately. The more frequently seen, but still uncommon vulvar lesions, molluscum contagiosum, pediculosis pubis, and scabies, are most frequently seen in urban, poor young women. In the United States, these women have limited or no access to the private health care system. These patients are more likely to be seen in hospital emergency rooms, gynecologic clinics, or STD clinics. In the referral vulvovaginitis clinic at Cornell, an occasional patient is seen with molluscum contagiosum, and patients with pediculosis pubis are rarely encountered. These are not common entities for the average physician in practice.

Patients with ulcerative diseases of the vulva have a variety of presentations that requires specifically directed laboratory testing to determine the diagnosis. For the doctor in a private office or surgery, the most common pathogens encountered in patients with small vulvar ulcerations will be herpes simplex virus 1 and 2 (HSV-1, HSV-2). The vagaries of clinical presentations and the basic laboratory work-up have been covered in Chapter 8. A rare viral isolate from a genital ulcer is cytomegalovirus (CMV), which was isolated from a vulvar ulcer in a woman positive for human immunodeficiency virus (HIV)[1] (**99**). Physicians caring for this patient were certain this was genital herpes, but the culture proved otherwise. The remainder of the

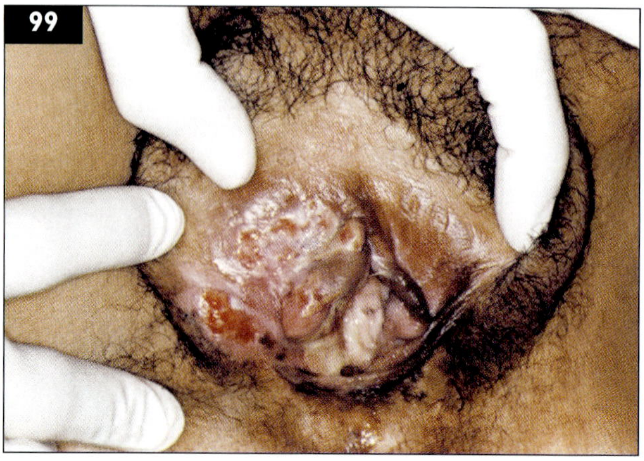

99 Ulcerative disease of the vulva in a human immunodeficiency virus- (HIV) positive patient. Clinically, the infection appeared to be due to HSV-1 or HSV-2, but culture grew cytomegalovirus.

genital ulcers, chancroid, granuloma inguinale, lymphogranuloma venereum, and the chancre of syphilis must each be considered in the evaluation of women with genital ulcers, and the clinician must always keep in mind that more than one pathogen can be present. Chancroid presents as painful genital ulcers, with inguinal adenopathy. If the adenopathy becomes suppurative, this is pathognomonic. The aspiration of a tender inguinal mass in such women can result in the collection of a copious amount of purulent material. The possibility of an HSV-1 and HSV-2 and *Treponema pallidum* as a primary or concomitant infection should be considered in every one of these patients. Granuloma inguinale presents with painless progressive ulcerative lesions without inguinal adenopathy. These lesions are highly vascular and bleed easily on contact. There is good evidence that the presence of these ulcers increases the risk both of the HIV-negative patient acquiring the virus and the HIV-infected patient being more likely to transmit the virus.

Patients with a lymphogranuloma venereum infection present with a history of a self-limited ulcer at the site of inoculation with unilateral tender inguinal nodes. Delayed or inadequate treatment can result in buboes being formed with rupture and associated inguinal or femoral ulcerations. The diagnosis of syphilis should be considered in every patient with a genital ulcer. Chancres classically are painless, but a secondary infection with other pathogens can result in discomfort at the lesion site.

Women with STDs of the vagina and lower genital tract are another matter. They usually have vague or no symptoms, and detection requires physician vigilance in obtaining a history and attention to the physical findings at the time of examination, so that appropriate laboratory tests can be obtained to establish the diagnosis. Part of the history obtained from these women should include information on whether the patient has had unprotected sex with a new partner. This can be an important clue from an asymptomatic patient, despite the fact that there is still a great divide about its importance among physicians. Many still believe that a patient with *Neisseria gonorrhea* will have symptoms of a pelvic infection and are only alert to the possibility of a pelvic infection if the patient is febrile or has pelvic pain. In an older, but still important study, Curran *et al.* showed that a significant portion of sexually active women with a positive culture for *N. gonorrhea* had either symptoms suggestive of a lower urinary tract infection, abnormal uterine bleeding, or a new vaginal discharge[2] (*Table 14*). All of these patients had negative urine cultures, and all had no pelvic examination abnormalities that suggested an anatomical cause for the bleeding. For the sexually active woman with this history and any of these findings, the physician should screen for the presence of *N. gonorrhea*. The physician's index of suspicion for *Chlamydia trachomatis* should be even higher in young, sexually active women, not in a monogamous relationship. There is good clinical evidence that many *Chlamydia* infections resulting in tubal damage have not been accompanied by clinical symptomatology enough to warrant the patient seeking medical care[3]. Wolner-Hanssen has suggested that many of these women in fact do have symptoms, which in his study were obtained by history retrospectively, many weeks or months after these patients were diagnosed with an infection[4]. Careful past-event questioning of these patients did reveal recalled symptomatology of an increased discharge or urinary burning, but these symptoms were not severe enough for the patient to seek medical care at that time. Because of the paucity of symptoms with *C. trachomatis* infections, it is now recommended by the Centers for Disease Control (CDC) that this population of young sexually active women have annual screening for an unsuspected *C. trachomatis* infection[5]. There is much support for this initiative, although one recent study raised the concern of false-positive gonorrhea test results in populations with low frequency of infection when very sensitive testing techniques are employed[6]. Despite these concerns, polymerase chain reaction (PCR) testing for both

Table 14 *N. gonorrhea* culture results by diagnostic category

Diagnostic category	Positives	(%)	Negatives	Total	Comparison with Group 5, no symptoms ($\times^2$)
1 Suspected *N. gonorrhea* infection, PID, or Bartholin's disease	42	(82.4)	9	51	<0.001
2 Abnormal uterine bleeding, undetermined cause	7	(43.4)	9	16	<0.001
3 Urinary tract infection	10	(35.0)	25	35	<0.001
4 Cervicitis or vulvovaginitis	6	(26.1)	17	23	<0.01
5 Other patients, no symptoms	8	(5.8)	129	137	

PID: pelvic inflammatory disease.

C. trachomatis and *N. gonorrhea* seems appropriate in this population, with the recognition that a few patients will have false-positive tests. The upside is that infected aymptomatic patients will be detected. Which screening test used – culture, DNA probe, or PCR testing – will be dependent in part upon the local economics of medical care.

Although less frequent now, an occasional patient will be seen with painful vulvar swelling, a Bartholin's abscess. Appropriate PCR testing for *N. gonorrhea* and cultures for anaerobic bacteria can be obtained when incision and drainage are accomplished.

MICROBIOLOGY AND IMMUNOLOGY

A multitude of sexually transmitted microorganisms causes vaginal and vulvar diseases. The probability a clinician will ever see a woman with any of the microorganisms discussed below will depend on the location and type of their medical practice. Nevertheless, a familiarity with the signs and symptoms of the various STDs is essential to be able to perform an accurate differential diagnosis.

Molluscum contagiosum is a sexually transmitted poxvirus and the cause of papular skin and mucosal lesions. It is a double-stranded DNA virus enclosed in a lipoprotein coat. Autoinoculation from the genital tract to other body sites is common. This infection is more common in females and is becoming an increasing problem in HIV-infected individuals. Many individuals with no known exposure to this virus are, nevertheless, positive for anti-molluscum contagiosum antibodies. molluscum contagiosum lacks most of the immune defense-related components present in other poxviruses. Nevertheless, it persists within lesions in the host for prolonged periods of time. Two of the viral proteins have been shown to inhibit apoptosis of infected cells. Other molluscum contagiosum proteins inhibit phagocytic cells from migrating to the site of infection and block the activity of interleukin-18, an inducer of interferon production[7].

Hepatitis B virus is a member of the hepadnavirus family, a class of viruses that infect hepatocytes and elicit acute and chronic liver disease. In addition to its presence in semen and blood, the virus has also been identified in saliva and breast milk. The hepatitis B genome is unusual in that it consists of a small, circular DNA molecule that is partially double stranded, along with a linear single-stranded region of variable length. The virus is double coated with two lipoprotein envelopes. Infected cells release a large excess of particles containing only the envelop glycoproteins and lipids into the circulation, as compared to complete DNA-containing virions. The majority of hepatitis B infections are acute and self-limiting, and result in immunity to reinfection. However, in a small percentage of cases a chronic infection develops with a variable concentration of virions persisting in the bloodstream. Interestingly, individuals that have successfully cleared hepatitis B as well as those with a chronic infection, have comparable sustained anti-viral antibody responses. Cytotoxic T cell responses, however, differ between the two groups and appear to be the main anti-viral defense mechanism. The hepatitis B virus does not appear to be directly cytotoxic to hepatocytes. Rather, it is the extent of the host's immune response to the infection that determines the degree of liver damage[8].

Haemophilus ducreyi is a short, nonmotile Gram-negative rod and the cause of chancroid, with painful and foul smelling genital and rectal ulcers. It is a predominant cause of genital ulceration in tropical and sub-tropical climates, and in regions with poor personal hygiene. Many *H. ducreyi* infections are resistant to antibiotics due to carriage by the microbe of one or more plasmids containing antibiotic resistance genes. A lesion in the skin or mucous membrane, due to abrasion during sexual intercourse, a concomitant infection or other irritation, is the portal of entry for *H. ducreyi*. An infiltration of polymorphonuclear leukocytes and subsequent ulceration form the characteristic lesions.

Genital ulcers also result from infection by *Calymmatobacterium granulomatis*, a Gram-negative encapsulated bacterium and the causative agent of donovanosis. Like chancroid, donovanosis is most prevalent in warm climates. However, the two diseases differ in that the lesions of donovanosis are painless.

Three serovars of the obliate intracellular microbe *Chlamydia trachomatis*, L1, L2, and L3, are other genital ulcer-causing microorganisms. The disease caused by these bacteria is called lymphogranuloma venereum. In infected women, a painless papule which subsequently ulcerates appears on the vulva, vaginal wall, or cervix. The secondary stage of infection, appearing predominately in men, is characterized by the appearance of painful inguinal lymphadenopathy. If untreated, lymphatic obstruction and elephantitis of the genitalia can develop.

Yet another cause of genital ulcers is *Treponema pallidum*, the spirochite bacterium responsible for syphilis. *T. pallidum* passes through microscopic genital tract abrasions and induces formation of genital ulcers known as chancres (primary syphilis) on the vulva, vaginal wall, or cervix. Following their replication, the microbe disseminates through the circulatory and lymphatic system resulting in formation of a rash, low-grade fever, and lymph node enlargement (secondary syphilis). These symptoms resolve and a latency period ensues. Untreated syphilis may then progress to a tertiary stage characterized by central nervous system (CNS), vascular system, and/or skin and bone involvement. The outer membrane of *T. pallidum* lacks lipopolysaccharide and is also largely devoid of transmembrane proteins. Thus, the microbe is poorly immunogenic and infected and treated individuals remain susceptible to reinfection[9].

Neisseria gonorrhea, the causative microorganism of gonorrhea, is a Gram-negative diploid bacterium. In women, it primarily infects columnar epithelia in the urethra, cervix, and rectum. However, the vulva and vagina are also sites of infection in prepubescent girls. Some sexually active women will develop a Bartholin's abscess casused by *N. gonorrhea*. Subsequent recurrent Bartholin's abscesses are usually associated with the recovery of anaerobic bacteria. Unlike in men, gonococcal infections in women are typically asymptomatic. The lack of detection or misdiagnosis has serious consequences, since untreated infections ascend to the fallopian tubes and cause pelvic inflammatory disease. Treatment of *N. gonorrhea* is becoming increasingly difficult due to the presence of plasmids that carry antibiotic resistance genes.

The ectoparasite, *Phthirus pubis*, infects pubic hair and is the cause of pubic lice. After sexual transmission from an infected to a noninfected individual, the female *P. pubis* lays an egg that becomes firmly attached to the base of a hair follicle. After a 7-day incubation period, the emerging parasite induces a skin lesion, secretes saliva and then ingests a mixture of saliva and blood. The severe itching that ensues is due to an immediate hypersensitivity reaction to allergens in the saliva.

DIAGNOSIS

The key to the care of the patients with STDs of the vulva, vagina, or lower genital tract is an awareness of the wide variety of different clinical presentations and the knowledge of appropriate laboratory tests necessary to confirm the diagnosis.

Molluscum contagiosum has a characteristic appearance, a central umbilicated area filled with a semi-solid white material. These lesions can present in a number of forms. Figure **100** shows a single lesion. These lesions can spread rapidly. Figure **101** shows a patient with multiple molluscum contagiosum lesions. Figure **102** shows the lesions immediately after local treatment when central white material has been removed. If local treatment fails to clear the lesions, a biopsy should be obtained to confirm the initial clinical impression.

Patients with pediculosis pubis seek medical attention for intense and continuous vulvar itching. On questioning, they may have noticed lice or nits on their pubic hair. This is a population in whom a few minutes surveillance of the pubic region with a colposcope will pick up the visible, moveable ectoparasites. Under magnification, these are ugly creatures; their appearance and movement makes many an examiner's skin crawl (**103**). Patients with scabies present for care, because of unbearable vulvar pruritis. Again, surveillance with a colposcope often reveals the presence of the *Sarcoptes scabiei* (**104**). These women will often have a vulvar rash, reflective of their contact dermatitis.

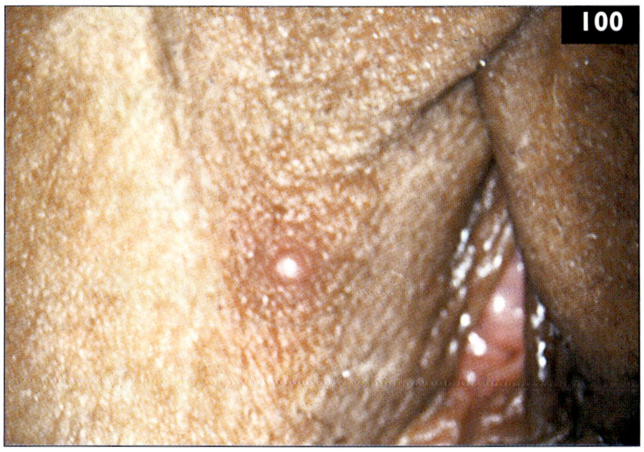

100 A patient with a solitary molluscum contagiosum lesion.

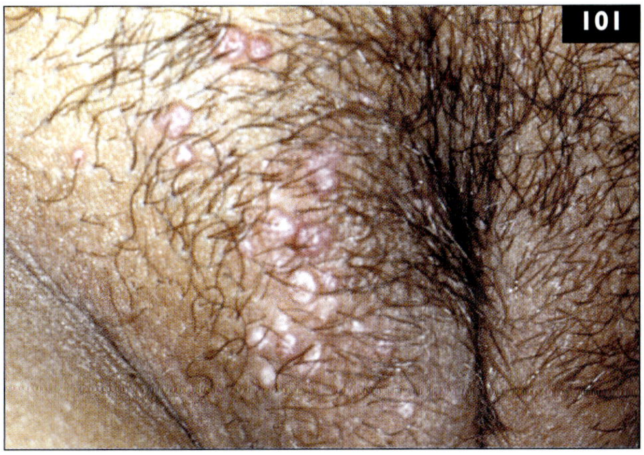

101 A patient with a field of multiple molluscum contagiosum lesions.

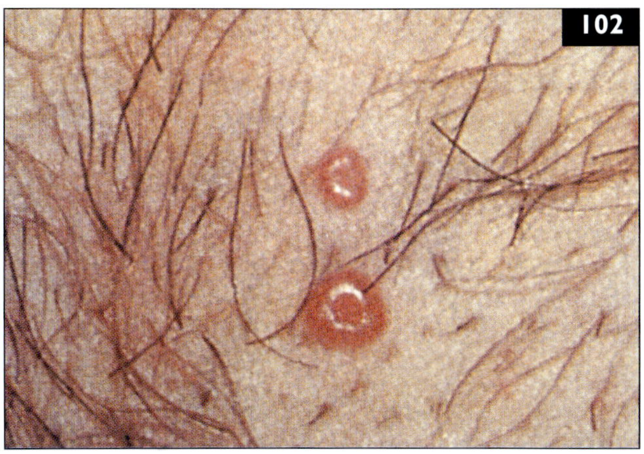

102 A patient with molluscum contagiosum after local treatment has removed the central white core.

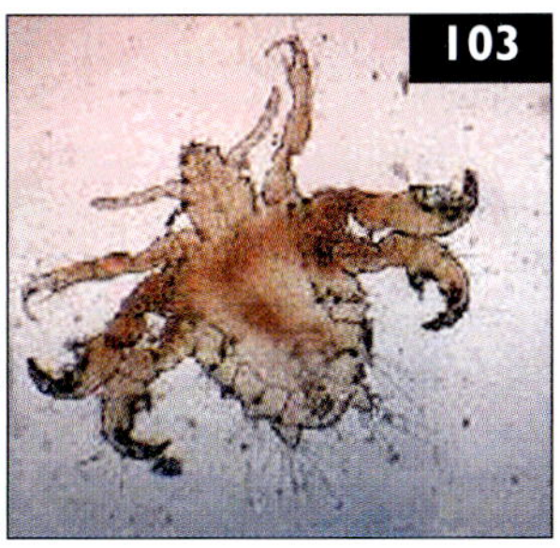

103 A magnified picture of a body louse.

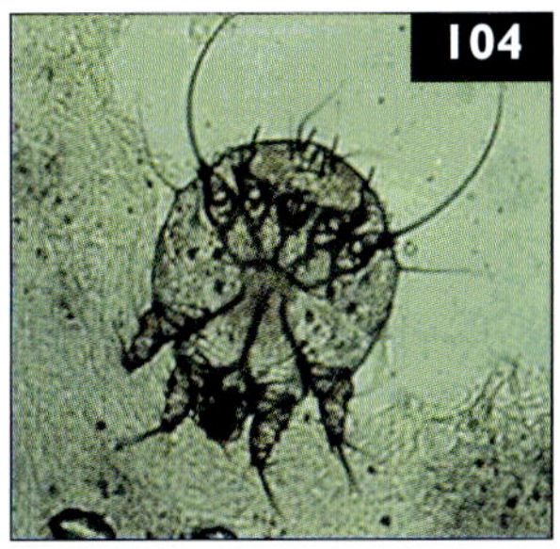

104 A magnified picture of a *Sarcoptes scabiei*.

Patients with ulcerative disease of the vulva have a variety of clinical manifestations that require appropriate laboratory testing to determine the pathogen involved. Persistent or recurrent vulvar ulcers may not have an infectious etiology. The physician must not stint on the use of biopsy to check for skin cancer, Behçet's disease, aphthous ulcers, vulvar Crohn's disease, or vulvar pemphigoid. This is a situation whose review of the biopsy by a dermatopathologist is needed to achieve an accurate diagnosis. Half the biopsy sample should be sent in special media for immune staining and the other half in formalin. These conditions will be discussed in more detail in Chapter 15. Knowing the diagnosis, the appropriate therapy can be prescribed.

Viruses will be the cause of most of the vulvar ulcerations seen by practicing physicians. For the doctor in a private office or surgery, the most commonly encountered pathogens in patients with small vulvar ulcerations will be HSV-1 and HSV-2. The vagaries of clinical presentation and the necessary laboratory testing to confirm the diagnosis has been presented in Chapter 8. In immunosuppressed women, unexpected viral pathogens can be confirmed by culture. In one such patient, the viral culture of the lesion grew CMV (**99**).

The remainder of these genital ulcer diseases (chancroid, granuloma inguinale, lymphogranuloma, and syphilis) are caused by bacteria. To make an accurate diagnosis requires linking the clinical findings with appropriate laboratory testing. Of this group of bacteria-caused ulcerative disease of the vulva, chancroid is probably the most common in the United States. Despite this, it is still rare. These women usually present with painful vulvar ulcers that are not indurated and usually have unilateral inguinal lymphadenopathy (**105**). There should be caution in making the diagnosis for other vulvar infections can have a similar presentation. Every possible confirmatory test should be ordered. To confirm the microbiologic diagnosis of chancroid requires plating exudates from the lesion on a special agar media within 1 hour of the patient's examination. If this can be done, there is the potential for isolating the offending organism, *Hemophilus ducreyi*. The sensitivity of this testing is 80%. There is a twofold problem in this approach for most practitioners: they cannot get the specimen to the laboratory for plating within this time frame, and some commercial laboratories may not have this culture media available. If there is an urban hospital nearby, a referral to the emergency room or a STD clinic may be the best option to obtain this diagnostic study. Other infections can masquerade as chancroid. In one study in Atlanta, 80% of the patients thought to have typical chancroid lesions were found to be culture-positive for HSV-1 and HSV-2[10]. With this in mind, another portion of the exudate should be sent for culture for HSV-1 and HSV-2 and a blood sample tested for HSV antibody. Not every chancre is painless. If possible, a dark field examination of ulcer exudate should be done as well as blood reagin testing, 7 days or more after the first appearance of the ulcer. If both of these alternate tests are negative, the diagnosis of chancroid is likely, even if *H. ducreyi* is not isolated on culture attempts. Since chancroid ulcers facilitate the spread of HIV infections, serologic testing for HIV should be done in these patients.

Granuloma inguinale is a very uncommon disease in the United States and western Europe. Because it is endemic in some tropical and developing areas, for example, India, Papua New Guinea, central Australia, and southern Africa, a history of travel or intimate contact with someone from that area should be obtained[5]. The primary lesion is an indurated papule, but these women usually present to the physician when it ulcerates. These lesions visually show gross infection with necrosis and purulence. Surprisingly, they are not painful and usually there is no inguinal adenopathy. The ulcerative lesions are highly vascular and bleed easily. The causative organism, *Calymmatobacterium granulomatis*, is a Gram-negative rod that is difficult to culture. A PCR test has been devised, but it is not clinically available. There is no serologic test for this infection. The diagnosis can definitively be made by either a scraping of the lesion or a biopsy tissue section stained with a Wright or Giemsa stain, in which Donovan bodies can be seen (**106**). There can be other causes for these indurated lesions. Figure **107** shows the site biopsied the day before in a woman who frequently visits southern Africa. Using selective staining, she was determined to have mycosis fungoides. In patients with granuloma inguinale, there are bipolar black clusters of bacteria in the cytoplasm of large histiocytes. Again, in dealing with patients with this vulvar ulceration, screening tests should be done for HSV, and *Treponema pallidum*. Often, these lesions are extensive and a tissue biopsy is also indicated to rule out the presence of cancer. Since a concurrent HIV infection can delay healing, HIV testing should be done in these women.

Lymphogranuloma venereum is such a rare disease in the United States that most private practitioners will probably never see it. There are less than 600 cases reported annually, and diagnosed infection is ten times more common in men than women. It has a variety of clinical presentations. The primary lesion is a self-limited genital ulcer at the site of inoculation, which usually does not cause patients to seek medical care[5]. If this is not treated, patients usually develop inguinal adenopathy with overlying brawny vulvar skin (**108**), and the abscesses within the nodes coalesce and drain from one or more sinus tracts (**109**). This later stage of the disease is the time when most patients present to the physician for care. The microbiologic pathogens for lymphogranuloma venereum are *Chlamydia trachomatis* serovars L1, L2, and L3. Two clinical care realities usually prevent a microbiologic confirmation: it is an uncommon disease, and a DNA probe or PCR to confirm the diagnosis is often not available to the practicing physician in a private office. These serovars can be grown on tissue culture, but tissue culture is usually not available in clinical laboratories. This leaves one available alternative to confirm the diagnosis: a serological blood test for complement fixation titers that are 1:64 or greater. In common with other sexually transmitted genital ulcer diseases, infections with HSV and *Treponema pallidum* should be ruled out by concomitant testing. HIV testing should be performed as well.

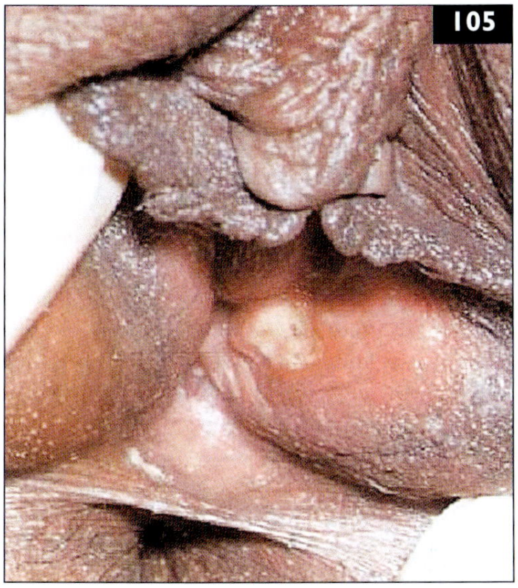

105 Ulcerative lesion of patient with chancroid.

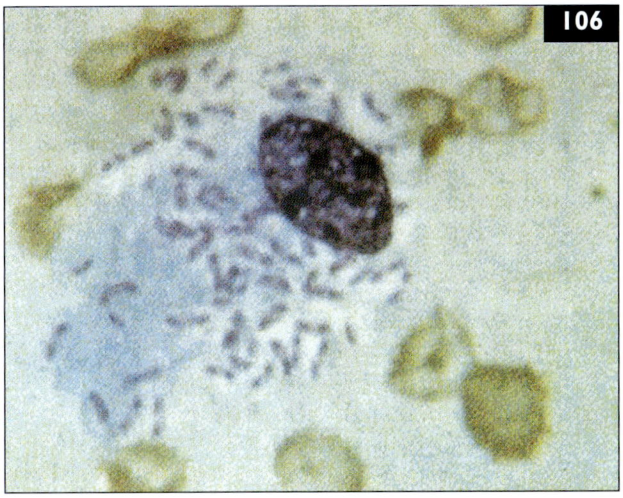

106 Donovan bodies. Bacteria are found in the cytoplasm of macrophages, and assume the shape of a safety pin.

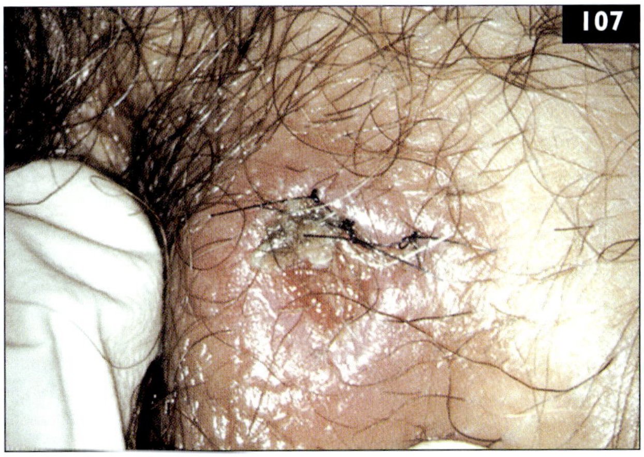

107 Solitary vulvar lesion of a patient suspected of having granuloma inguinale. Special staining confirmed the diagnosis of mycosis fungoides.

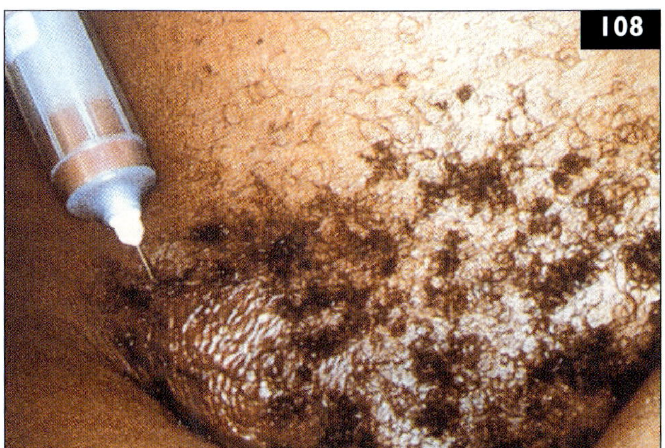

108 The brawny vulvar lesion of a patient with lymphogranuloma venereum.

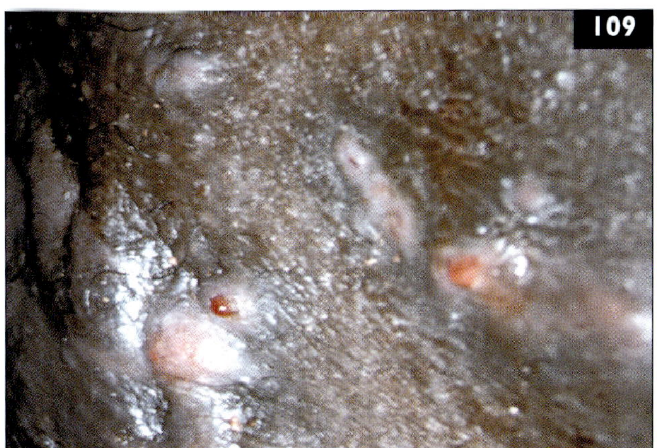

109 Draining sinus tracts in a patient with lymphogranuloma venereum.

The primary lesion of an infection due to *T. pallidum* is a chancre. This lesion starts as a small papule that breaks down to form a superficial, painless ulcer. More than one lesion can be seen. These lesions are painless, and they go away without systemic antibiotic treatment, suggesting to the patient that whatever caused the infection has been eliminated by her body's host defense mechanism. If the physician encounters an indurated painless ulcer, syphilis should be at the head of the list of differential diagnoses. The diagnosis can be confirmed by the presence of the corkscrew-shaped pathogen, *T. pallidum*, on a dark field microscope examination of serum obtained by scraping the surface of the lesion. The difficulty will be to find both the equipment and the medical personnel trained to do the dark field study. As an alternative, a biopsy can be taken from the rim of the lesion with a request to the pathology department to stain with silver salts in an attempt to visualize these spirochetes. If an accurate dark field examination cannot be obtained, the diagnosis can be established by obtaining a positive reagin test from blood obtained taken 7 days or more after the lesion was first noted by the patient. This positive reagin test is not specific. The diagnosis of a *T. pallidum* etiology can be confirmed by a positive specific treponemal test, fluorescent treponemenal antibody absorbed (FTA-ABS) test or *T. pallidum* particle agglutination (TP-PA) test[5]. These patients with a painless genital ulcer should also be tested for granuloma inguinale and herpes. Again, in this population HIV testing should be done.

A much more common cause of vulvar discomfort caused by infection is a Bartholin's abscess. It presents as a painful unilateral swelling (**110**). Under local anesthesia in an outpatient setting, incision and drainage (I&D) are performed. The free flow of purulent material is obvious. Patients with a recurrent Bartholin's abscess should have a more extensive operation performed. After I&D drainage with a cruciate incision, a drain is left in place to maintain ostia patency (**111**). Although first episodes of a Bartholin's abscess can be caused by *Neisseria gonorrhea*, recurrences usually are associated with the recovery of anaerobic bacteria.

The first hint to the physician that a patient might have a STD of the vagina or lower genital tract will be garnered from the history. When these young women, who are sexually active without using any barrier protection, respond to the question that they have a new sexual partner, the physician's level of concern should increase. This is elevated further when they also note the recent onset of a troublesome, but not serious set of symptoms that includes urgency and frequency of urination, vaginal spotting, or an increased vaginal discharge. These symptoms are so slight that they usually will not be volunteered until the physician asks specific questions. On vaginal examination, vaginal secretions are obtained for microscopic study with a saline and potassium hydroxide (KOH) prep, vaginal pH is measured from the lateral wall of the vagina, and a PCR test is obtained for *Neisseria gonorrhea* and *Chlamydia trachomatis*. Suspicions of a sexually transmitted bacterial

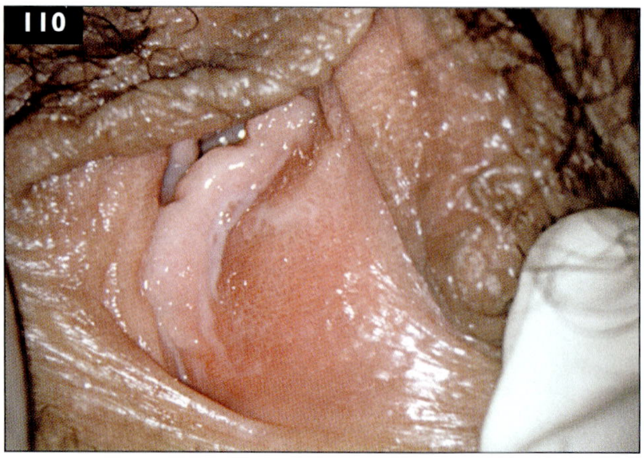

110 Unilateral vulvar swelling associated with a Bartholin's abscess.

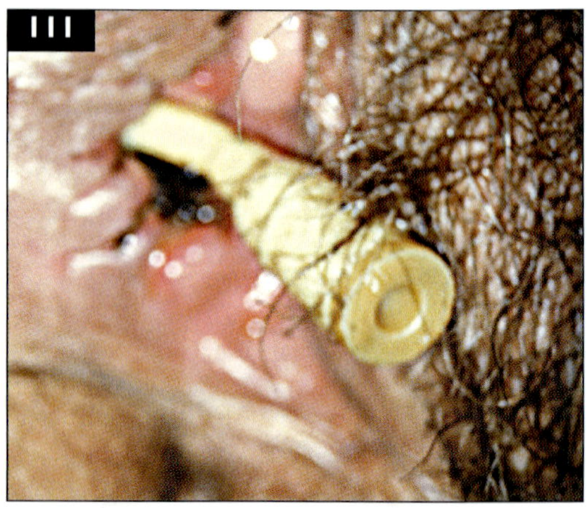

111 Bartholin's abscess after incision and drainage, with drain in place.

infection should be further heightened by an alkaline vaginal pH and the presence of large numbers of white cells (WBCs) on the microscopic examination of the saline prep. This presence of WBCs in the vaginal smear is the most sensitive test to determine if the patient has upper genital tract infection[11]. There are other important points to note during the pelvic examination. It is difficult to make a diagnosis of cervicitis, based upon the gross appearance of the cervix, either with a naked-eye view or the added magnification of a colposcope. A large field of columnar epithelium on the face of the cervix is common in these young sexually active women, and it has a bright red appearance (**112**). If cervicitis is suspected, a cotton swab is placed in the endocervical canal, allowed to remain there for a few seconds, and when withdrawn and held against a white background, yellow mucopus can be seen in positive cases. The diagnosis is more certain when a drop of the mucopus is added to saline, and on microscopic examination, myriads of WBCs are seen. This is the best office test available to confirm the diagnosis of cervicitis[12] (**113**). On the bimanual examination of the patient with this history, these office laboratory findings, the presence of cervical motion, and adnexal tenderness should confirm the diagnosis of an upper genital infection.

Concerns about four other sexually transmitted viral diseases should lead to diagnostic testing in the sexually active young woman, not in a monogamous relationship who also is not using any barrier methods of protection. The most commonly sexually transmitted virus is the human papilloma virus (HPV) (Chapter 9). For the patient not previously immunized, blood tests can be performed for hepatitis B antibodies and, if she is pregnant, the hepatitis B surface antigen as well. For the woman planning a pregnancy, or when seen early in pregnancy, blood should be drawn to test for CMV antibodies. With the patient's permission, blood should be drawn for HIV antibodies.

TREATMENT

There are a variety of effective treatments for molluscum contagiosum. A tried-and-true quick method for most gynecologists is to unroof the central core of each lesion with a needle or a scalpel and then apply silver nitrate to the base. The dermatologist's approach of using a freezing nitrous oxide spray to each lesion is preferable. It is well tolerated and results in a small scar. Imiquimod cream, applied directly three times a week to each lesion by the patient, is also effective. There are three problems with this approach, however: (1) imiquimod can irritate the tissue around the lesion, (2) it takes weeks or months to eliminate the lesion, and (3) there is a failure rate, which is very distressing to these young patients who have carefully followed a treatment regimen for what seems to them to be a long period of time.

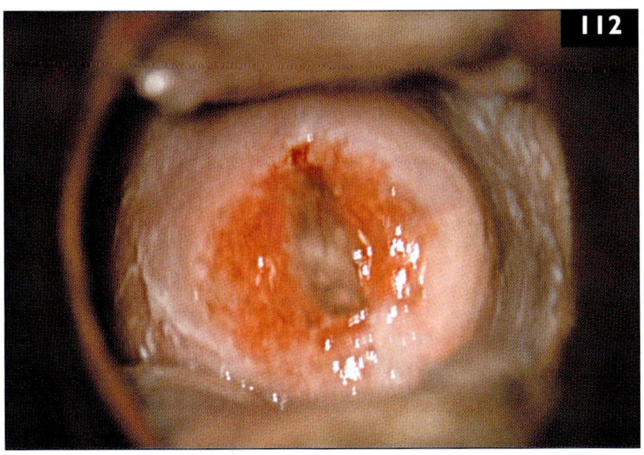

112 Face of cervix. The columnar epithelium has a bright red appearance.

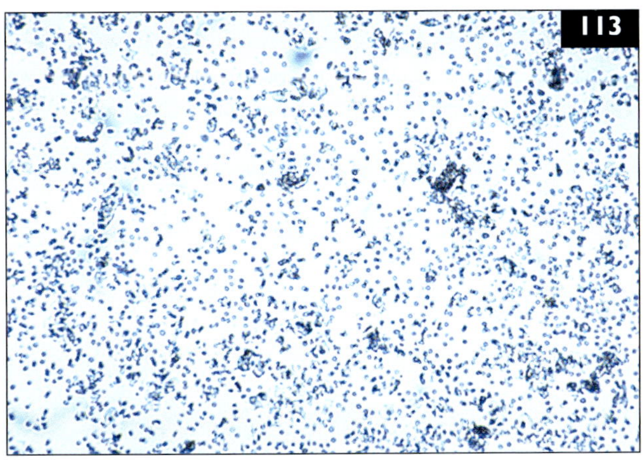

113 Microscopic examination of a saline preparation of vaginal fluid. The field is covered with white blood cells.

Pediculosis pubis is an easily managed infection, because there is a variety of treatments, there is a short duration of treatment, and the follow-up occurs within 1 week of treatment. There are three different treatment regimens recommended by the CDC[5] (*Table 15*). The patient should be re-evaluated 1 week later if symptoms persist, with a careful colposcopic survey of the areas in question. Any sexual partners of this patient within the last month should be treated as well. Bedding and clothing should be decontaminated by machine washing and drying or dry cleaning.

Scabies also has a variety of treatment options. The regimen recommended by the CDC is the total body application of permitrin cream (5%) from the neck down, to be washed off in 8–14 hours[5]. There are alternative treatments, but strict guidelines of care must be followed to avoid complications. Lindane (1%) either 1 oz of lotion or 30 g of cream is applied in a thin layer to the entire body from the neck down to be washed off in 8 hours. If too much is absorbed, this drug has toxicity. Seizures have been reported when applied after a hot bath or when the patient has an extensive dermatitis. It should not be prescribed in pregnant or lactating women, or in children 2 years of age or younger. The reports of aplastic anemia after lindane administration have eliminated this drug as an option for many practicing physicians. Alternatively, ivermectin 200 mg/kg orally can be given, to be repeated in 2 weeks[5]. In addition, bedding and clothing should be machine washed and machine dried, or dry cleaned if machine washing is not recommended for the clothes.

There is a wide variety of CDC-recommended antibiotic regimens for the treatment of the patient with chancroid[5]. The single-dose options have appeal, for these are the regimens that patients are most likely to comply with and therefore receive the full intended antibiotic dose. They can be given a single oral dose of 1 g of azithromycin or single-dose intramuscular 250 mg of ceftriaxone. If the patient balks at the single-dose regimen, more extended oral regimens can be used, either ciprofloxacin 500 mg orally twice a day for 3 days, or erythromycin base 500 mg orally three times a day for 7 days. There can be patient problems with either of these latter two regimens. Ciprofloxacin increases the half-life of caffeine. Patients should be made aware so they decrease their caffeine intake during the 3-day treatment interval and hopefully avoid sleepless nights. Oral erythromycin can cause abdominal distress, bloating, and discomfort, to the extent that some patients will not complete the 7-day course of treatment. The earlier the diagnosis is made and treatment initiated, the better. In far advanced cases, despite successful antibiotic therapy permanent scarring can occur. At the onset or during therapy, any fluctuant buboes should be aspirated, drained, or removed. Another underlying concern in these patients is that the presence of these ulcers facilitates both the acquisition and the spread of HIV infection.

Patients with granuloma inguinale present a more complicated therapeutic problems. The CDC treatment regimens are prolonged and often must be continued beyond the recommended 3-week intervals until all of the ulcer lesions have completely healed[5]. Relapses occur in 10–20% of patients 6–18 months after seemingly effective therapy and will require another course of therapy. All of the treatment regimens are given by the oral route. The two recommended regimens are doxycycline 100 mg orally twice a day for at least 3 weeks or one double strength trimethoprim–sulfamethoxazole (800 mg/160 mg) twice a day for at least 3 weeks. It is important to know the HIV status of these patients.

Patients may not be able to avoid the sun for 3 weeks or are allergic to either of these drugs. Fortunately, there are three alternative regimens: ciprofloxacin 750 mg twice a day for at least 3 weeks, erythromycin base 500 mg four times a day for at least 3 weeks, or azithromycin 1 g each week for 3 weeks. Again ciprofloxacin users need to be cautioned about caffeine intake, and many women will not be able to tolerate the erythromycin regimen because of gastrointestinal (GI) distress. The azithromycin regimen is popular, for it is a less patient-demanding dosage regimen. A clinical response is usually evident within 7–10 days. In an HIV-positive patient, parenteral gentamicin can be added to the regimen, particularly if the initial response to therapy is unsatisfactory.

Table 15 Treatment regimens for pediculosis pubis

- Permethrin 1% cream rinse applied to affected areas and washed off after 10 minutes

Or

- Lindane 1% shampoo applied for 4 minutes to the affected area and then thoroughly washed off. Not recommended for pregnant or lactating women or for children aged 2 years or younger

Or

- Pyrethrine with piperonyl butoxide applied to the affected area and washed off after 10 minutes

When the diagnosis of lymphogranuloma venereum has been made, there are two oral treatment regimens recommended by the CDC[5]. One is doxycycline 100 mg twice a day for 21 days. If the patients are allergic to doxycycline or are pregnant, an alternative regimen is erythromycin base 500 mg four times a day for 21 days. Patients receiving doxycycline should limit their exposure to the sun and those receiving erythromycin should be counseled about possible GI distress. If buboe formation occurs, either aspiration or incision and drainage should be employed. The earlier treatment is begun the less likely the patient will have permanent scarring. Again, the HIV status of these patients should be determined.

For the patient with a Bartholin's abscess, the key to treatment is adequate incision and drainage, with appropriate operative techniques to maintain an opening for the gland. This can be achieved by suturing the edges of the gland to the cruciate incision or by the use of a drainage catheter (**111**). Antibiotic therapy for 3–5 days is indicated, with the use of antibiotics effective against *Neisseria gonorrhea* and anaerobic bacteria.

There are many treatment options for the patient with a chancre, the lesion of primary syphilis. The antibiotic of choice is penicillin, but the strategy of antibiotic administration is different from the usual physician selection. *Treponema pallidum* replicates slowly, every 24–26 hours, so that antibiotics need to be in the tissue for days to ensure a cure. Penicillin is the best option, for it has proven effective and has been the most studied of all treatment regimens. A long-acting penicillin, benzathine penicillin G 2,400,000 units given intramuscularly as a single dose is the drug of choice[5]. For the nonpregnant patient allergic to penicillin, a good choice is doxycycline 100 mg orally twice a day for 14 days, because it is better tolerated by patients and they are more likely to complete the full course of therapy. The problem with this 14-day treatment schedule is compliance. As an alternative, it has been suggested that a single 2 g oral dose of azithromycin is effective, but the data are limited. There are two groups of patients that pose additional therapeutic problems. Pregnant women allergic to penicillin should be desensitized and treated with penicillin. As is true with all patients with a genital ulcer, these patients should be tested for HIV. There is concern about inadequate treatment of early syphilis in an HIV-positive patient with the subsequent development of CNS syphilis. There are two acceptable treatment strategies, either treat with a longer treatment regimen, benzathine penicillin G, 2,400,000 injected intramuscularly weekly for three doses, or standard treatment with pre-treatment spinal fluid analysis, close follow-up at 3-month intervals, and a repeat spinal fluid analysis at 6 months. The clinical superiority of the latter approach has not been proven.

The treatment of women with suspected lower genital infection with *N. gonorrhea* or *C. trachomatis* requires some assessment of the potential extent of the infection. The patient with assumed lower genital tract disease can be treated as an outpatient. The various options are noted in *Table 16*[5]. The single-dose oral medication combination of azithromycin plus cefixime, ciprofloxacin, ofloxacin, or levofloxacin has great appeal. Some young women, however, regard an intramuscular injection as being sufficient and do not bother to take the oral medication. If there is cervical motion and uterine tenderness present on examination, the physician's concern should be that there has been upper genital tract extension of the disease,

Table 16 Suspected uncomplicated lower genital tract infections with *Neisseria gonorrhea* or *Chlamydia trachomatis*

- Cefixime 400 mg orally in a single dose

Or

- Ceftriaxone 125 mg IM in a single dose

Or

- Ofloxacin 400 mg orally in a single dose

Or

- Levofloxacin 250 mg orally in a single dose

Plus

- Azithromycin 1 g orally in a single dose

Or

- Doxycycline 100 mg twice a day for 7 days

particularly if the saline prep vaginal smear is loaded with WBCs. In this instance, it should make no difference to the physician that the patient is afebrile. These patients can be admitted and given parenteral antibiotics, cefoxitin 2 g plus doxycycline 100 mg intravenously every 12 hours. Twenty-four hours after the patient improves, the patient can be switched to oral doxycycline 100 mg orally, twice a day for 14 days, and metronidazole 500 mg orally twice a day for 14 days. The alternate clindamycin and gentamicin parenteral regimen requires a switch to oral doxycycline, and this is a conversion to a different antibiotic than the ones that were initially effective. The reality in the United States, at least, is that most insurance companies will not approve admission for such patients. They base this on the large study comparing admission and intravenous antibiotics to oral outpatient antibiotic therapy, which showed no difference in results[13]. This study was flawed, for over 70% of the patients already had well established infections with symptoms for more than 3 days when they were admitted to this study. Patients with well established infections tend to not respond as well to antibiotic care[14]. Most of these relatively asymptomatic patients will prefer outpatient treatment. A popular ambulatory regimen is ofloxacin 400 mg twice a day for 14 days, plus metronidazole 500 mg twice a day for 14 days. This provides effective coverage of *N. gonorrhea*, *C. trachomatis*, and Gram-negative anaerobes. These women need to be seen in follow-up to be sure that they have responded to this care.

The therapeutic approaches to sexually transmitted viral infections involve both prevention and treatment. Strategies for HPV care and prevention have been presented in Chapter 9. For the patient who is not immune to hepatitis B, there is a vaccine available. For the pregnant woman susceptible to CMV, some personal health precautions can reduce the risk of infection. For the sexually active woman not in a monogamous relationship, condom use should be encouraged. For the woman with exposure to young children, there should be avoidance of their saliva or urine. For the woman discovered to be HIV-positive, multi-drug antiretroviral therapy can be prescribed by an infectious disease doctor familiar with the most effective combination regimens as well as the individual drug toxicities.

CHAPTER 11

STAPHYLOCOCCUS AUREUS AND GROUP A STREPTOCOCCAL INFECTIONS OF THE VAGINA AND VULVA

BACKGROUND

These staphylococcal and streptococcal infections remain under the clinical radar screen for most practicing obstetricians–gynecologists around the world. There are no descriptions of early lower genital tract staphylococcal and streptococcal infections in obstetric–gynecologic textbooks and physician awareness of the clinical significance of these organisms is limited to a late-stage disease, toxic shock syndrome (TSS), serious post-partum endomyometritis, or a breast abscess. To give examples of this lack of awareness, obstetric and gynecologic patients have been seen in consultation at the referral vaginitis clinic at Cornell for a persistent symptomatic vaginal discharge in whom there was no physician reaction to the fact that the vaginal culture obtained had a heavy growth of *Staphylococcus aureus* or the Group A streptococcus. In one case, the vaginal and rectal screening culture for Group B streptococcus at 36 weeks gestation yielded an isolate of the Group A streptococcus. Since this was not Group B, no note was made of this; this culture report was discovered when the patient with a persistent irritating vaginal discharge came to the referral vaginitis clinic for a consultation. In this case, the isolation of the Group A streptococcus had been ignored because of the mistaken assumption that Group B was the only streptococcal isolate of significance for an obstetrician. Despite this critique of early-stage awareness, most physicians know about late-stage streptococcal and staphylococcal disease.

It is interesting that TSS caused by *Staphylococcus aureus*, which gynecologists equate with menstruation and tampon use, was first definitely described and named by James Todd, a pediatric infectious disease expert. His report, published in 1978, is a description of seven children and adolescents of both sexes, none of whose cases was associated with either menstruation or the use of vaginal tampons[1]. Following this description of a new clinical entity, there was a plethora of cases culminating in a peak incidence of TSS cases reported in 1980[2]. Nearly every one of these cases occurred in menstruating women using tampons. All physicians in the United States, and the Centers for Disease Control (CDC) in particular, focused upon this entity, and over a period of years, there has been a diminution in the number of reported cases[3] (**114**). There were many factors contributing to this decline. The super-absorbent tampon which could remain in place for long periods of time was withdrawn from the market, even though TSS has been reported with all tampons, and physicians, more aware of this syndrome, diagnosed this entity in the early stages of the disease and initiated antibiotic treatment before multiorgan involvement was encountered. TSS is still seen today, but for most gynecologists, it is a rarely encountered clinical entity.

Nearly all cases of menstrual and nonmenstrual TSS in women caused by *Staphylococcus aureus* require a series of unrelated events to coalesce that then culminates to spawn this serious clinical syndrome. First, the woman must have

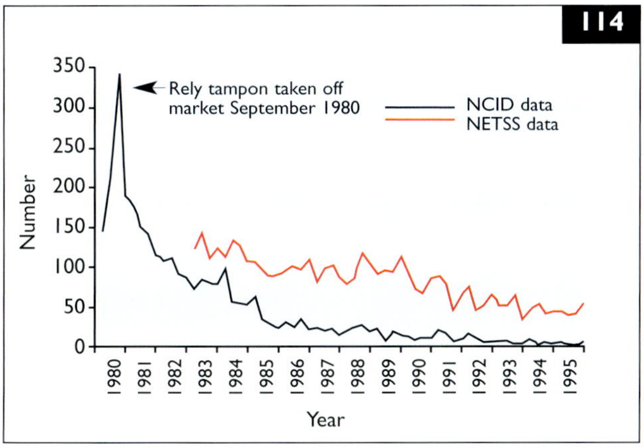

114 Toxic shock syndrome by year United States 1980–1995.

vaginal colonization with a toxigenic strain of *S. aureus* that produces the toxic shock syndrome toxin (TSST-1). In view of the predominance of staphylococcal TSS cases in the midwest and far west of the United States, as compared to the paucity of cases in the New England and mid-Atlantic states, this must be related in part to environmental seeding of this organism. One obvious question: could this be influenced by the widespread use of antibiotics in animal feeds in these farm state areas? Next, conditions in the body must enhance the proliferation of these toxigenic strains of *S. aureus* that subsequently increase the production of TSST-1. In the vagina, tampon use, particularly when in place for long periods of time, facilitates this increased TSST-1 production in menstrual TSS. There is evidence that tampons increase the oxygen content of the vagina to the point that toxin production of these staphylococcal strains is induced[4]. The role of intrauterine devices, diaphragms, and the vaginal sponge in nonmenstrual TSS is not clear. Host factors are the next piece in this disease complex. The patient fulfilling all of these aforenoted disease prerequisites finally must also lack protective levels of antibody to TSST-1. The vast majority of women in the United States and Europe have this antibody present, so this is a clinical situation that is the exception, not the rule. Clearly, this unfortunate combination of events can result from any skin or body cavity infection in a woman caused by a TSST-1-producing strain of *S. aureus.* In menstrual and nonmenstrual TSS, the TSST-1 crosses the vaginal wall and begins an immunologic cascade that, if not checked, results in full-blown TSS.

Although TSS has also been reported with various strains of streptococci, the dominant pathogen is the Group A streptococcus. There are differences in the presentation and pathophysiology of streptococcal and staphylococcal TSS. Nearly all of these streptococcal cases occur in women with soft tissue infections. For the obstetrician–gynecologist, the concern should be focused upon post-partum episiotomy infections or vulvar abscesses. Although these TSS cases are uncommon, there are signs that the overall incidence of Group A streptococcal infection is increasing and, as a result, more streptococcal TSS cases will probably be seen in the future[5]. The Group A streptococcus produces pyrogenic toxins and other factors that contribute to soft tissue necrosis that can proceed in some women to full-blown necrotizing fasciitis. That is a very serious late-stage infectious disease development. There is a high risk of mortality and the life-saving immediate operative debridement too often results in a horribly disfigured patient who will face months or years of restorative plastic surgery. Even if they survive, their lives will be forever changed.

MICROBIOLOGY

S. aureus and the Group A streptococcus, *Streptococcus pyogenes*, are Gram-positive cocci that typically exist as harmless commensal microorganisms on mucosal surfaces but have the potential to become serious human pathogens. *S. pyogenes* can cause necrotizing fasciitis and TSS. It is sometimes confusing that while *S. pyogenes* is classified as a Group A streptococcus, it is nevertheless beta-hemolytic, producing clear zones of hemolysis when incubated on blood sugar plates. *S. aureus* is a second cause of TSS as well as such hospital acquired infections as post-operative abdominal wound abscesses and post-partum breast infections. The two microbes are easily differentiated in the laboratory because only the staphylococci are catalase-positive.

S. pyogenes is a frequent cause of inflammatory vulvovaginitis in prepubertal girls[6]. It is rarely detected in vaginal cultures from reproductive age women or during pregnancy[7]. However, rare cases of Group A streptococcal puerperal sepsis have been reported. In contrast, *S. aureus* is a frequent vaginal isolate, being detected in 5–20% of cultures from healthy women. However, the application of gene amplification assays to the detection of *S. aureus* indicates a greatly increased carriage rate of this microorganism in the vagina. It may contribute to a type of vaginitis termed 'aerobic vaginitis' by European investigators[8]. Most strains of *S. aureus* carry at least one temperate bacteriophage as well as one or more plasmids. The staphylococcal phages carry genes for virulence factors such as enterotoxin A (a cause of food poisoning) and exfoliative toxin A (the cause of scalded skin syndrome). The gene responsible for skin infections and boils, *PV-luk*, is also carried by a staphylococcal phage. The staphylococcal plasmids carry genes responsible for resistance to antibiotics, antiseptics, and heavy metals.

IMMUNOLOGY

Both *S. pyogenes* and *S. aureus* have a multitude of mechanisms to prevent their detection and/or elimination by the host's immune system. The major immune defense against *S. pyogenes* is recognition, phagocytosis, and killing of the microorganism by polymorphonuclear leukocytes. One of the *S. pyogenes* proteins, known a M protein, has potent anti-phagocytosis properties. It binds to factor H and C4b-binding protein, components of the complement system, and prevents complement deposition on the streptococcal surface and subsequent opsonization. Similarly, fibronectin binds to M protein, thereby masking the bacterial surface from recognition. Streptococcal-derived C5a peptidase, endoglycosidase, and Mac1-like protein also limit complement activation, as well as antibody binding and leukocyte recruitment. Streptolycin O, a streptococcal virulence factor, also blocks phagocytic functions[9].

A major immune-related virulence factor common to both *S. pyogenes* and *S. aureus* are superantigens. Superantigens are protein enterotoxins that bind to the major histocompatibility complex class II molecules on the surface of antigen-presenting cells and interact with receptors on the surface of T lymphocytes. This results in a very large polyclonal T cell activation and a massive release of pro-inflammatory cytokines. The net effect of the stimulation of a large fraction of the host's T lymphocytes is a precipitous lowering of blood pressure and multiorgan failure, hallmarks of TSS. There are at least 11 streptococcal and 15 staphylococcal superantigen genes[9,10]. Two of the staphylococcal superantigens, SEG/SEI, appear to be unique to female genital tract isolates, suggesting a role for these enterotoxins in microbial adaptation to this site[10].

DIAGNOSIS

The diagnosis of early vaginal staphylococcal and streptococcal infections is difficult. These are uncommon cases, and the clinical signs are subtle. At Cornell, approximately one patient a year is seen with these problems. There are a few clinical tips that should lead the physician to suspect this Gram-positive coccal infection as a possibility. All of the Cornell patients with an early Group A streptococcal vaginitis have complained of an excessive irritating vaginal discharge and grossly have an inflamed vulvovaginitis. The pH of this copious serous vaginal discharge is alkaline. The whiff test is negative, and the saline vaginal smear is riveting because of the sheer number of white cells (WBCs) (**115**). This should alert the microscopist to take a close look with higher power at the bacterial flora. Under higher power of both saline (**116**) and potassium hydroxide (KOH) (**117**) preparations, there are cocci present. Figure **117** shows an overwhelming number of cocci on a KOH preparation in a woman with a Group A streptococcal vaginitis. Cultures should be obtained and antibiotic therapy begun immediately.

The women with a *Staphylococcus aureus* vaginitis have the same complaint of an irritating vaginal discharge, but the amount of discharge is less than with streptococcal infections. The most striking clinical sign in menopausal and post-partum patients is the heightened inflammation of the vaginal wall. These women have a grossly red, inflamed vagina. One memorable post-partum patient with this vaginal inflammation had been prescribed an estrogen vaginal cream by her obstetrician the day before for the mistaken diagnosis of an estrogen lack vaginitis. When seen the next day in our referral vaginitis clinic, this woman's mucosal inflammation far exceeded any of the usual post-partum vaginal changes. Again, the vaginal pH was alkaline, the whiff test was negative, and the microscopic examination of the saline preparation showed a field loaded with WBCs, and high-power field examination of the saline and KOH preparation showed a dominance of cocci. With this scenario, antibiotic therapy should be instituted immediately.

TSS as a result of a staphylococcal infection is a solution to a diagnostic puzzle that is feared by all obstetrician–gynecologists. A missed early diagnosis can mean the difference between an uncomplicated cure and the frighteningly rapid downward spiral of a once healthy patient into the morass of intensive unit care for multiple organ system failure. It is a difficult diagnosis to make for a number of reasons. It is an uncommon disease, and most obstetrician–gynecologists are not familiar with it. Clinical experience plays an important role in early recognition. At Cornell in the early 1980s, with a national focus upon this new dreaded TSS, only one case of menstrual TSS was recognized. In contrast to this New York City experience, at

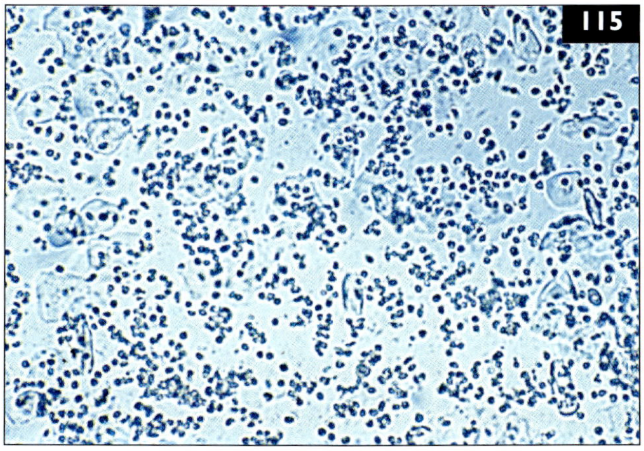

115 Low-power microscopic examination of a saline preparation showing an abundance of white blood cells.

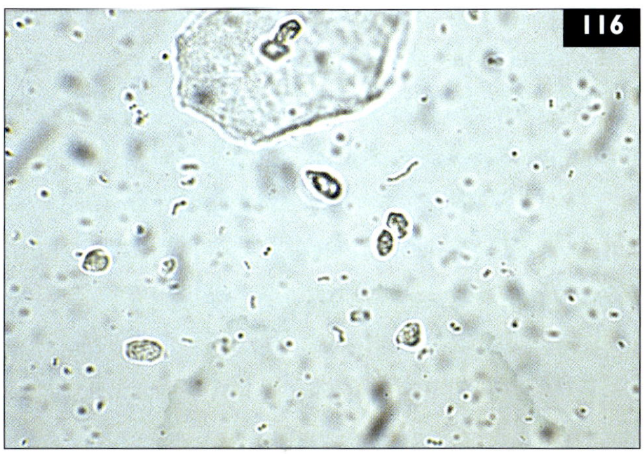

116 High-power microscopic examination of a saline preparation showing cocci in pairs and chains.

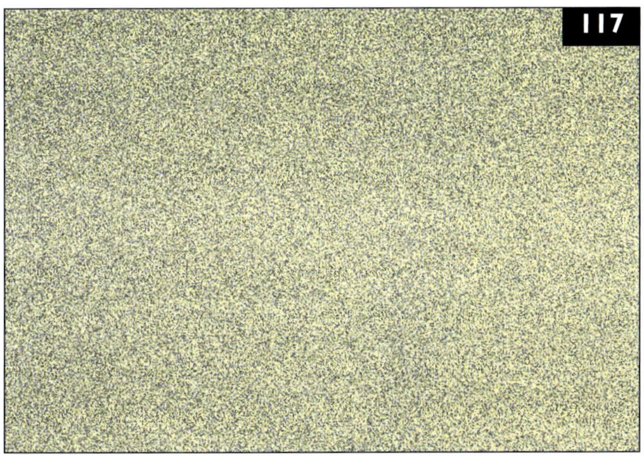

117 Microscopic examination of a potassium hydroxide preparation showing multitudes of cocci in a patient with a Group A streptococcal vaginitis.

the University of Iowa case after case of TSS was recognized or treated. Physicians there were suspicious of TSS at the first sight of a distressed young woman's reddened face across the room as they walked toward her to begin their consultation in the emergency care department. From this initial impression, the patient had TSS until proven otherwise.

There are other diagnostic difficulties. TSS is a syndrome with a wide range of clinical manifestations also seen with a number of other infections that are not familiar to obstetrician–gynecologists, such as measles, leptospirosis, and Rocky Mountain fever. *Table 17* details the diagnostic criteria for staphylococcal TSS[3]. Early in the course of the infection when the diagnosis can dramatically change the prognosis, the clinical signs can be very vague. The patient may exhibit only gastrointestinal symptoms, and the skin rash may be subtle, only detected by close evaluation under a good light source. In many instances, the initial work-up of this patient with a fever of undetermined origin (FUO) has been by an internist; if called to evaluate a young woman with a FUO, a rash, and hypotension, the physician should perform an immediate pelvic examination and remove the tampon if present. This simple intervention may be life-saving for the patient. Cultures should be obtained and blood laboratory screening tests done to determine organ system involvement. There are some women who will be seen in the early stages of TSS who do not meet the criteria noted in *Table 17*. These women can have a fever and a rash, but no organ system involvement. These are the cases in which early antibiotic treatment stops the progression to the full-blown syndrome. Nonmenstrual TSS can occur with any soft tissue infection of the vagina or vulva in which a TSST-1-producing *Staphylococcus aureus* is involved.

TSS caused by the Group A streptococcus is another diagnostic nightmare for obstetrician–gynecologists. If an early diagnosis is not made, the underlying concern is always that the infection can progress to that life-threatening entity, necrotizing fasciitis. The clinical manifestations of this disease are protean. *Table 18* lists the diagnostic criteria for streptococcal TSS[11]. In the vagina and vulva, streptococcal TSS usually follows a soft tissue infection, such as a post-partum episiotomy infection or a vulvar abscess in a diabetic. The physician's suspicion for necrotizing fasciitis should be heightened to the equivalent of a security 'red alert' when the patient complains of severe pain in the area of infection. A quick diagnostic test should lead the physician to transport the patient to the operating room for soft tissue debridement, using a sterile intravenous needle to pierce the surface of the skin overlying the site of infection. If the patient has no pain and there is no blood flow from the needle site, a detailed operative site evaluation should be done in the operating room to be sure there is no rapidly progressing tissue necrosis.

Table 17 Diagnostic criteria for staphylococcal toxic shock syndrome

- Temperature >38.9°C
- Systolic blood pressure <90 mmHg for adults, less than the fifth percentile for children, or >15 mmHg orthostatic drop in diastolic blood pressure or orthostatic dizziness/syncope
- Diffuse macular rash with subsequent desquamation
- Three involved organ systems:
  Liver: bilirubin, ALT, AST >twice the upper normal limit
  Blood: Platelets <100,000/mm^3
  Renal: BUN or creatinine >twice the upper normal limit or pyuria without urinary tract infection
  Mucous membranes: hyperemia of the vagina, oropharynx, or conjunctivae
  Gastrointestinal: diarrhea or vomiting
  Muscular: myalgias or CPK >twice the normal upper limit
  Central nervous system: disorientation or lowered level of consciousness in the absence of hypotension, fever or focal neurologic deficits
- Negative serologic studies for measles, leptospirosis, and Rocky Mountain spotted fever. Blood or CSF culture results negative for organisms other than *Staphylococcus aureus*

ALT: alanine aminotransferase; AST: aspartate aminotransferase; BUN: blood urea nitrogen; CPK: creatine phosphokinase.

Table 18 Diagnostic criteria for streptococcal toxic shock syndrome

- Isolation of group A streptococci:
  From a sterile site for a *definite* case
  From a nonsterile site for a *probable* case
- *And* two of the following:
  Renal dysfunction
  Liver involvement
  Erythematous macular rash
  Coagulopathy
  Adult respiratory distress syndrome
  Soft tissue necrosis

TREATMENT

The treatment for the patient with either an early *Staphylococcus aureus* or the Group A streptococcus vaginitis is straightforward; clindamycin vaginal cream alone for 10 days, if the patient is afebrile. The women should be followed day by day to be sure there is no progression of symptomology with fever, rash, and so on, the culture results should be monitored closely, and Gram-positive aerobic isolate should be identified with antibiotic susceptibility testing done to be sure there is no resistance to clindamycin.

There are levels of severity of disease in women with staphylococcal or streptococcal infections of the vagina or vulva. Some women will present with fever and a rash, but have no evidence of organ system involvement or necrotizing fasciitis. These are patients seen early, who will respond to oral or intravenous beta-lactam antibiotics or clindamycin. These febrile patients with a rash should be admitted and given parenteral vancomycin and clindamycin. For the patient fulfilling the criteria for TSS noted in *Tables 17* and *18*, again intravenous antibiotics with a combination of a beta-lactam antibiotic, usually vancomycin, and clindamycin is probably appropriate. The vancomycin should not be considered overtreatment. These patients are seriously ill and the disease will rapidly progress if the staphylococci are resistant to the first choice of antibiotics. A recent study from Los Angeles documented 14 community-acquired cases of necrotizing fasciitis caused by methicillin-resistant *Staphylococcus aureus*[12]. In the author's opinion, clindamycin is the antibiotic centerpiece of treatment. With staphylococcal TSS, it inhibits TSST-1-production. In Group A streptococcal TSS, it is a more effective antibiotic than one of the penicillins. The Group A streptococcus is highly susceptible to penicillin in the laboratory, but at the site of infection, the Eagle phenomenon occurs with a decrease in the penicillin-binding proteins on the wall of the Group A streptococcus with an increasing colony count[13]. In febrile patients, this accounts for the delay between the initiation of penicillin therapy and the patient's becoming afebrile. Figure **118** shows such a temperature response in a post-partum patient with endomyometritis and bacteremia due to Group A streptococcus in the pre-clindamycin era. Note the number of days before the temperature returned to normal[14]. Time is of the essence in the care of these patients. These women require intensive care, beyond this selection of antibiotics. Any foreign body in the vagina should be immediately removed. If there is an abscess, it should be drained. The patient with staphylococcal TSS requires intravenous fluids in every case and often needs plasma expanders, inotropic agents, and vasopressors to maintain blood pressure and urine output. These women need intensive care unit therapy with close attention to urine output. Through this care, careful cardiovascular and respiratory monitoring needs to be done. Some of these women will require intubation to maintain respiratory function. Many of these women will also receive adrenal corticoid steroids and intravenous gamma globulins (IVIGs), in attempts to protect the organ systems from the toxins released by these organisms. One multi-center study compared high dose IVIG in 21 patients with streptococcal TSS to a cohort of 32 patients who did not receive IVIG in the previous 3 years[15]. The survival figures were significantly better. To help confirm the diagnosis of TSS, any *Staphylococcus aureus* isolates should be assayed for TSST-1 production and blood studies should be done to demonstrate the absence of anti-TSST-1 antibody.

The patient with necrotizing fasciitis is an operative emergency. She will require extensive debridement until bleeding viable tissue is reached with the dissection. At times, this is an extensive and mutilating procedure. Although life-saving, it will often be followed by months of plastic surgery intervention.

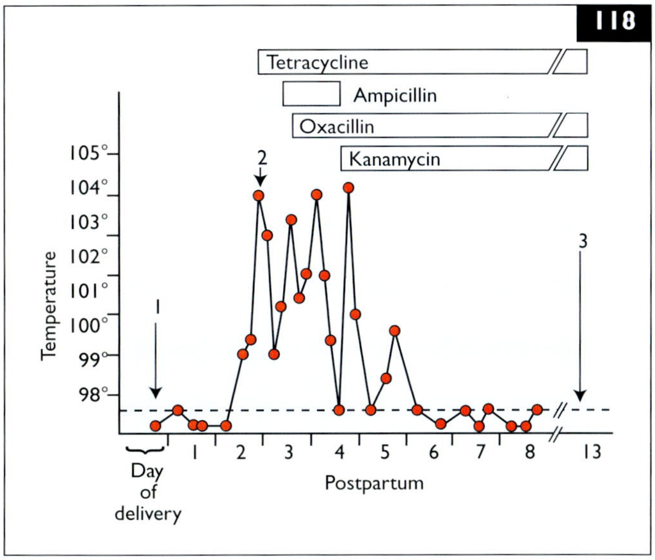

118 The post-partum course of a patient with endoparametritis due to the Group A hemolytic streptococcus. The delivery occurred at point 1, a positive blood culture for *Streptococcus pyogenes* was obtained at point 2, and the patient was discharged at point 3.

CHAPTER 12

ALLERGIC VULVOVAGINITIS

BACKGROUND

The term 'allergic vulvovaginitis' is thought by some to be a misnomer, better labeled as an irritant dermatitis, for it often is a mucosal reaction, not confirmed by skin testing on cornified squamous skin. However, immunoglobulin E (IgE) has been found in the vaginal fluid of patients with those reactions[1], and the term 'allergic vulvovaginitis' has been widely used to describe these patients. This is the terminology that will be employed in this chapter.

The discussion of this entity, vulvovaginal allergy, is an enigma. At the referral vaginitis clinic at Cornell, there is a steady stream of patients with either a chronic recurring vaginitis or chronic vulvar inflammation. For many of these women with symptomatology that has persisted for months or years, a major component of their problem is what we call allergic vulvovaginitis. A laboratory test marker of this is the presence of IgE in the vaginal fluid. Indeed, in one subgroup of patients with vulvar vestibulitis, 43 of 161 (26.7%) of those tested for vaginal IgE had this finding[1]. In another study of women with recurrent vaginitis, 25% had IgE in the vaginal fluid[2]. Allergic vulvovaginitis is a daily practice reality in the author's referral clinic that provides care for patients with chronic problems. In contrast, most physicians and patients are not aware that this entity exists. Physicians have had the concept ingrained into their minds in medical school and residency that all vulvovaginal problems are caused by one of three infectious entities, bacterial vaginosis, *Candida* vaginitis, and *Trichomonas* vaginitis.

This narrow view is apparent as patients with a chronic vaginal problem are evaluated. A common scenario unfolds when a history is obtained. The first doctor seen for this problem gave the patient an anti-fungal cream for presumed *Candida* vaginitis. When the symptoms persisted or got worse, she was then given a vaginal antibiotic preparation for presumed bacterial vaginosis. Still without relief, she was then prescribed an oral anti-fungal medication for the suspected vaginal yeast infection caused by the vaginal antibiotic medication. When this failed, she was given oral metronidazole, because by the physician's process of elimination, this persistent problem must be *Trichomonas*. When all of these treatment interventions have failed, the physician throws up his/her hands and says the cause is unknown and there is nothing more they can do for these women. The patients in frustration go on to another physician and, unfortunately, often repeat this cycle of misguided therapy, sometimes with longer and higher dosage regimens. In addition to these treatment shortcomings, physicians have also falsely counseled women in the United States to believe that constant or recurring vulvovaginal problems are usually due to a vaginal yeast infection. Many physicians erroneously tell patients they have a chronic vaginal yeast infection not confirmed by vaginal culture. In addition, in their homes women are bombarded by television advertisements with the simplistic theme that patients can recognize the presence of a vaginal yeast infection and, when these symptoms are present, relief will be obtained by using the over-the-counter product of the firm sponsoring the advertisement. This myth of recurrent vaginal yeast infections is firmly ingrained in the psyche of the female American consumer. It can make history taking a difficult task. When a new patient is seen in consultation and asked, 'What is your problem', frequently the terse reply is, 'I have a yeast infection'. A disconnect between the physician and the patient usually follows this initial disclosure as physicians probe for details, 'How does it bother you?' The repeated response is, 'I have a yeast infection'. The patient repeats this diagnostic mantra, for she believes that if she can recognize the symptoms of a vaginal yeast infection, then the physician should know this as well. Unfortunately, the physician's reality is that the majority of these women with an assumed yeast infection, when tested by culture, will not have this confirmed. This American myth of frequent recurrent or chronic vaginal yeast infections is difficult to eliminate. After a work-up on more than one occasion in the past, which has never detected a positive culture or polymerase chain reaction (PCR) test for *Candida*, patient messages still come to the clinic stating, 'I have another yeast infection. Can you call in a medication for me?' This physician and patient re-education will be a long, slow process.

The task in this chapter is therefore to educate the practicing physician about the existence of this entity we call allergic vulvovaginitis. A primer on how to recognize and treat it will follow. Over time, hopefully, this information will be diffused from newly aware physicians to their patients.

MICROBIOLOGY

The concept of a local allergic reaction in the vagina as a cause of vaginal symptoms is totally foreign to the majority of practicing gynecologists. Nevertheless, published data detailing the existence of this entity has been slowly accumulating and its existence is no longer debatable. An important emerging concept is that vulvovaginal microbial infections might arise as the secondary consequence of an underlying local allergic response. In these cases, antimicrobial treatment of the infection might temporarily clear the microorganism and result in the alleviation of symptoms. However, without addressing the underlying allergic component the patient remains highly susceptible to recurrences of the infection. This appears to be especially true for women with recurrent vulvovaginal candidiasis[2,3]. The presence of condyloma acuminatum due to a human papillomavirus (HPV) infection has also been associated with a vaginal allergic reaction[4].

Allergic vaginitis may result in symptoms that are indistinguishable clinically from a vaginal infection. A patient fulfilling the Amsell criteria for bacterial vaginosis – elevated vaginal pH, positive whiff test for volatile amines, a homogeneous, white, malodorous discharge – was shown to not have this syndrome, but instead be suffering from a local vaginal allergic response to contraceptive spermicides[5].

IMMUNOLOGY

An allergic reaction is characterized as an immediate hypersensitivity response to antigens (allergens) that are typically benign to most individuals. A simplified diagram of an allergic response is illustrated in Figure **119**. Basophils and mast cells contain surface receptors for IgE antibodies. Each

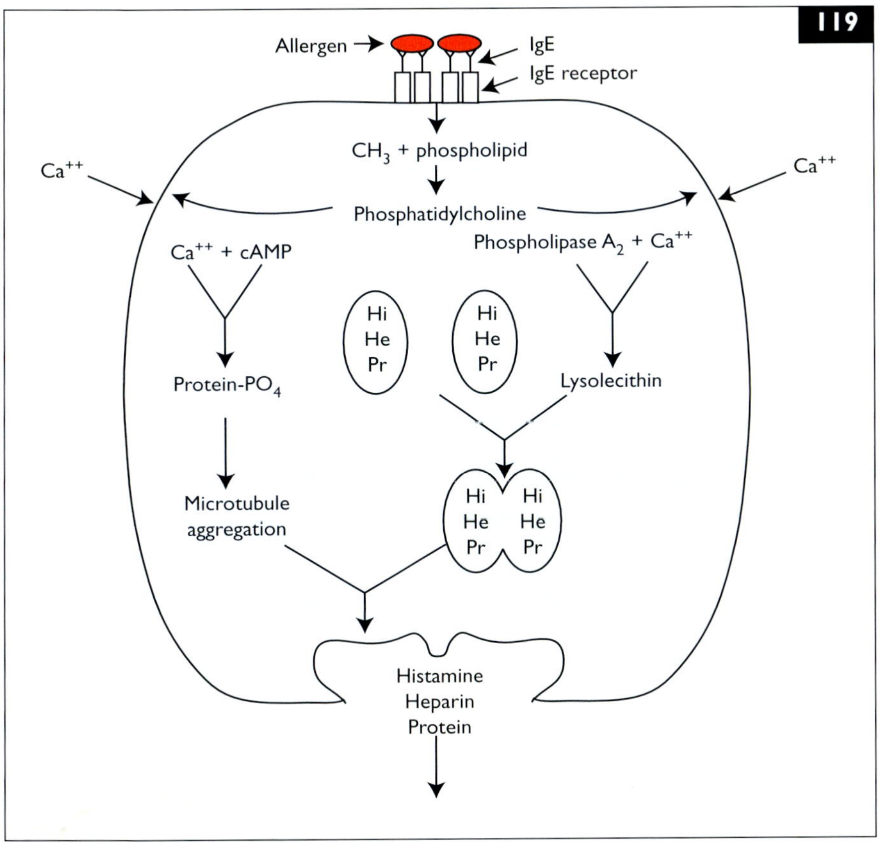

119 Mechanism of histamine release from basophils and mast cells. Immunoglobulin (Ig) E antibodies specific for a particular allergen are bound to IgE receptors on the surface of basophils and mast cells. When the corresponding allergen is present, it binds to the IgE and triggers a sequence of events leading to the joining together of vacuoles containing histamine (Hi), heparin (He), and other proteins (Pr). The vacuoles are transported to the cell surface and their contents are released into the lumen.
Ca: calcium; cAMP: cyclic adenosine monophosphate.

IgE molecule bound to these receptors is specific for a single antigen. When the corresponding antigen is encountered within the vaginal lumen, the antigen couples to the surface-bound IgE antibody and initiates a sequence of intracellular events, culminating in the release of histamine and other protein mediators. This results in a localized inflammatory reaction. In addition, the extracellular histamine binds to specific receptors on T lymphocytes, inducing them to release a factor that stimulates the release of prostaglandin E_2 (PGE_2) from macrophages. This further promotes inflammation and, furthermore, markedly inhibits cell-mediated immunity. PGE_2 inhibits the release of interleukin-2 (IL-2), the cytokine that is essential for T lymphocyte replication[6]. In the absence of IL-2, the proliferation of T cells that recognize microbial components cannot occur and antimicrobial defense mechanisms are severely limited. Should *Candida albicans* or a bacterial or viral pathogen be present at low levels in the vagina at the time of induction of an allergic reaction, the block in cell-mediated immunity will allow the microorganism to proliferate to levels capable of inducing clinical symptoms. PGE_2 also stimulates B lymphocytes to produce more IgE[7], thereby further amplifying the allergic response. *C. albicans* has been shown to synergize with histamine to amplify the quantity of PGE_2 released from macrophages greatly[8]. This suggests that a vaginal allergic response may be more severe in those women who harbor *Candida* in their vagina as a commensal microorganism.

The possibility of inducing a vaginal allergic response in a nonallergic female has been demonstrated[9]. If the male sexual partner has an allergy in his genital tract and both IgE and the corresponding allergen are present in his ejaculate, the IgE can bind to IgE receptors in the female genital tract after sexual intercourse, the allergen can associate with the IgE, and an immediate hypersensitivity response will be initiated.

A wide variety of substances has been shown to be capable of acting as allergens in the female genital tract. These include components or products of *C. albicans* or other microorganisms, intrinsic semen components present in all ejaculates, components such as medications or foods ingested by a particular male partner and present in his ejaculate, components of spermicide preparations or locally applied medications, chemicals present on clothing, fingers, or toiletry products as well as environmental or seasonal allergens that are transferred from fingers or clothing to the vagina. The clinician needs to be aware of these possibilities and be a good detective to attempt to uncover the offending compound.

There have been no double blind, randomized placebo-controlled trials to evaluate the efficacy of various treatments for allergic vaginitis. However, oral or local anti-allergy treatments appear to be helpful in a variable number of patients.

DIAGNOSIS

Making the diagnosis of allergic vulvovaginitis is a difficult task. In most cases, it becomes a product of exclusion for the diagnosis is rarely confirmed at the time of the first patient contact. There are hints that allergy is part of the problem when the initial history is obtained from these women with a chronic vulvovaginal problem. Their response to the question, 'What is your problem?', is a recurrent or constant set of symptoms, either an excessive vaginal discharge and/or vulvar itching and burning that has not responded to a variety of local and systemic medications. The next step in the attempt to unravel the source of these symptoms is to focus upon any possible precipitating cause, such as were symptoms initiated or made worse by any local medications, a new sexual partner, or associated with a different method of contraception? Inquiry should also be made about the patient's general history of allergy, whether the intensity of symptoms varies with the seasons, or whether the ingestion of a specific food or class of foods triggers the problem.

The physical examination proceeds as described in Chapter 3, with vaginal secretions obtained for pH, the whiff test with the potassium hydroxide (KOH) suspension, microscopic examination, and appropriate cultures. There are no distinguishing findings on physical examination to confirm this diagnosis. These women can have vulvar inflammation, there is no vestibular gland tenderness, and no common form of vaginal discharge. The vaginal secretions in these women can be minimal, moderate, or excessive. The vaginal pH is usually acidic, the whiff test is negative, and the microscopic examination often shows moderate to increased numbers of white cells, no yeast forms, and lactobacilli are present. The most striking finding on microscopic examination is the presence of sheets of squamous epithelial cells. Usually, individual squamous cells can be seen in low-power (**120**) or high-power (**121**) microscopic examinations of a saline preparation. In contrast, sheets of epithelial cells are seen in low-power (**122**) and high-power (**123**) microscopic examinations. Figure **124** shows a massive sheet of epithelial cells. In the initial evaluation of these patients, it is important to obtain a culture to rule out a *Candida* infection, for occasionally it is positive despite the lack of yeast forms on microscopic examination. If these patients have had repeated tests to rule out a *Neisseria gonorrhea* or *Chlamydia trachomatis* infection, it often is not necessary to do a DNA probe or a polymerase chain test (PCR) test for these organisms. The most sensitive test for a local vaginal allergy is the presence of immunoglobulin E (IgE) in the vaginal fluid[2]. Unfortunately, this test is seldom available in United States or European laboratories. Alternative tests have been used. Some reports have equated allergic vaginitis with the presence of excessive number of eosinophils detected by eosin staining of a smear of vaginal fluid[10]. This test should be available on physician request to clinical laboratories. In most cases, the initial microbiologic cultures show no evidence of a specific pathogen associated with this vulvovaginitis.

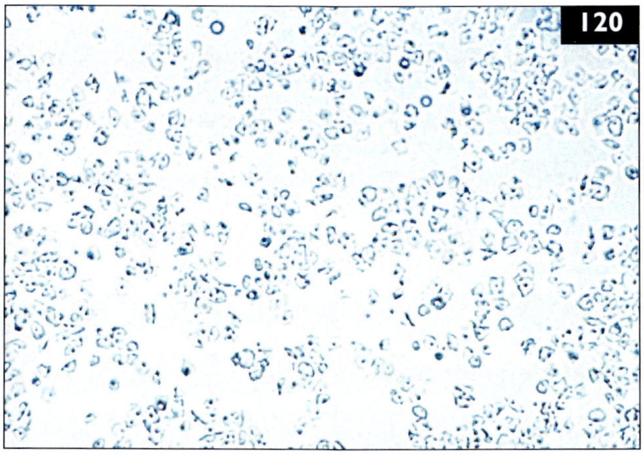

120 Normal exfoliated squamous cells seen on microscopic examination of a saline preparation.

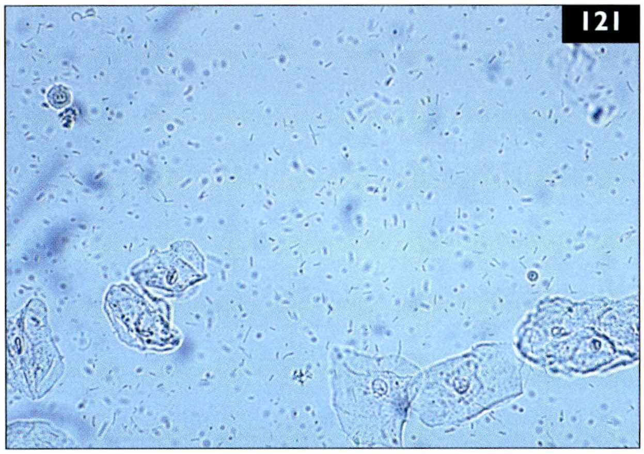

121 Another view of individual exfoliated squamous cells on a saline preparation.

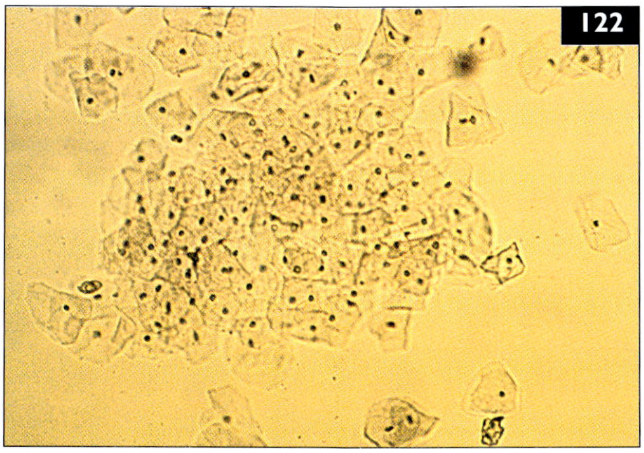

122 Microsheets of vaginal epithelial cells seen on microscopic examination of a saline preparation.

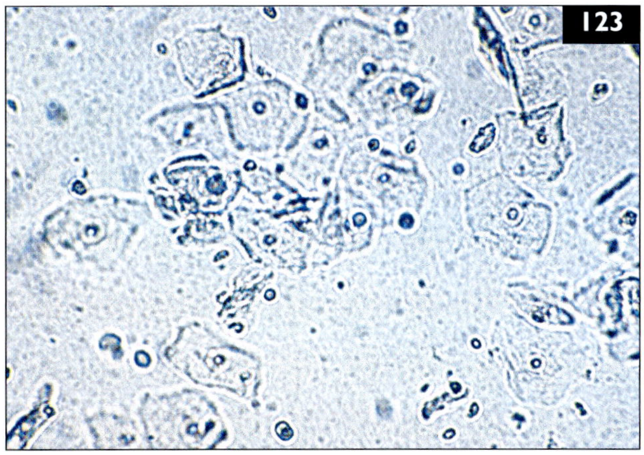

123 Another view of sheets of vaginal epithelial cells seen on a saline preparation.

124 A massive sheet of epithelial cells.

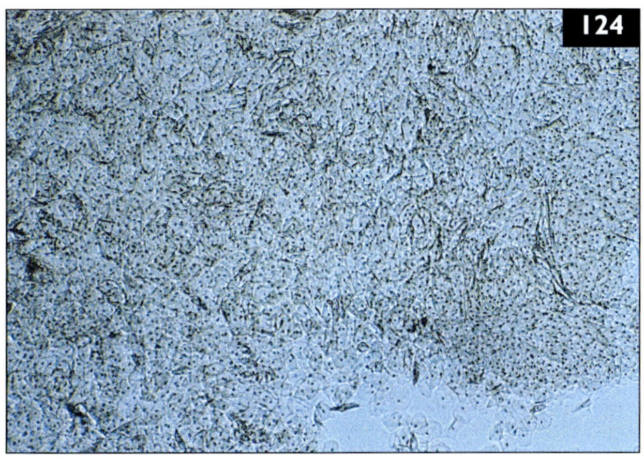

There is a number of specific tests that can be done if the history reveals that the patient's vaginal symptoms are exacerbated with intercourse and exposure to ejaculate fluid. Studies should be initiated to see if the woman is allergic to the seminal fluid of the male ejaculate. Physicians who order these tests should do so with the awareness that these tests vary from more common studies of allergy in couples with infertility in which the focus is upon the women's reaction to spermatozoa. In contrast, in the woman with a suspected allergic vulvovaginitis her reaction to the seminal fluid (SF), not spermatozoa, is monitored. This will be documented by the presence of the specific anti-SF IgE in the vaginal fluid and/or the patient's serum. There is another unique group of patients in whom the woman's reaction to the ejaculate is not associated with IgE in the vaginal fluid. Instead, there are high levels of IgE present in the ejaculate[9]. This combined with allergens also present in the ejaculate causes an immediate hypersensitivity reaction when these components bind to mast cells and/or basophils in the vaginal mucosa.

There are also specific tests that can be used to determine if allergy is an added component to vaginal infections caused by *Candida*. Anti-*Candida albicans* IgE can be detected in the vaginal fluid[10]. Summers, from the University of Utah, has noted flaking of the genital epithelium manifested by microsheets in the saline wet preparation as a characteristic of patients with this *Candida* allergy. Figures **120** and **121** show the appearance of normal exfoliated squamous cells in an asymptomatic healthy woman. Figures **122** and **123** show a sheet of cells in a saline wet preparation. The correlation between allergic rhinitis and recurrent vaginal candidiasis seems to be based upon history and not specific testing[11].

Food allergy testing remains controversial, for the correlation between testing and patient symptoms is poor. The diagnostic approach to most of these women is based upon careful history-taking, and disciplined method of eliminating one food at a time from the patient's diet.

TREATMENT

The physician interventions for this complex clinical problem are diverse. A starting point is to redirect personal hygienic attitudes of some of these patients. Misguided ideas of care can add to the persistence and severity of symptoms. The mindset of many of these women is that these chronic local symptoms can be equated with genital uncleanliness that will be relieved by thorough and frequent washing of the genitals. Unfortunately, soap is used repetitively, and this is a skin and mucosal irritant. No matter how thoroughly a patient rinses after the application of soap, a residue is left on the skin and mucosa that continues to act as an irritant. Patients will often show resistance to the suggestion that they stop applying soap to this area when they shower until the vulvar inflammation can be brought under control. This runs contrary to their beliefs of personal care.

There are novel therapeutic interventions that can be helpful in selected patients. For immediate relief of symptomatic vulvar irritation, the local application of a solid cooking fat, Crisco® in the United States, or one of the solid vegetable oils available in the British Isles or Europe can be helpful. It is soothing, contains no chemical preservatives, and protects the mucosa from any irritation from urine. It is not as occlusive as petroleum jelly, and thus is less likely to macerate mucosa or the skin. The mainstay of treatment for these women is the elimination of any future exposure of the patient to the allergen or the irritant causing her symptoms. Often this results in treatment schemes that vary from the usual norm in medicine of identifying a problem and then prescribing appropriate medications to ensure the most rapid cure possible. For most women with an allergic vulvovaginitis, an opposite strategy is needed: less medication is usually better than more. Continued patient exposure to local medications containing substances that exacerbate the patient's symptomatology delays rather than accelerates the road to the elimination of the symptoms.

The physician's initial focus when obtaining a history is to determine if the patient has had an untoward response to any local medications. This is easy to document. It is not a subtle, nuanced possibility. Instead, it is an instantaneous inflammatory response manifested by extreme vaginal burning that follows the vaginal insertion of an anti-fungal or antibiotic cream, gel, or suppository and persists. An awareness of this phenomenon is important. In the author's clinic, some patients report a prior experience that in response to their call of distress to a physician's office when this reaction occurs, a healthcare worker had erroneously advised them that this response meant the medication is really working and they should continue to use it. When this advice was followed, it markedly increased the degree of vaginal inflammation and prolonged the time the patient was inflamed and symptomatic. A similar history of an immediate deleterious response can be obtained from women reacting to a cream, gel, or ointment locally applied to the mucosa of the vestibule of the vagina. When prescribing any local vaginal or vulvar medications, the patient should be advised that an instant intense burning reaction that persists is abnormal and, if it occurs, the medication should be washed off or flushed from the area, not to be applied again.

The next step in history-taking is to pinpoint the medication used. The anti-fungal azoles themselves can be irritating and cause local reactions. However, by far the most common source of a local inflammatory reaction is due to the chemical preservative propylene glycol. It is ubiquitous. It is present in all local vaginal anti-fungal preparations in the United States except Gynelotrimin® and nystatin vaginal tablets. It is also present in the vaginal antibacterial medications, metronidazole gel and clindamycin vaginal cream. In contrast, the newly marketed clindamycin vaginal ovules have no propylene glycol. Most adrenocorticoid creams and some ointments have propylene glycol as well. It is also present in some locally applied lidocaine products. This results in a therapeutic paradox. The locally applied adrenocorticoids to reduce inflammation instead produce an accentuated inflammatory response, because of the local tissue reaction to the propylene glycol. Estrogen creams, given to decrease local tissue inflammation and to build up the integrity of the vulvar or vaginal mucosa, can also cause an acute local inflammatory reaction due to the presence of propylene glycol. It is often helpful to have a compounding pharmacist mix an equivalent estrogen ointment in a nonirritating base, such as solid vegetable oil. Some lidocaine preparations applied to the vulvar vestibule to decrease pain, unfortunately increase it, because of this reaction to propylene glycol.

The patients describe an intense local burning with the application of the medicine that persists. If the reaction occurs with a medication containing propylene glycol, the physician should document this on the record so this woman will not be prescribed another propylene glycol-containing preparation in the future. If this patient subsequently needs a local vaginal anti-fungal agent, Gynelotrimin® products, nystatin vaginal tablets, or boric acid capsules are alternatives. If a vaginal anti-bacterial agent is needed, the vaginal clindamycin ovule is a possibility. If topical adrenocortical steroids are to be prescribed, ointments that do not contain propylene glycol are readily available. If local estrogen treatment is appropriate, a compounded ointment, a vaginal estradiol tablet, or vaginal estradiol ring can be used, none of which contain propylene glycol.

In addition to the future avoidance of local exposure to allergens, the use of anti-histamines often has an immediate impact on symptomatology. Given orally, these are histamine H1 receptor antagonists and block with varying degrees of effectiveness the deleterious effects of histamine released locally as the vaginal or vulvar mucosa reacts to allergens or irritants. Hydroxyzine 10 mg, or a newer anti-histamine, fexofenadine hydrochloride 60 mg at bedtime, can be prescribed. This usually helps reduce tissue swelling due to inflammation and reduces the symptoms of itching and burning associated with these tissue changes and the formation of new tissue. If this is not effective, cromoglycate preparations have been employed by some physicians. They stabilize the mast cells in the vaginal tissue and lower the release of histamine. A major problem is the lack of a specific vaginal preparation. These same compounds were also evaluated in a trial in patients with vulvar vestibulitis. No therapeutic advantage was found with their use (J Sobel and P Nyirjesy, personal communication).

There is a number of possibilities if the patient's symptoms are triggered by intercourse. If this history is obtained, the patient should be asked if this is related to a new male sexual partner. The physician also wants to know if the patient is being exposed to the male ejaculate. If the vaginal reaction begins after the male ejaculates, there are two quick physician endeavors that have proven helpful. The couple should use a condom to see if the lack of exposure to the ejaculate eliminates the symptoms, and more detailed information should be obtained on the patient's history of allergies and the male sexual partner's medication and dietary history. Occasionally, this exposes a direct cause-and-effect. Two uncommon examples from the author's vulvovaginal clinic demonstrate this. One patient, allergic to tetracycline, was sexually involved with a male taking a low daily dose of an oral tetracycline product for adult acne. When the antibiotic was discontinued, the symptoms lessened and then completely disappeared over time. Another couple's pattern of sexual activity included the male drinking large quantities of beer before the initiation of intercourse. When the beer drinking stopped, so did the vaginal symptoms. These two cases are the exceptions, not the rule. Most women require continued use of the condom to avoid recurrence of symptoms. This is an effective diagnostic trial and can be an effective short-term solution for the couple. When testing reveals this incompatibility to seminal fluid, however, immunotherapy with the male's purified seminal plasma protein fraction, although still experimental and not standardized, has been reported to help some patients[12].

There are other potential sources of difficulty for coitus-related vaginitis. Some women with an unrecognized latex allergy have symptoms related to the use of a latex condom or diaphragm. After eliminating the patient's exposure to latex and seeing symptoms diminish, the physician can refer the patient to an allergist for skin testing and serologic testing. This is an important diagnostic exercise, and provides support for the plan of avoidance of latex products. To date, however, no desensitization protocols for latex are currently in use. Nonoxynol nine contact allergy is another possibility. This detergent is used to coat most latex condoms and is the main ingredient in most gels placed in a diaphragm cup. Again, eliminating exposure to this preparation has been highly effective.

There is a small number of men who have large amounts of IgE present in their ejaculate, and it is theorized that the presence of IgE and an allergen in the ejaculate triggers the acute inflammatory reaction when the seminal fluid makes contact with the vaginal mucosa[9]. Interestingly, the majority of these men have previously undergone a vasectomy. This is one situation in which exact scientific information does not elicit a warm patient response. The physician monologue usually follows this pattern: 'We have discovered the source of your problem. You have an allergic element in the ejaculate. The solution is simple: wear a condom'. The male response is instantaneous and a bit hostile: 'That's why I had a vasectomy after years of avoiding this operation. The deciding factor was I wouldn't ever have to wear a condom again!'

The rapid recurrence of symptoms in women whose treatment of vulvovaginal candidiasis has resulted in a microbiologic cure has always been of interest to investigators. Many of these women have an allergic response to *Candida albicans.* In one study, 31.4% of women with a history of recurrent *Candida* vulvovaginitis had anti-*Candida* IgE present in their vaginal secretions[10]. A vaginal IgE-mediated immediate hypersensitivity reaction to *C. albicans* results in the release of histamine and prostaglandin E_2[10]. This produces local inflammation and a localized vaginal immunosuppression, which provides an ideal environment to foster the growth of *C. albicans* and other opportunistic microorganisms. Anti-histamines have been employed with success in some of these patients. The oral use of prostaglandin synthesis inhibitors has not been effective. Immunotherapy with a *C. albicans* extract has also been tried by some doctors. Summers has found a relationship between allergic vulvovaginitis and asthma, hay fever, and eczema[13]. He postulates that Th2 cytokine-mediated flaking of the vulvovaginal mucosa compromises the normal epithelial barriers and facilitates yeast adherence. He suggests that topical steroids would suppress this response and result in a clinical cure. There should be no reluctance to use steroid preparations on the vulva when needed. Long-term use of steroids on the vulva may cause subdermal atrophy and neovascularization, but these cosmetic effects are much less consequential in the vulvar area, in contrast to cosmetic changes on exposed areas of the body, such as the face.

Some women develop vaginal symptoms after exposure to certain foods. Skin testing for food allergies is usually inconclusive. These women are managed by a selective reduction of the intake of one food item at a time, while gauging the patient's response.

Chapter 13

Menopausal Vulvovaginitis

BACKGROUND

As the baby boom generation ages, physicians are seeing increasing numbers of women with body function changes related to a drop in endogenous estrogen production. The most obvious symptoms are those of vasomotor instability, the 'hot flashes', a warning signal to some women that they have lost some control of their bodies. The most publicized medical concerns are the associated thinning of the bones, osteopenia and osteoporosis, and cardiovascular and cerebrovascular disease. Concerns about the lack of protection against cardiovascular and cerebrovascular disease, by the WHI study[1] and the development of nonhormonal drugs, such as alendronate sodium for the prevention of osteoporosis and statins to lower cholesterol and protect against heart attack, have given physicians and patients preventive medicines other than hormones to lessen the risk of these potentially serious medical problems. None of these medications addresses the quality-of-life issues that result from changes in lower genital tract tissue from the lack of estrogen.

There are demonstrable alterations in the lower genital tract of menopausal women. There is a loss of tissue elasticity and turgor. This can be manifested in some women by thinning of the vulva and retraction of the labia majora, and a decrease in the size and capacity of the vagina. A common complaint of menopausal women is vaginal dryness when intercourse is attempted. The reason for this is apparent to the physician doing a speculum examination where there are limited vaginal secretions to ease the entry of the speculum and the decreased capacity can make it difficult to visualize the cervix, which is in turn more retracted and flush against the vaginal wall. Getting an adequate endocervical sample for the Pap smear can be a painful experience for the patient and a frustrating exercise for the physician. Examination of the vaginal secretions of an asymptomatic woman in this estrogen-lack state reveals an alkaline pH, a negative whiff test when vaginal fluid is added to a drop of 10% potassium hydroxide (KOH), and the microscopic examination of a saline suspension of vaginal secretions shows immature squamous cells, a moderate number of white cells (WBCs) and decreased numbers of lactobacilli.

Many women have symptoms due to this estrogen deprivation. The thinning of the vulvar tissue makes it less resilient to the daily stresses to that skin. This is particularly true in the winter season of countries away from the equator. The cold, dry air outside and the warm, dry air with central heating in the home or office dry the skin and make it more prone to cracking. The thinning tissue can split and separate with the resulting tissue break, a source of burning and pain. The thinning tissue can acquire a thickened squamous cell cover (lichen sclerosis) and the whitened tissue can be a source of constant burning and itching. This altered epithelium is a fertile site for the growth of *Candida*, which increases the local vulvar inflammation. The thinning and retraction of the tissue around the urethral orifice, may contribute to the increased frequency of urinary tract symptoms that are more common in menopausal women.

These hormonal changes can also contribute to vaginal symptoms. The altered pH and decreased numbers of lactobacilli can tip the microbiologic balance in the vagina, allowing an overgrowth of Gram-negative bacilli. These women are often symptomatic, and the colonization with increased numbers of Gram-negative aerobes is the most important factor in the increased risk of urinary tract infections (UTI) in post-menopausal women[2].

Lifestyle changes for many of these menopausal women can result in a new group of vulvovaginal disorders. Married women with husbands undergoing the mid-life crisis face the possibility of acquiring a sexually transmitted disease from their male's extramarital sexual adventures. Alternatively, these men can become enamored of drugs like sildenafil citrate that enhance the possibility of an erection and increase the frequency and duration of sexual intercourse. This is good for the male ego and pleasure satisfaction, but the women's estrogen-deprived vagina can be ill-equipped for this sudden increase in activity. The result often is vaginal soreness, vulvar swelling, an increased discharge, or vulvar and vaginal tissue tears with symptoms of burning and discomfort.

There is another new risk factor for this age group of women. Divorce, which is the end-point of approximately 50% of marriages in the United States and western Europe, is usually followed by a period of increased sexual activity with new partners by both men and women. As an added risk for the menopausal woman in whom pregnancy is no longer a concern, this means intercourse with no barrier methods of protection. This can have a deleterious effect for many women, because it is a perfect scenario to acquire an infection that may not be recognized. Often, these menopausal women have not been sexually active for months or years before this exposure and assume the irritation, burning, and pain is the result of vaginal irritation or vulvar mucosal tears. These patients do not have an awareness that they can acquire a sexually transmitted disease (STD). This can be an immediate and apparent problem to them with the appearance of the painful lesions of genital herpes simplex virus (HSV)-1 and HSV-2, or an immediate increased vaginal discharge as a result of bacterial vaginosis, *Trichomonas* vaginitis, or lower genital tract *Neisseria gonorrhea*, or *Chlamydia trachomatis* infections. The infections have subtler presentations over time: new growths on the vagina or vulva, condyloma acuminata, due to low-risk human papillomavirus (HPV) infection or Pap smear abnormalities due to a high-risk HPV infection. Other viral exposures can result in subsequent laboratory abnormalities that have major health care implications, such as blood antibody testing that indicates a recent hepatitis B or human immunodeficiency virus (HIV) infection.

Menopausal women also have an increased risk of the presence of pre-cancerous or cancerous lesions of the vulva or vagina. Although their complaints can be a constant vulvar burning or itching they assume is due to *Candida*, tissue changes should not be ignored and biopsies should be obtained of any vulvar or vaginal abnormalities no matter how minimal they appear. What grossly seems benign, too often is an area of altered cellular growth that could lead to, or already is, cancer.

MICROBIOLOGY

The decrease in vaginal estrogen concentrations following menopause leads to dramatic changes in the vaginal flora during this period. As mentioned in a prior chapter, estrogen stimulates glycogen deposition in vaginal epithelial cells. The metabolism of glycogen to glucose and then to lactic acid results in vaginal acidification and preferential colonization by lactobacilli. Vaginal glycogen levels become greatly reduced or are absent following menopause and the vaginal epithelia become very thin. These changes are minimized in women who receive exogenous estrogen.

A study of post-menopausal women aged 55–79 years, with a mean age of 67 years, using quantitative culture techniques demonstrated that although lactobacilli could be isolated from about half of the women, the concentrations were 10- to 100-fold lower than those present in reproductive-age women. Lactobacilli was the dominant vaginal species in only 13% of the subjects[3]. The predominant bacterial species isolated were anaerobic Gram-negative rods in 89% of women and Gram-positive peptostreptococci from 88% of women. The concentration of these microorganisms was similar to levels present in pre-menopausal subjects. The frequency of vaginal colonization by *Gardnerella vaginalis*, genital mycoplasmas, and yeast species was also much reduced following menopause. Utilization of gene amplification techniques rather than bacterial cultures has demonstrated that over 90% of post-menopausal women do in fact remain colonized with vaginal lactobacilli, but at low concentrations[4].

Comparisons of post-menopausal women who were not, and those who were, using systemic or topical hormone replacement therapy (HRT) demonstrated large increases in vaginal lactobacilli colonization in the latter subjects[5,6]. Vaginal colonization with *Escherichia coli* also occurs at an increased incidence in post-menopausal as compared to reproductive-age women, and the rate of colonization is inversely associated with the presence of lactobacilli[6]. These observations suggest that the relative absence of lactobacilli in post-menopausal women may explain the increased rate of vaginal colonization by *E. coli* and the increased incidence of UTI in this population.

The decrease in lactobacilli in post-menopausal women causes problems in the interpretation of scoring systems for bacterial vaginosis. The Nugent scoring system for determination of the presence of bacterial vaginosis is based upon an analysis of vaginal lactobacilli. Therefore, application of this system to post-menopausal women may lead to a false-positive diagnosis of bacterial vaginosis. The decrease in vaginal lactobacilli in post-menopausal women is not associated with an increased rate of bacterial vaginosis.

IMMUNOLOGY

The decline in ovarian function at menopause also results in immune alterations. Estrogen compounds are mediators of pro-inflammatory cytokine production. Basal as well as induced levels of interleukin-1, interleukin-6 and tumor necrosis factor-α are elevated in post-menopausal women as compared to women of reproductive age[7]. This increased production of cytokines that induce inflammation is undoubtedly a component of the pathogenic mechanism responsible for diseases associated with aging. Post-menopausal bone loss has also been related to an elevated release of these cytokines. HRT has been shown to prevent this selective increase in pro-inflammatory cytokines and to restore the physiological balance between pro-inflammatory and anti-inflammatory immunity[8].

DIAGNOSIS

Obtaining an accurate history in these menopausal women is not an easy task. Accurate history-taking requires patience and an attentive ear for the frequently muted concerns of these women. Many are reticent to voice any of their deeply held fears, and the elucidation of any new symptomatology is usually not straightforward. After questioning about health problems and a review of symptoms that has revealed no problems, the woman will ask, as an aside just before the pelvic examination, 'Will you look down there? I have a new lump I'd like you to check'. This is an age group that has been touched by the awareness of friends newly discovered to have breast, skin, or ovarian cancer and finds it hard to address this issue as a personal possibility. If a lesion has been identified, details about how long it has been noticed by the patient can be obtained. The other area of delayed information is the symptom of vaginal dryness or discomfort with intercourse that too often is broached after completion of the exam. To avoid this, vaginal pH should be measured, and secretions placed in saline a whiff test performed on vaginal secretions mixed with 10% KOH. If patients have tardily addressed concerns about vaginal symptoms, there is then the opportunity to view the saline and KOH mount under the microscope.

Many menopausal women in this first decade of the 21st century are very private about their personal affairs and are not forthcoming about their recent sexual history. At some point during the interview, the subject should be broached indirectly with a variety of phrasing fashioned to elicit a response. For the newly widowed or divorced patient, it can take the form of a reference to their personal life, 'How are you doing?', followed by an unhurried pause in which sometimes important medical information will be shared. Many of these women have had to deal with the disapproval of their children for any social activities with someone of the opposite sex. Alternatively, a response can sometimes be achieved by a seemingly off-hand query, 'How's your social life?' This can hopefully set the stage for a more open discussion. In every case, the physician's willingness to listen is more important than any history-taking ritual. Any information obtained will specifically target a physical examination focus with appropriate laboratory studies.

In this diagnostic evaluation, it is also important to get a detailed medical history and current use of drugs by these patients. Women with a history of breast or endometrial cancer will not ordinarily be candidates for systemic or local estrogens. Some liver illnesses, such as cirrhosis from a chronic hepatitis B or C infection, can preclude the use of oral estrogens as a treatment option. Tamoxifen citrate can cause vaginal symptomatology for patients under care for breast cancer. Any history of allergy is important. If local estrogens have been used, inquiries need to be made to see if the patient has had any adverse reactions to them. They can cause severe vaginal or vulvar burning after the application of an estrogen cream that contains propylene glycol as a preservative. In these situations, the vaginal estrogen tablet that has no propylene glycol would seem an ideal choice, but women with reduced vaginal secretions can develop vaginal or vulvar irritation within a day or two of inserting the vaginal estrogen tablet.

The physical examination of the menopausal woman should be a cooperative effort of the doctor and patient. Physicians want patients to point out any perceived lump, bump, or irritation, and patients want physicians to conduct an unhurried, gentle examination that will not hurt them. The colposcope or a magnifying glass can be used to view any perceived abnormalities of the vulva. It magnifies any lesion. A camera picture provides a baseline for comparison when the patient comes back for follow-up after treatment. A number of anatomic lower genital tract changes alarm some patients who have used a hand mirror, for example, a new, red introital lesion, a urethral caruncle. These can vary in size and degree of inflammation from slight to extreme (**125–127**). The patient in Figure **127** had burning after urination. These women can be immediately reassured that

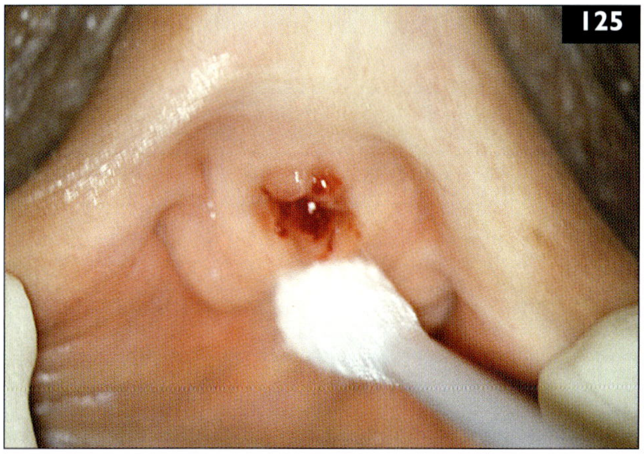

125 A small urethral caruncle in a menopausal patient.

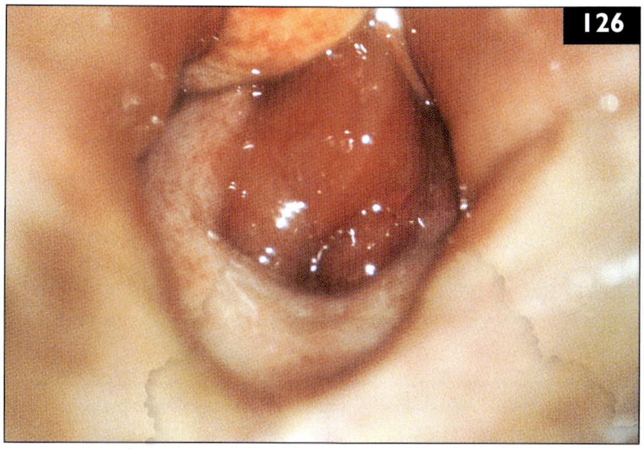

126 A larger urethral caruncle.

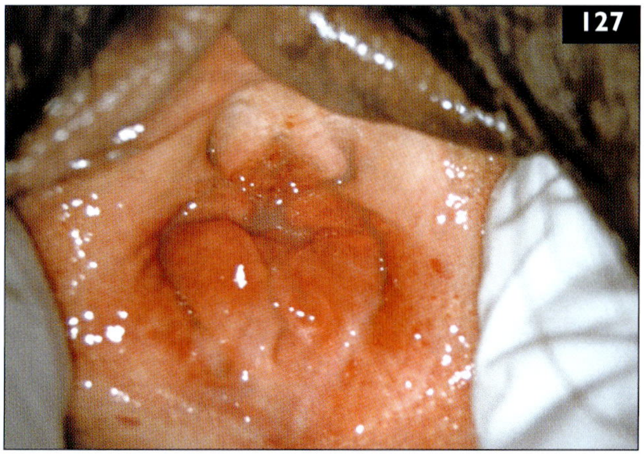

127 A large urethral caruncle. This patient had burning after urination.

this is due to estrogen lack and not a new tissue growth. The entrance to the vagina, the vulvar vestibule, can also become very inflamed and result in pain and burning after urination (**128**). A careful examination should be performed and appropriate tests obtained before a diagnsosis is made.

In contrast, the vulvar tissue in menopausal women is often thinned and becomes paler in color with retraction of the labia majora (**129**). The retraction can be accompanied by a split in the surface epithelium, which can be painful for the patient. These problems occur more often in the winter months, with cold air outside and the warm, dry air of central heating. They can take many forms (**130–132**). Some women complaining of painful intercourse describe a tearing pain during intimacy and lower genital tract discomfort that persists afterwards. Upon inspection, a mid-line introital tear is apparent (**133**), and touching it gently with a cotton-tipped applicator stick elicits a pain response. If untreated, this area is prone to tear again with every attempt at intercourse (**134**).

Vulvar vestibulitis is an infrequent cause of vulvar pain in post-menopausal women. The diagnosis can be made by a careful examination of the vulva with cotton tip applicators touching the painful vestibular glands (**135**). In other patients, the skin can become whitened with a crust, lichen sclerosis, a diagnosis that should be confirmed by biopsy (**136**). This crusted tissue can also become very inflamed, because of a *Candida albicans* infection, an organism that finds this altered surface epithelium a favorable site for colonization and multiplication, with resulting tissue inflammation and patient symptomatology (**137**).

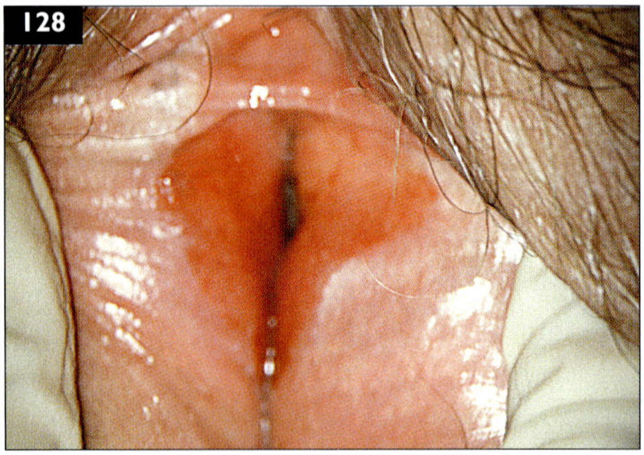

128 An inflamed vaginal entrance in a post-menopausal woman not taking hormone replacement therapy.

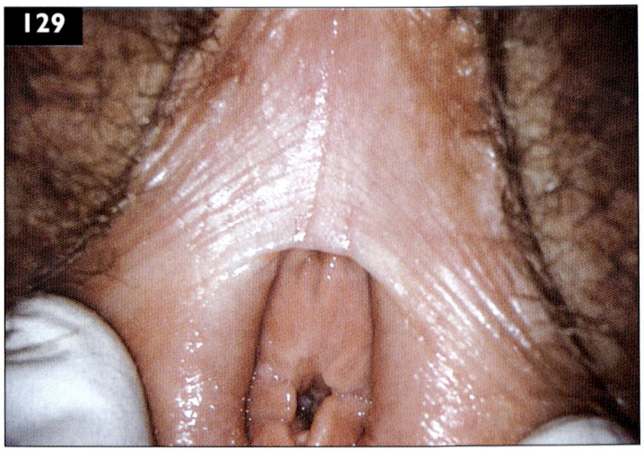

129 Thinning vulvar tissue, very prone to epithelial surface tears.

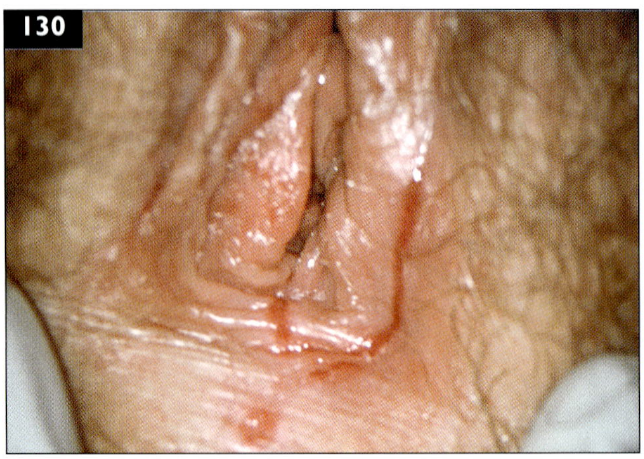

130 Thinning vulvar tissue with a surface epithelium tear.

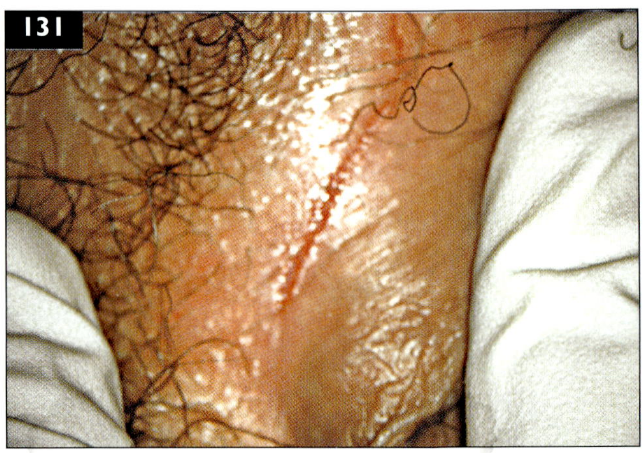

131 A vulvar epithelial tear on the skin fold of the retracted vulvar skin near the clitoris.

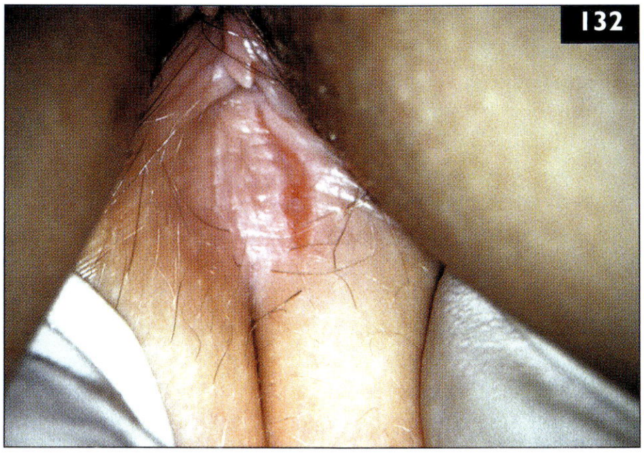

132 A perineal skin tear near the rectum.

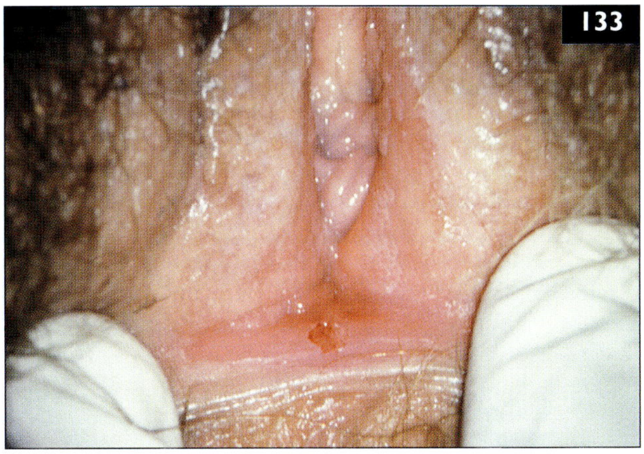

133 A mid-line introital epithelial tear discovered after painful intercourse.

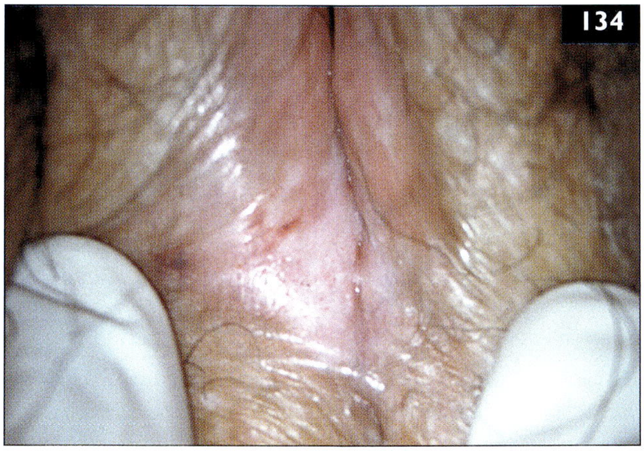

134 A healed mid-line introital tear, prone to tear again with attempts at intercourse.

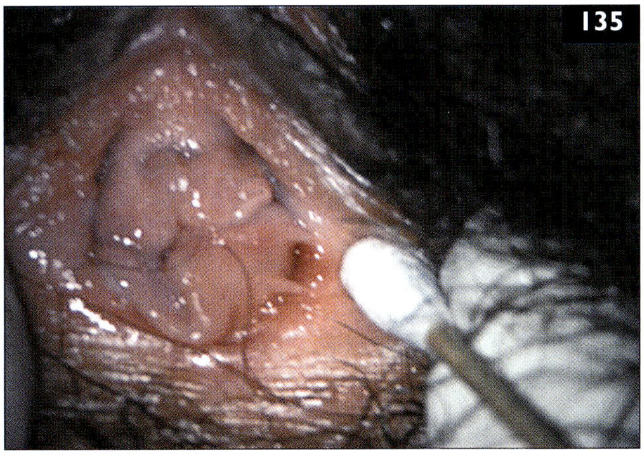

135 A post-menopausal woman with vulvar vestibulitis.

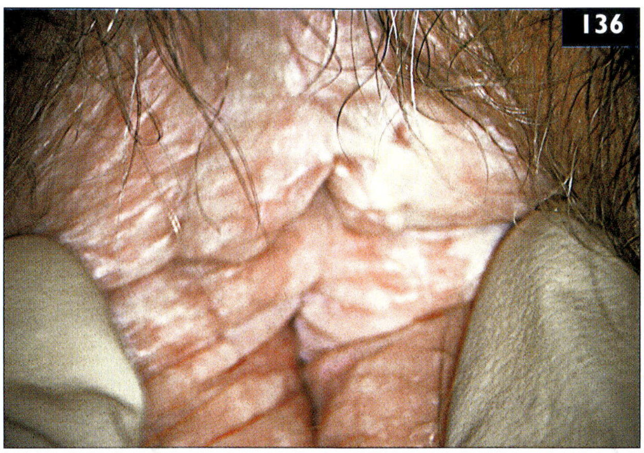

136 Thickened white vulvar tissue. Biopsy confirmed lichen sclerosis.

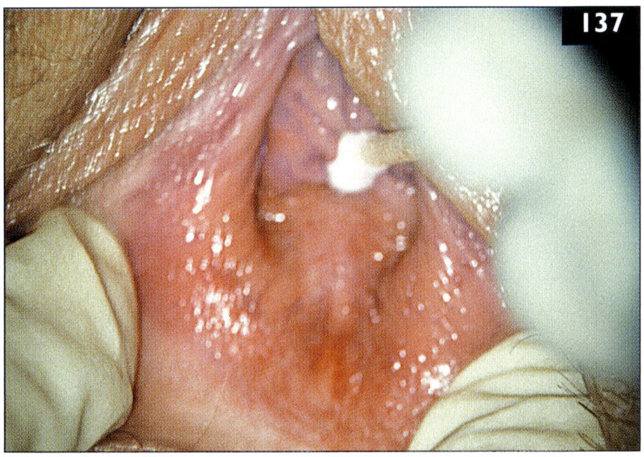

137 Inflamed thickened white vulvar epithelial tissue. A scraping placed in potassium hydroxide showed the presence of pseudohyphae.

A KOH preparation of surface scraping revealed pseudohyphae (**138**), and the culture grew *Candida albicans.* An occasional patient complaining of perineal pain 1–3 days after intercourse has a painful cluster of lesions, which on culture in this case grew HSV-1 (**139**). In another post-menopausal woman with sudden onset of vulvar irritation, only inflammation and none of the classic findings of a genital herpes infection was found (**140**). She was culture-positive for HSV-2 and had IgG antibodies to HSV-2 only and no IgM antibodies. This was a clinical outbreak that had been preceded by an asymptomatic primary infection. Another patient complaining of new growths was found to have a field outbreak of condyloma acuminata (**141**). New infectious vulvar ulcers can be found, and these are discussed in Chapter 10.

Alternatively, there is abnormal tissue growth, pre-cancerous vulvar intraepithelial neoplasm-3 (VIN-3) (**142**) and invasive vulvar cancer. These patients have ignored new growth for months or years before coming to the gynecologist (**143, 144**). The clinical diagnoses of lichen sclerosis, condyloma acuminatum, and pre-cancerous and cancerous changes in the vulva are made by biopsy. This diagnostic intervention must be done in women with chronic vulvar changes in whom a long duration of therapy is contemplated to obtain symptomatic relief.

The vaginal examination should be thorough, with the slow introduction of a small speculum followed by careful visual perusal and appropriate use of miscroscopic studies. Occasionally in menopausal women complaining of an increased vaginal discharge, an endometrial polyp can be

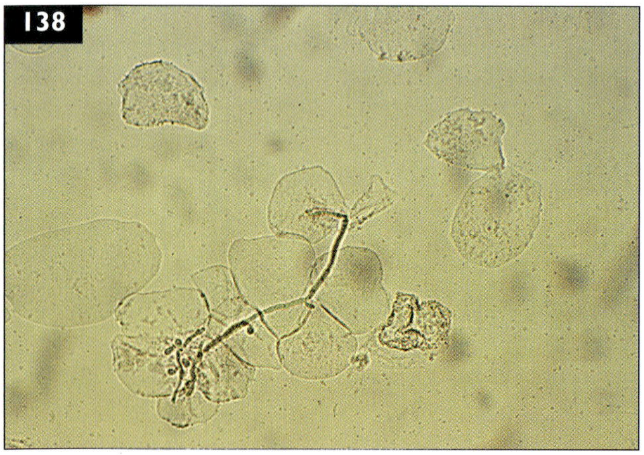

138 Microscopic examination of potassium hydroxide preparation of vulvar scraping. Pseudohyphae are present.

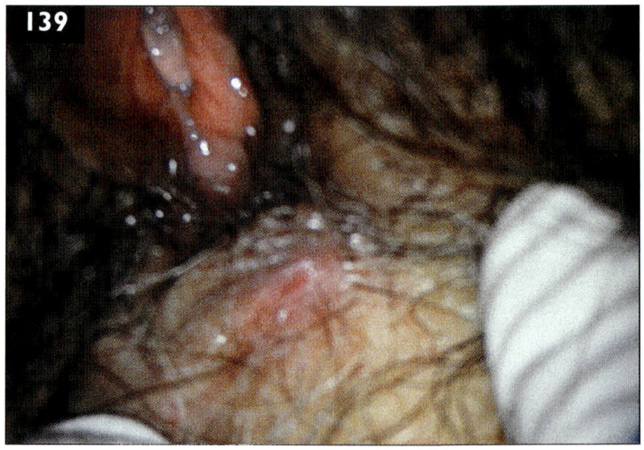

139 A painful cluster of lesions, culture positive for herpes simplex virus-1.

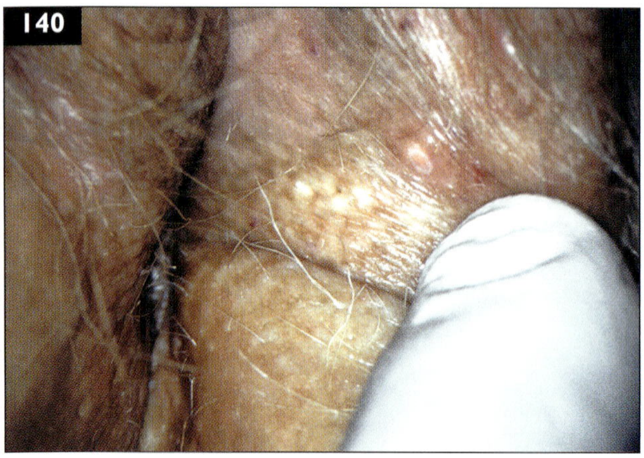

140 Vulvar inflammation, recurrent 'cut'. This was culture positive for herpes simplex virus -2.

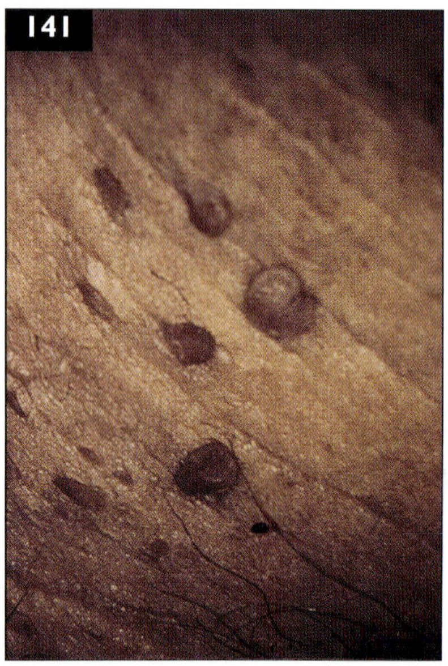

141 New growths found in the vulva. Biopsy diagnosis was condyloma acuminata.

seen protruding through the cervical os (**145**). These fragile vascular structures are sometimes the source of an increased discharge. In other patients, the pattern of examination involves the use of a plastic spatula to obtain vaginal secretions, which are added to a drop of saline, and to a drop of 10% KOH where a whiff test is performed; a vaginal pH is determined by using a swab that had been applied to the lateral vaginal wall. In women not taking estrogen systemically or locally, the pH is usually alkaline. Then, the microscopic examination is performed. The saline preparation often shows immature squamous cells, and many WBCs (**146**). These WBCs are

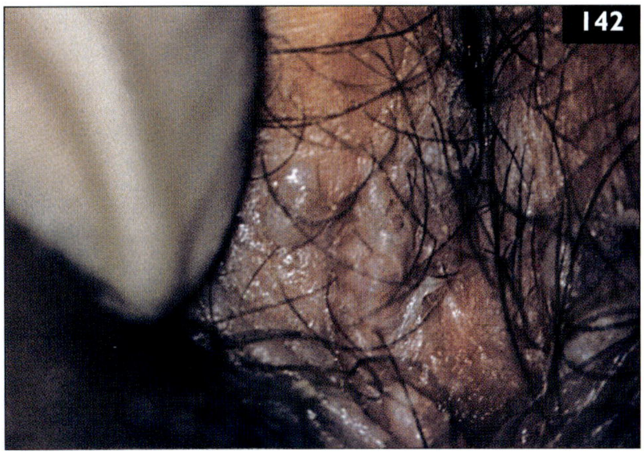

142 Vulvar lesion on biopsy found to be vulvar intraepithelial neoplasm-3.

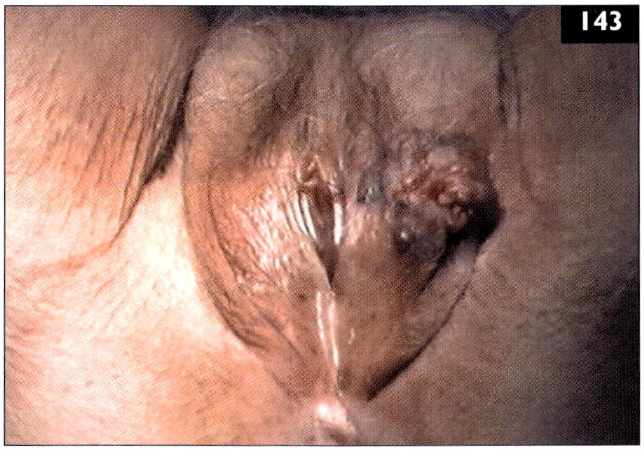

143 Vulvar lesion ignored by the patient. On biopsy, invasive squamous cell cancer of the vulva was found.

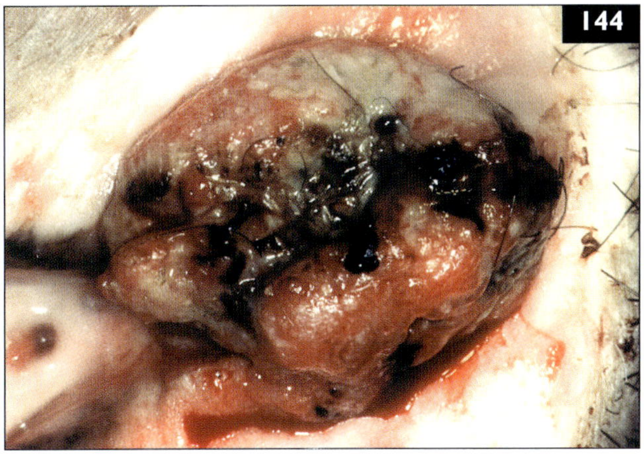

144 Vulvar lesion. Biopsy diagnosis was invasive squamous epithelial cancer of the vulva.

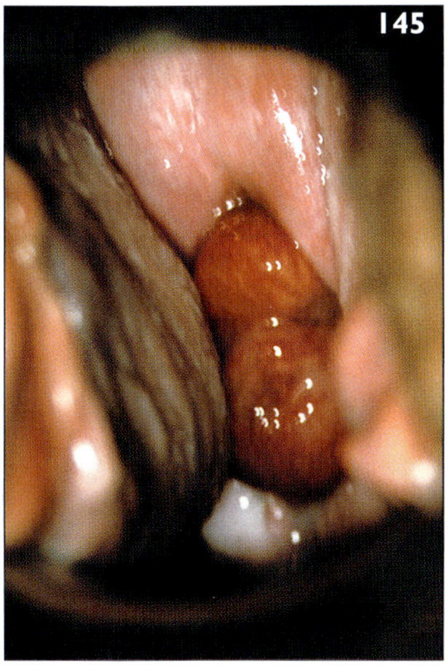

145 An endometrial polyp found protruding out of the cervical os.

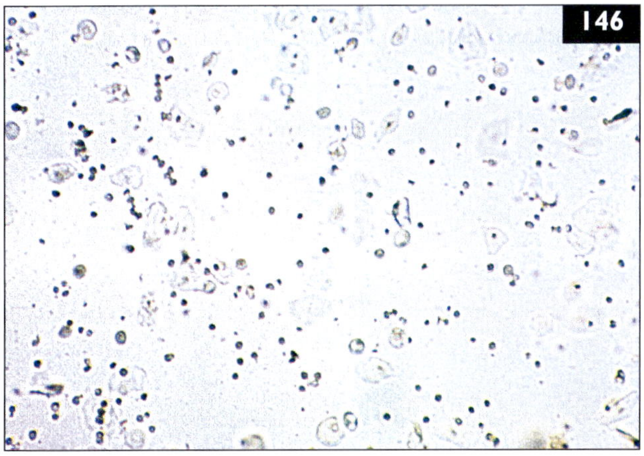

146 Microscopic examination of the saline preparation shows immature squamous cells and many white blood cells.

eliminated when the KOH suspension is examined and a decreased number of lactobacilli are seen (**147**). Women with a history of breast cancer who are taking tamoxifen citrate have immature squamous cells present and an increased number of WBCs (**148**).

Laboratory testing should be individualized to fit the diagnostic needs of each patient. For the woman with an inflamed, irritated vulva (**137**), a surface scraping should be obtained with a plastic spatula, placed in a drop of 10% KOH, and examined under the microscope. The presence of hyphae confirms the clinical suspicion that this is a *Candida* vulvitis (**138**). Women with introital lesions that appear to be herpetic (**139**) should have a viral culture performed to determine the type of herpes present. The greater sensitivity of the polymerase chain reaction (PCR) test makes it a better choice in women seen a few days after the onset of new vulvar lesions[9]. Blood should be drawn for HSV-1 and HSV-2 antibodies to determine if this is a primary outbreak. The patient, not sexually active, with a vaginal discharge, should have both the saline suspension (**149**) and the KOH suspension (**150**) examined for the presence of pseudohyphae. A vaginal culture will determine the exact *Candida* species present and screen for other bacterial pathogens. Current guidelines for the use of Pap smear and HPV testing are based upon the patient's history of normal Pap smears for 3 consecutive years, followed by future screening at 3-year intervals. There can be exceptions: the ending of a monogamous relationship by either the male or female can expose the patient with no history of an abnormal Pap to the acquisition of a high-risk HPV infection. Three years may be too long to wait in post-menopausal women who have had this exposure.

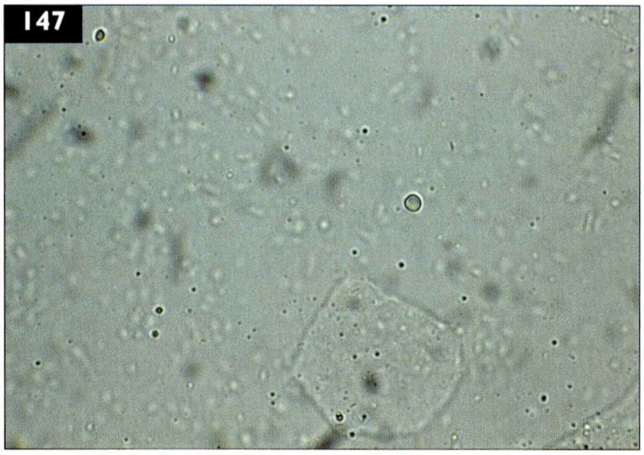

147 Microscopic examination of a potassium hydroxide preparation shows a decreased number of lactobacilli.

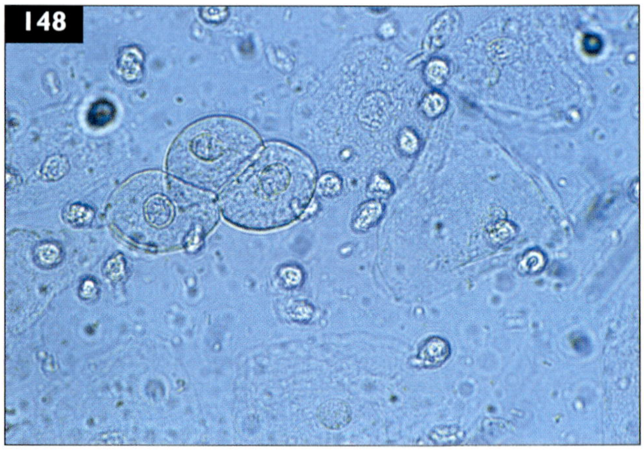

148 The microscopic examination of a saline preparation from a post-menopausal woman with a history of breast cancer who is taking tamoxifen shows immature squamous cells and an increased number of white blood cells are present.

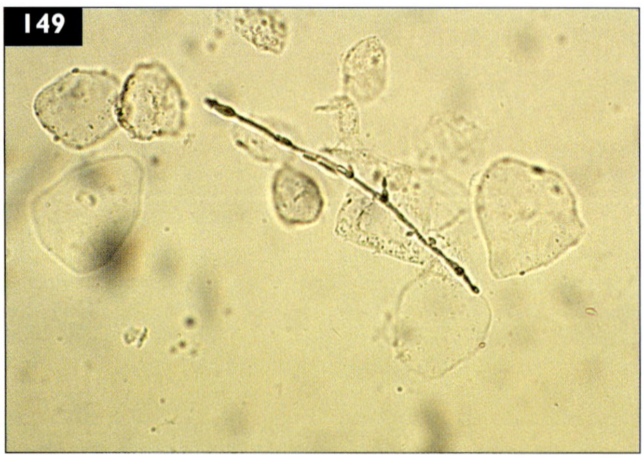

149 Microscopic examination of a saline preparation showing pseudohyphae.

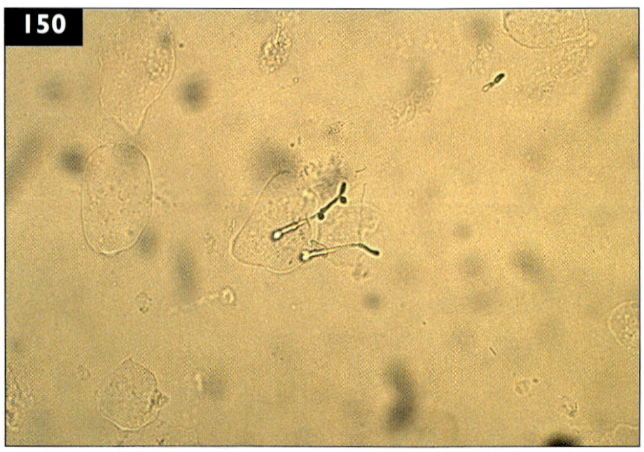

150 Microscopic examination of a potassium hydroxide preparation from the same patient, showing the presence of pseudohyphae.

TREATMENT

For many of these women, the cornerstone of care that will reduce or eliminate symptoms is estrogen, given either locally or systemically. This can be a problem, because of the recent heightened concerns about systemic hormone therapy raised by the WHI study that demonstrated increased risks of breast cancer, cardiovascular disease, and stroke[1,9]. Systemic HRT is not recommended for women with urogenital symptoms alone, but local preparations can be used in most of these patients[10]. Unless there is an absolute medical contraindication, such as a history of breast or endometrial cancer, estrogen therapy can be a useful therapeutic choice.

The first anatomical area of therapeutic concern is the vulva and the entrance to the vagina, the vulvar vestibular region. Patients present with persistent vulvar burning and itching with an increase in their symptomatology every time they urinate. On examination, they are noted to have an inflamed vulva (**128**). These symptomatic patients' concerns about a STD can be ruled out by microbiologic studies. Patients are also seen complaining of persistent vulvar discomfort because of a split in the vulvar epithelium (**130**) or a mid-line introital tear that surfaced after intercourse (**133**). These women are excellent candidates for local estrogen therapy after a *Candida* infection is ruled out by microscopy and culture. This is also true for the post-menopausal woman with vulvar vestibulitis (**135**). An estradiol cream can be applied to the inflamed vulvar area once or twice a day. If the patient has an immediate inflammatory reaction to the application of the cream or does not improve after 2 or more weeks of care, a vaginal estrogen tablet twice a week can help. Patients usually respond to one or the other of these two treatment choices and usually have the symptoms resolve after 1 or 2 months' treatment. Local adrenocorticoid creams or ointments are indicated if the diagnosis is lichen planus or lichen sclerosis. These diagnoses are made by biopsy.

Not every patient is a candidate for estrogen therapy. Some have a history of breast or endometrial cancer while others refuse to use any estrogens because of a family history of breast cancer or their fear of the relationship of HRT to breast cancer. They are candidates for the local use of a hydrocortisone ointment or the more active clobetasol preparations for specific time intervals of treatment.

Other vulvar problems are seen in which a different therapeutic approach is more appropriate. Patients complaining of constant vulvar itching and burning are seen in whom thickened and whitened vulvar skin is seen (lichen sclerosis) (**136**). The diagnosis should be confirmed by biopsy. This is a clinical situation in which a potent local adrenocorticoid (clobetasol) can effectively reduce the local inflammation. If this thickened vulvar epithelium is inflamed with a white discharge on the surface (**137**), a scraping obtained with a plastic spatula and then placed on a KOH drop should be examined under the microscope. If pseudohyphae are present (**138**), at least a portion of the inflammation is due to the *Candida* infection. The use of a local anti-fungal cream can result in a local contact dermatitis, which increases the local inflammation. Oral fluconazole is an alternative, with 150 mg tablets taken orally every 4 days. After this treatment, local steroids can be prescribed.

Post-menopausal women with infections of the vulva should be managed with specific care directed towards the pathogen identified by laboratory studies. Post-menopausal women complaining of the sudden onset of vulvar pain should be seen as soon as possible, for they may have genital herpes. These may be clinically obvious lesions (**139**) or simply a new onset of vulvar inflammation without the presence of the recognizable clinical signs of herpes (**140**). This latter case demonstrates the importance of obtaining a herpes culture in any new lesions of the vulva, no matter the age of the patient. Herpes culture for HSV-1 and HSV-2 should be obtained with blood antibody studies as well to determine if this is a primary infection. If herpes is suspected on clinical examination, a variety of anti-viral agents can be immediately prescribed while waiting for the lab report. Some women will complain of new growths in the perineal area, which on biopsy are shown to be condyloma acuminata (**141**). A variety of ablative techniques or the use of locally applied immunoenhancers can be used to eliminate these lesions on this tough, cornified, squamous epithelium. Vulvar ulcers should have appropriate cultures, biopsy, and blood tests done to determine the diagnosis (see Chapter 10).

In addition to the readiness to culture any inflammatory lesions, the physician must be prepared to biopsy any new suspicious growths on the vulva. If a vulvar intraepithelial lesion is found (VIN-1, -2, -3), a variety of treatment options are available to the physician and patient. The usual course is close observation over time with repeated biopsies to be sure there has been no progression of the lesions in this area. Interferon injection in the base of the VIN-3 lesion noted in Figure **142** was performed. This intervention was based upon the observations that a locally applied immunoenhancer, imiquimod, can accelerate the elimination of high-risk HPV associated with these tissue changes[11], and the Cornell experience with the successful use of local interferon injections in eliminating HPV infections of the vulva (M. Geneç, personal communication 2001). The effectiveness of this intervention has not been subjected to a prospective clinical trial. If invasive squamous cell carcinoma of the vulva is found by biopsy (**143, 144**), then the patient should be referred to a gynecologic oncologist so that appropriate vulvar resection and appropriate decision be made about the necessity for node dissection in these women.

The care of a post-menopausal woman complaining of a vaginal discharge or vaginal burning requires an accurate diagnosis for there can be unusual etiologies for these symptoms. Symptoms can be due to the presence of an endometrial polyp (**145**). Often, these patient complaints will cease when the polyp is removed. There are other, uncommon, benign causes of an increase in vaginal symptoms in this population of women. Rarely, a foreign body is found, and when it is removed, the patient becomes asymptomatic. In addition, any new growth should be biopsied to rule out the possibility of any vaginal pre-cancer or cancer.

In most cases, the care of these menopausal women will be based upon the diagnosis made by the history and laboratory findings. *Candida* infections occur in these patients. Some menopausal women will be found to have pseudohyphae and/or spores present on the wet mount (saline and KOH) microscopic examination (**149, 150**), or will have a vaginal culture positive for *Candida*, usually *C. albicans*. If *C. albicans* is present, treatment with a single 150 mg dose of oral fluconazole is effective in women not taking any form of estrogen supplementation. If the isolate is *C. krusei* or *C. glabrata*, local or oral azoles are not indicated and a regimen with local boric acid is begun for a 2-week treatment interval (see Chapter 4).

Women with a history of breast cancer taking tamoxifen citrate often complain of an irritating vaginal discharge. The microscopic examination of the saline preparation shows immature squamous cells and an inflammatory response with an increased number of WBCs. Cultures show no yeast and no abnormal bacteria. Local estrogen, which should reverse this process, is not indicated. The periodic use of an acidic vaginal gel helps some patients, but relief comes when the tamoxifen citrate therapy is terminated. The introduction of new, more effective therapeutic agents, such as exemestane, should reduce the overall use of tamoxifen[12].

A large group of symptomatic post-menopausal patients complain of either an irritating vaginal discharge or vaginal dryness and burning. On examination, they have an alkaline vaginal pH, a negative whiff test and, on microscopic examination, immature squamous cells, an increased number of WBCs, and a diminution in the number of lactobacilli (**147, 148**). If the cultures show no *Candida* and no bacterial pathogens, a local form of estrogen will help. One study found that local estrogen given to post-menopausal women increased the number of lactobacilli, reduced vaginal pH, and reduced vaginal colonization with enterobacteriaciae[2]. Although this estrogen therapy improved the bacterial flora of these women, it was not as effective as a daily dose of oral nitrofurantoin in preventing UTIs in this population[13]. However, the vaginal estrogen pessary[13] did not normalize the vaginal pH as the estrogen cream had done previously[2].

For women with vaginal symptoms, 2 g of intravaginal estradiol cream given daily for 2 weeks is usually effective. If the patient has had a reaction to the cream in the past, or has a reaction with current therapy, a vaginal estradiol tablet once or twice a week is often helpful. For the woman who cannot or will not take estrogen, vaginal acid gels can be employed, supplemented with the vaginal use of boric acid gelatin capsules once or twice a week. This maintains the normal acid state of the vagina for a time and does result in a diminution of the vaginal symptoms in many of these women. Few of these women have either bacterial vaginosis or *Trichomonas* vaginitis but, if present, they should be appropriately treated (see Chapter 5 and Chapter 6). If the patient has had unprotected sex with a new sexual partner, cultures or PCR for *Neisseria gonorrhea* and a PCR for *Chlamydia trachomatis* should be obtained. If either is positive, then appropriate antibiotic therapy should be prescribed.

Some asymptomatic post-menopausal women present with an abnormal Pap smear and are found by testing to be positive for a high-risk HPV. Current care utilizes colposcopy examination and biopsy to determine whether there are more severe tissue changes than noted in the cytology report. Since the squamo-columnar junction in many of these women has receded from the face of the cervix into the endocervical canal, it is important to get a sample of endocervical tissue from these patients.

Chapter 14

Vulvodynia

BACKGROUND

Vulvodynia is a concept that is difficult for most clinicians to grasp. To provide some clarity, the International Society for the Study of Vulvovaginal Disease has provided one definition of vulvodynia. They describe it as burning pain, occurring in the absence of relevant visible findings or a specific clinical neurologic disorder[1]. Attempting to define such a variable clinical syndrome obviously is difficult. For example, the author believes there are visible findings in these women that can be recognized at the time of the first physician examination. In addition to this definition, the Society subclassifies this syndrome on the basis of the site of the pain, whether it is generalized or localized, and whether it is provoked, unprovoked, or mixed. There are other components in this attempt to bring some order to the wide variety of clinical presentations seen in women with vulvar pain. It can be primary, pain presenting with the first attempt at intercourse, or secondary, pain developing after prior months or years of intercourse with discomfort. Is the pain provoked, i.e. only present with attempts at intercourse or tampon insertion, or is there constant vulvar burning, which has been given the name dysesthetic vulvodynia?

The subset of vulvodynia that will be focused upon in this chapter is what has been previously called vulvar vestibulitis syndrome (VVS). VVS is a condition characterized by point tenderness of at least 6 months' duration, demonstrable when vestibular gland openings are touched with a cotton-tipped applicator. The result of this pain response is that these women do not experience pain-free vaginal penetration. Vaginal intercourse is impossible for many, and the pain is so severe for some that they cannot even tolerate the insertion of a tampon. The original three criteria for diagnosis proposed by Dr. Friedrich included severe pain during attempted vaginal entry, tenderness to pressure localized in the vulvar vestibule, and erythema of the vulvar vestibule[2]. This erythema obviously lies outside the definition of vulvodynia by the Vulvovaginal Disease Society[1]. There can be a wide range of inflammation noted in these patients from severe (**151, 152**) to minimal (**153**). Despite these anatomic

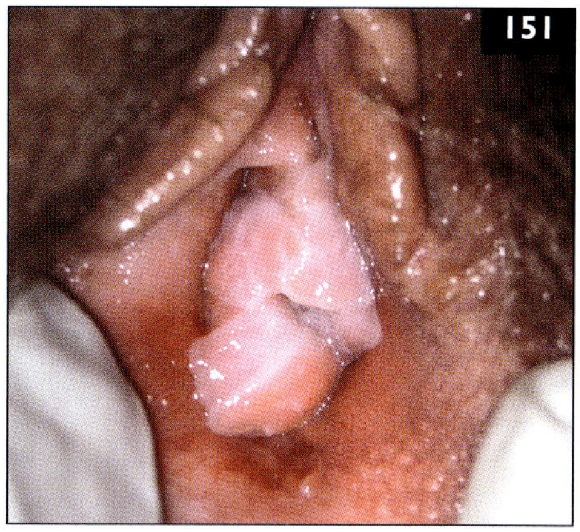

151 Marked introital inflammation in a patient with vulvar vestibulitis.

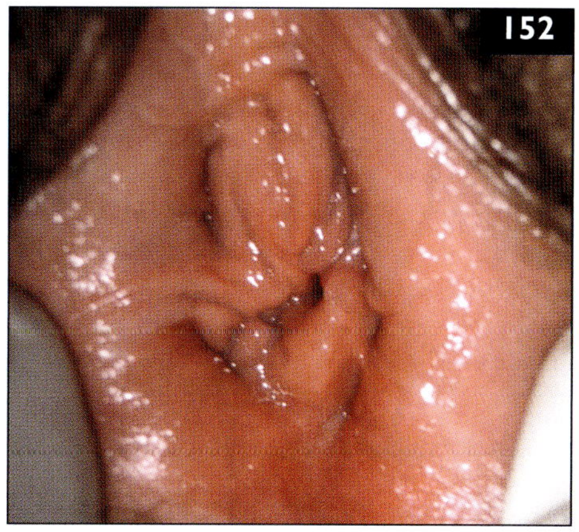

152 Another vulvar vestibulitis patient with introital inflammation.

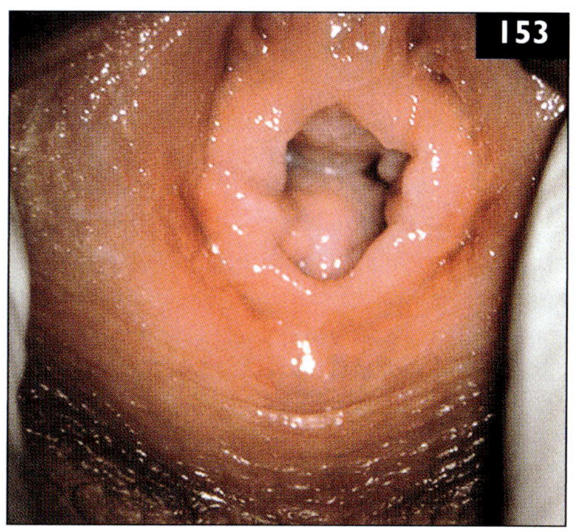

153 Minimal introital inflammation in a patient with vulvar vestibulitis. This patient had exquisite pain when the vestibular glands were touched with a cotton-tipped applicator. She was unable to have intercourse because of the pain with insertion, and she could not use a tampon because of the discomfort.

differences, all of these women had excruciating pain when a cotton-tipped applicator was applied to the vestibular glands, particularly at 4:30 o'clock and 7:30 o'clock. Neither was able to have intercourse, because of the pain. Some women will have the pain localized to one side (**154–156**). Again, the pain was specific when pressure was applied to these single vestibular gland sites. Women with VVS have other symptoms as well, including an increased frequency of vaginal discharge (75%), as well as urinary frequency and urgency (10–40%)[3]. Every physician should recognize that women with VVS have varying histories and different physical findings. This is a complex clinical picture.

The true frequency of VVS is not known. Harlow and Stewart, using a patient questionnaire technique and Goetsch, evaluating patients in a general gynecologic practice, have proclaimed this to be a common problem for adult women, affecting 15% of the total population[4]. This figure seems much too high. The most distressing characteristic of VVS is its persistence, with the result of a totally dysfunctional personal and social life. The symptoms of VVS take over their lives. With the instant availability of e-mail to request consultation that results from the Cornell listing on the National Vulvodynia Association website, which names a small cadre of American physicians who will care for these patients, the author's clinic phone has not been bombarded with inquiries from the huge population base in the New York City area. It is more likely there are thousands, not millions, of women in the United Sates with VVS. It is a syndrome seen in Europe as well. During a 3-year period at the Radboud University Medical Center, Nijmegen, the Netherlands, 275 women with vulvar vestibulitis underwent operative treatment for this disorder[5].

A major problem for women with this syndrome is that most physicians in practice do not recognize it. Physicians caring for these women subsequently can have the surprising experience of women crying with joy when told at their consultation visit that they have vulvar disease, VVS. Their past experience with doctor after doctor has been the physician response that they have no reason for their pain. It is either a problem 'in their head', or they have a yeast or bacterial vaginal infection. None of these responses addressed their problem of pain. There are many reasons for this. Physician hearing is too often selective. Patients with VVS, in addition to the vulvar pain, often have urinary tract symptoms and/or an excessive vaginal discharge[3]. Physicians shy away from pain. They don't understand it, they don't know how to treat it, and the easiest course is to deny its existence. A urinary tract infection (UTI) or a vaginal infection are different entities. Doctors can deal with these problems for they are known clinical syndromes that can be routinely solved in the outpatient practices. The result is repeated treatments for UTI when the urine culture has no significant growth of bacteria, anti-fungal treatments for vaginal candidiasis when the vaginal culture shows no growth of *Candida*, or antibiotic treatment of unconfirmed vaginal bacterial infections when the anti-fungal treatment fails. Other factors add to physician confusion. The ritual when performing a pelvic examination

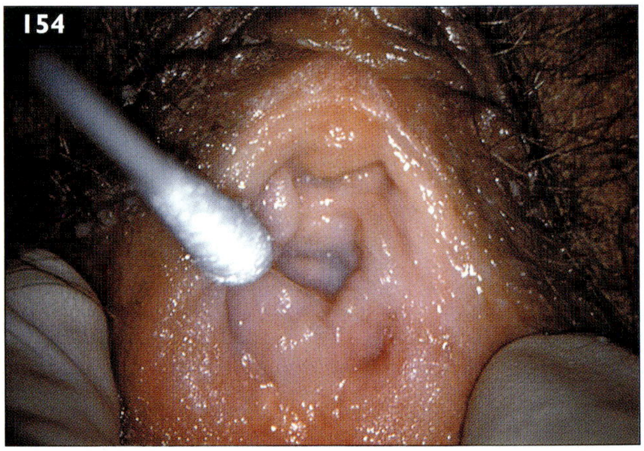

154 Patient with vulvar vestibulitis limited to the left side at 4:30 o'clock.

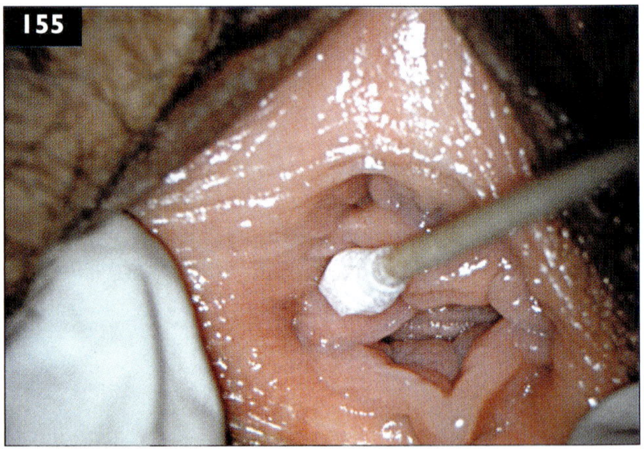

155 Patient with vulvar vestibulitis limited to the right side at 7:30 o'clock. Grossly, this appeared less inflamed than the left side.

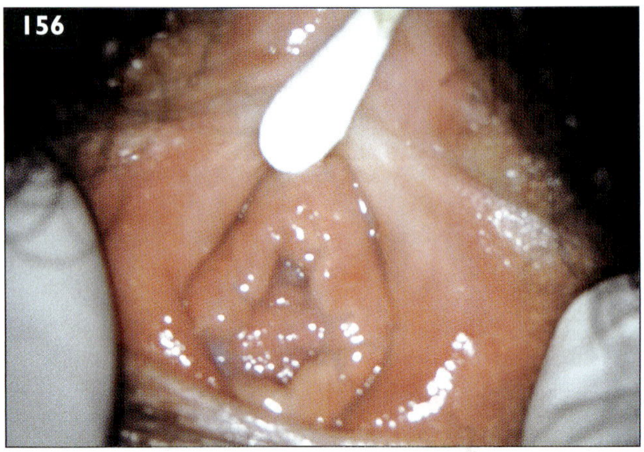

156 Patient with vulvar vestibulitis limited to the right left side at an uncommon site, 10 o'clock.

begins with the insertion of the speculum. This obviates the chance for a proper examination of the introitus. Even when the examination of the introitus occurs, it may not be diagnostic for many practitioners. Patients with VVS do not have the visible pathology that physicians associate with other vulvar pathologies that cause pain, such as a Bartholin's cyst or abscess.

There is a common thread in the evolution of the symptomatology of women with VVS. Many can pinpoint the onset of symptomatology to a specific event. In one study, pain occurred in 20.4% of the women the first time they tried to have intercourse, and following a vaginal infection in 24.7%[6]. There can be other events separate from the vulva that some patients relate to the onset of symptomatology, such as a laparotomy for a pelvic operation or a distant intervention such as a colonoscopy or liposuction of the thighs. The difference between these women with VVS and the vast majority of women who have vulvar symptomatology is that the symptoms persist in women with VVS.

Other factors can contribute to the persistence of symptomatology. Misdiagnosis of nonexistent UTIs leads to repeated exposures of the patients to systemic antibiotics with no benefit and the possible unfavorable result of an allergic reaction to the antibiotic or an alteration in the vaginal flora, resulting in more symptoms than existed before this misguided therapy. A similar scenario exists for women repeatedly treated locally with vaginal creams or suppositories for nonproven *Candida* or bacterial infections. Women can develop a local allergy or a contact dermatitis to either the anti-fungal medication or, more often, to the chemical preservative propylene glycol present in most creams and suppositories. Instead of helping, these local agents produce a severe local inflammatory reaction that intensifies and prolongs the discomfort. Similarly, women are often given steroid or estrogen creams to apply locally to the vulvar vestibule. The same local allergic reaction, again usually due to the propylene glycol present in these preparations, increases the local inflammation, aggravating the inflammation. The most important thing for the patient and the physician to keep in mind is that VVS is a chronic process. There are no quick therapeutic fixes. Usually, a cure will not be achieved with the first treatment regimen and eventual resolution of symptomatology can require months of treatment with higher than initial doses or a different regimen than the first one prescribed.

Despite the persistence of symptoms, there can be variations in patient discomfort. Some women have resolution of symptoms for months or years, only to have them return. The most dramatic responses occur during pregnancy. Most patients have symptoms decrease during gestation. This can be attributed to the dramatic increase in estrogen and adrenocortical steroid production during pregnancy, both of which have anti-inflammatory effects. This hypothesis obviously falls apart with the occasional exception, the patient whose VVS symptoms increase during pregnancy. Despite the usual improvement during pregnancy, most patients are more uncomfortable and more sensitive immediately after delivery. This is a common event for all post-partum women. Over time, these same patients usually end up with less intense vulvar symptomatology than they had before the pregnancy. This is attributed to the stretching of the perineum with vaginal delivery and the associated disruption of some of the extra nerve plexuses that these patients possess[7]. Because of this, it does not seem wise to favor elective cesarean section for the pregnant women with VVS. On the other hand, long-term post-partum improvement has been seen in women delivered by cesarean section. Obviously, there is still much that is not understood about these women.

MICROBIOLOGY

The microbiology of VVS has still not been satisfactorily resolved and remains a controversial subject. One case-control study noted that a self-reported history of a physician-diagnosed vaginal yeast or human papillomavirus (HPV) infection, as well as bacterial vaginosis, was more prevalent in women with VVS than in controls[8]. A second case-control study reported an increased rate of physician-reported *Candida albicans*, *Trichomonas vaginalis*, and bacterial vaginosis, but not HPV, genital herpes, or *Chlamydia trachomatis* infection in women with VVS[9]. An earlier, larger study of 220 patients with VVS determined that 24.1% had a genital HPV infection and 11.4% were culture-positive for *C. albicans*[3]. An investigation of 135 women with VVS and 322 control women detected a similar prevalence of polymerase chain reaction (PCR)-positive genital HPV infections, 29.6% vs. 23.9%, in the patients and controls, respectively[10]. Numerous other investigations have been inconsistent in reporting possible relationships between a vaginal yeast or HPV infection and VVS. In general, it appears that VVS patients typically report a more frequent history of various vulvovaginal infections than do other women. However, it is difficult to rule out bias in these reports. Women seeking medical help for symptoms associated with VVS may be more likely to receive a nonculture-confirmed diagnosis of a vaginal infection by physicians and are more likely to recall the diagnosis of an infection than women without symptoms. In addition, symptomatic women are tested for infections or bacterial vaginosis more frequently than asymptomatic women. The frequency of these vaginal perturbations may be underestimated in the control groups.

Infection may be associated with the initial trigger that leads to symptom formation in vulvar vestibulitis, but may not play a role in symptom persistence. For example, a microorganism or microbial product may activate a cascade of events leading to increased localized nerve stimulation or sensitivity. The resultant alterations may become permanent or more readily induced by a variety of subsequent triggers. It has also been suggested that sensitization to *Candida* antigens may result in development of autoimmune responses to cross-reactive self antigens[11]. Therefore, negative results on microbial analyses of women with this syndrome may erroneously negate the relationship of specific microorganisms to this syndrome.

A further possible clue of microbial involvement in the pathogenesis of VVS has come from a study of mannose-binding lectin (MBL) genetic polymorphisms[12]. MBL is a protein present in the systemic circulation and a major participant in the innate immune defense against microorganisms, including *C. albicans*. Possession of a variant allele of the MBL gene results in formation of an unstable MBL protein, which is degraded in the circulation. Individuals possessing this MBL variant allele have a decreased defense against infection. Investigations of women in New York City and two cities in Sweden revealed that patients with VVS had over a 14% incidence of the MBL variant while only 5–6% of controls were positive. Possession of the variant MBL was associated with a 10-fold decrease in MBL concentrations in the bloodstream[12]. These results suggest that a subset of women with VVS are more susceptible to infection than are other women, and adds support to the hypothesis of an infectious component to this syndrome.

Many patients with a diagnosis of VVS have undergone various treatments for infections, regardless of the utility of this approach. In some cases symptoms are exacerbated by components within anti-microbial treatment agents that have been applied to the vulva or vagina. Clinicians encountering women with VVS, therefore, should not rely on clinical criteria to diagnose a possible vulvovaginal infection. Instead, laboratory results are essential to assure reliable diagnostic criteria and treatment modalities.

IMMUNOLOGY

A pronounced increase in pro-inflammatory immunity in the vaginal vestibule, due to a transient or persistent infection in a woman who is genetically predisposed to produce high levels of pro-inflammatory cytokines and/or low levels of anti-inflammatory mediators, could result in activation of dormant nerve fibers in the vestibule or at other body sites. This, in turn, could translate into increased sensitivity of the infected area and development of clinical symptoms consistent with a diagnosis of VVS. Support for an immunological component to this syndrome is accumulating. Concentrations of the pro-inflammatory cytokines, interleukin-1β and tumor necrosis factor-α were shown to be elevated in the vestibule from women with VVS relative to controls[13]. An elevated frequency of variant alleles associated with increased pro-inflammatory immune activity in the genes coding for interleukin-1 receptor antagonist[14] and interleukin-1β[15] has been demonstrated in the DNA of vulvar vestibulitis patients. Whole bloods from women with vulvar vestibulitis produce higher levels of pro-inflammatory cytokines, and lower levels of anti-inflammatory cytokines, than do control women, suggesting a relative inability to down-regulate inflammation[16].

A history of allergies has been associated with VVS in some women[3,6]. Immediate hypersensitivity reactions lead to increases in prostaglandin E_2, which also stimulates nerve fiber activity. Some vulvar vestibulitis patients have been shown to have IgE antibodies to seminal fluid[17]. The presence of these antibodies was most common in the subset of patients who reported an association between symptom onset and an act of sexual intercourse with a male partner.

It is becoming increasingly clear that more than one immunological pathway may predispose women to develop VVS. The challenge for the future is to develop accurate and sensitive means to determine the underlying problem in individual women, and to identify specific and effective treatments for each.

DIAGNOSIS

History-taking is a critical first step in making the diagnosis of VVS. It requires patience to allow these women to state freely all of their symptoms. The first question should be 'What is your problem?' Their key message is that they are either unable to have intercourse or it is so painful that they rarely even try to have any type of sexual intimacy. These women often have other symptoms, urinary frequency or burning, or an excessive vaginal discharge. These symptoms should not shift the physician's attention from the patient's main problem, the pain associated with any attempts at vaginal penetration. When the diagnosis of VVS is confirmed with a physical examination, it is helpful to have the patients fill out a questionnaire to provide more details about their clinical history. *Table 19* is the template that the authors have devised. There are a few historical details that should be focused upon, for they are helpful in planning subsequent therapeutic strategy. If the painful intercourse began after there had been no prior problems, it should be established if this was related to a new sexual partner or a new method of contraception. Also, a detailed history of the medications the patient has used to treat her symptoms should be obtained, and the patient questioned whether or not the medications have helped, made no difference, or worsened this problem. The physician should also be aware of what drugs the patient is currently taking and if the patient has had any direct vulvar treatments that could scar the vulva, including laser or trichloracetic acid for 'warts' or an operation to remove the inflamed vulvar tissue. These prior treatment failures are the most difficult in the VVS population to achieve any easing of vulvar pain.

The suspicion based upon history that the patient has VVS can be confirmed by the physical examination. There is a number of characteristics of this patient population. There are very few blacks, and the majority of the Caucasian women have a porcelain white skin, which with minimal tactile stimulation results in marked dermographism. The inquinal nodes are nearly always palpable and tender. The pelvic examination begins by spreading the labia majora with thumb and forefinger and scanning the vulva. A colposcope is helpful in the evaluation of these women for two reasons: the magnification is an aid and the picture obtained yields a permanent record of the appearance of the vestibule at this first visit. The vulvar introitus can be very inflamed (**151, 152**) or minimally inflamed (**153**). The small, inflamed vestibular glands should then be touched, using a cotton-tip applicator. The glandular pore is no bigger than the tip of a ballpoint pen. The most tender glands are usually at 4:30 and 7:30 o'clock, and sometimes the tenderness is limited to one side (**154, 155**). Rarely, the most tender gland will be at 10 o'clock (**156**). In addition, many of those women will have a tender healed vertical scar at 6 o'clock (**157**). As a

Table 19 Questionnaire for women with vulvar vestibulitis

Name: ______________________ Age: __________ Race: ________________ Ethnic group: ____________

No. pregnancies: ______ No. children: ________ Episiotomy: __________ Age at onset of symptoms: ________

Length of symptoms (years): ________

Was any event associated with onset of symptoms?

Did symptoms begin with first act of sexual intercourse?

Do you have a history of:

- ☐ Inflammatory bowel disease
- ☐ Arthritis
- ☐ Diabetes
- ☐ Autoimmune disease
- ☐ Gynecologic surgery
- ☐ Cancer
- ☐ Estrogen replacement therapy
- ☐ Gynecologic infections
- ☐ Hormonal dysfunction
- ☐ Allergy

Is there a family history of:

- ☐ Vulvodynia
- ☐ Inflammatory bowel disease
- ☐ Arthritis
- ☐ Autoimmune disease
- ☐ Diabetes

Were you ever treated for:

- ☐ Vulvar warts
- ☐ Recurrent candidiasis

Did you ever have:

- ☐ Laser surgery
- ☐ 5-flurouracil treatment

Is vulvar pain:

- ☐ Constant
- ☐ A period of time every day
- ☐ 1–2 days per week
- ☐ Sometimes
- ☐ Seldom
- ☐ Only with sexual intercourse

Can you tolerate vaginal penetration:

- ☐ Always
- ☐ Sometimes
- ☐ Never

Do you have a vaginal discharge?

Do you have symptoms associated with urination?

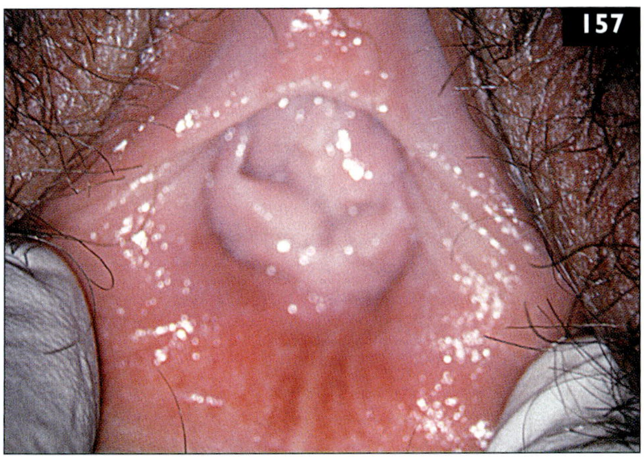

157 Paper cut scar at 6 o'clock in a patient with vulvar vestibulitis.

routine in these women, a sample of the vaginal fluid should be obtained with a plastic spatula to mix on a drop of saline and a drop of 10% potassium hydroxide (KOH) on glass slides. A whiff test of the KOH mixture for volatile amines (fish-like odor) should be performed before the cover slip is applied. A cotton swab is rubbed against the lateral wall of the vagina and applied to pH paper, and a standard vaginal culture can be obtained for *Candida* and aerobic bacteria isolation. The saline and KOH preparations should then be viewed under the microscope. The yield of an active vaginal infection in this population is very low. For example, in one study, *Candida* vaginitis was present in 11.4%, bacterial vaginosis in <1%, and no cases of *Trichomonas* vaginitis were present[3]. When a specific vaginal infection is recognized, it should be treated, for it can contribute to the persistent inflammation associated with this disease. However, successful treatment of the vaginitis alone seldom results in a cure. Finally, in the author's referral vulvovaginitis clinic, buccal smears are obtained to determine if this patient has one of the two gene polymorphisms that have been found to be associated with this syndrome[12,14]. One results in a low production of the blocker of the inflammatory cytokine, interleukin 1-β, that is, interleukin-1 receptor antagonist (IL1-ra). The second gene polymorphism is associated with a diminished production of mannose binding lectin (MBL)[12]. MBL is a substance produced by the body that is part of the first line of defense against microorganisms that can cause human disease.

TREATMENT

Clinical classifications have questionable long-term value in the care of these patients, for they might not be related to the different underlying etiologies of this multifaceted clinical syndrome. Attempts at classification of disease without full knowledge of the pathophysiology should not guide therapy.

Currently, the treatment of these patients begins with the post-physical examination interview. These women should be encouraged to be accompanied by their partner, for this is a relationship problem. Physicians should begin by stating, 'You have a vulvar syndrome that we call 'vulvar vestibulitis''. Both should be cautioned not to be afraid of the term, for it is only a descriptive phrase. Because of our English background, the entrance to the vagina is called the 'vestibule'; because there are tiny glands there, they are called 'vestibular' glands; and because they are inflamed in this syndrome, we call it 'vestibulitis'. It helps to sketch a diagram of the entrance of the vagina to give them a visual image of the vulvar problem. The physician should stress that this is a quality-of-life issue. Many of these women fear a yet-undetected serious infection, a sexually transmitted disease (STD) such as human immunodeficiency virus (HIV) infection. The author has never detected this in the clinic. The patients are also informed that in the majority of women, the cause of this problem is unknown. In some clinics, genetic testing is performed to determine specific underlying abnormalities that, if present, will help guide therapeutic strategies. Also this woman needs to be counseled that this is a chronic inflammatory process that will be treated empirically until the gene testing results are available. Physicians should measure success by any diminution in symptomatology. There is no magic therapeutic bullet that will achieve an instant cure, either medically or by operation. Finally, and most important, they must be given hope. Physicians should be able to help most of the patients seen with this condition.

The first step in planning therapy is a complete accounting of all medicines taken in the past and particularly all they are currently taking. For many women, less is better. This information gives the prescribing physician knowledge of what drugs they've previously used, makes the doctor aware of any adverse reaction to the drugs, or keeps them up-to-date on the current medications the patient is taking. The aim should be to avoid any medications that will flare vulvar symptoms or react unfavorably with any medications the patient is currently taking. In addition, if the patient is having a reaction to the male ejaculate or to the use of a latex condom with nonoxynol nine applied to the surface, alternate sexual approaches should be suggested.

One arm of an initial dual treatment strategy is to use a local medication to lessen vulvar inflammation. Even though topical adrenocortical steroids are effective anti-inflammatory agents, they are not the initial choice in most patients. Although they can provide temporary relief, there is the danger that patients with this chronic vulvar inflammation will use the medication over and over again and end up thinning the epithelium, making it more prone to persistent irritation and pain. Instead, treatment should begin with a commercial estradiol cream that the patient will apply with her fingertip to the vulvar vestibule each day at bedtime. History-taking is important, for if the patient has had a prior reaction to this medication, then this estradiol cream should not be used. To obtain local estradiol therapy, there are alternatives. Some pharmacists can compound an estradiol cream without propylene glycol. Alternatively, there is an estradiol vaginal tablet commercially available that the patient can insert in the vagina once or twice a week without a reaction.

The other arm of the initial therapeutic approach is to use an oral drug to moderate the assumed excessive vulvar nerve activity associated with the vulvar pain of this syndrome. There are at least four classes of drugs that have been used in this patient population, each of which has been effective for some patients. The underlying rationale for the use of these drugs has been their record of success in other pain syndromes such as fibromyalgia and post-herpetic neuralgia. There is a rhythm in the physician's prescription of these drugs, beginning with the agent that causes the fewest side-effects. A good initial drug is hydroxyzine, a member of the anti-histamine family, at a dosage level of 10 mg at bedtime. Patients should be counseled that they will probably sleep better with this drug and that their mouth may be dry in the morning when they awaken. A period of 3–4 weeks of observation will determine the initial impact. By then, the cultures and the gene polymorphism results will have been reported. If the patients do not require alternative therapy for an infection or for either of these gene polymorphisms, the original therapy can continue. If the patient notices improvement, not a cure, and is tolerating the medication, the dose of the hydroxyzine can be increased gradually. If improvement continues, the physician can increase the dose to 50 mg. Although improved, if they are still not able to have intercourse at this dosage, this is the time to use another drug.

The next group of drugs employed is one of the mood-elevators. It is a good strategy not to begin with these drugs, for many patients are nonplussed when, on the one hand, they are told they have vulvar disease and, on the other, they are being treated with a drug they think is aimed at their head, not their vulva. It should be emphasized these drugs are used to try to decrease the nerve-pain messages from the vulva to the brain, and the prescribed dose is much less than they would receive if they were being treated for depression. A wide variety of mood-elevators has been used, with some successes seen with all of the drugs. To date, there is not any one agent that provides better results than another. Amitriptyline, a tricyclic anti-depressant, has been widely used with an initial dose of 10 mg at bedtime. The dosage is increased incrementally at 3–4 week intervals if the patient has lessening of the pain and is having no problems taking the drug. Again, an alternate medication option should be chosen if the dosage has reached 50 mg a day and the patient has not reached the point where she can have intercourse. As patients improve, more comfortable vaginal penetration can be accelerated by the use of biofeedback techniques. For women who have constant burning, dysesthetic vulvodynia, amitriptyline might be more effective than hydroxyzine. For patients who are improving with amitriptyline, but who are too sedated with the drug, newer tricyclic anti-depressants such as desipranine and nortriptyline can be tried. Some physicians have tried another group of anti-depressants, those that inhibit the central nervous system neuronal uptake of serotonin, including sertaline and paroxetine.

Another drug used is the muscle relaxant, cyclobenzaprine. The patients should be informed they are not given this drug to relax their pelvic floor muscles, but instead to modulate the excessive nerve signaling from the vulva to the brain. This drug can markedly sedate some women, so that they remain groggy from the bedtime dose when they awaken in the morning to go to work. To obviate this, the patients should begin with the lowest dose, 5 mg at bedtime. If they tolerate this and show improvement, the dosage can be increased to 10 mg. There are concerns about the long-term use of the drug and infrequent liver toxicity has been reported. If the treatment regimen is extended beyond 1–2 months, it is prudent to check liver function tests. Again, there will be patients who do not respond to this drug.

Another drug that will be used empirically is the anti-epileptic drug, gabapentin. Again, the rationale is that this agent will lessen the impact of the excessive number of nerve signals sent from the vulva to the brain. The starting dose is 100 mg three times a day. To obtain symptom relief, the dosage is gradually increased. Some women require 1500–1800 mg per day for a response.

A number of local vulvar interventions have been used in these women with success, such as local injection of interferon alpha 2 beta, 1,000,000 units given three times a week for a total of 12 doses. The original target population was those women with vulvar inflammation noted histologically, with koilocytic cells and a DNA probe positive for a high-risk HPV type. In this group of women, the clinical response rate was high (77%)[3]. In a subsequent study at Cornell, using a positive polymerase chain reaction (PCR) for HPV from a Dacron swab rubbed against the vestibule as the indication for treatment, the interferon injection resulted in clearance of the virus in 95% of the patients, but a clinical response was achieved in only 40% of these women (MR Geneç, personal communication). Another study from Baltimore using interferon injections in all patients with VVS had a similar 40% response rate. How do we explain these results? There is evidence that this local injection of interferon stimulates the body to increase the local production of the inflammatory cytokine blocker, IL1-ra. However, it is a rarely used treatment because of the discomfort with multiple injections. The injections are given subcutaneously with a 26-gauge needle at alternating sites, i.e. 6 o'clock, 7 o'clock, 5 o'clock, and so on. These patients should be warned that each injection hurts and that they will have a 'flu'-like reaction to the first injection and will probably require acetominophen one or two times that night. Another new treatment is the placement of a cotton pledgelet soaked with lidocaine gel on the vestibule and kept in place for several hours. The rationale for this approach is a twofold patient response. It causes local numbing and can relieve the vestibular pain on that basis. It also stimulates the body to increase the production of IL1-ra. Some women have a local reaction to this gel, with an increase, not a diminution, of symptoms. Obviously, they have to discontinue this form of therapy.

Over the past two decades, there has been an emphasis in some quarters on the role of excess oxalate in urine as a source of the vulvar inflammation. The therapeutic approach has been the use of a very restrictive low oxalate diet, plus the daily ingestion of large numbers of calcium citrate tablets in the hope that the citrate will neutralize the oxalates. The author no longer screens for oxalates in the urine in the clinic, nor suggests the diet as the success rate was so low (14.3%)[3], and most women were miserable on the diet. Despite this, there is an occasional patient who has felt better on the diet and if it helps them, they can continue to follow this regimen.

For the patients positive for the gene polymorphism associated with a lower production of IL1-ra, the standard oral therapies are discarded and alternative approaches are tried. A cox-2 inhibitor, celecoxib, 100 mg twice a day is used initially, if the patient will agree due to the recent concern about an increased risk of heart disease. Cox-2 inhibitors provide no increase in IL1-ra production, but they do block the anti-inflammatory actions of the potent inflammatory cytokine, interleukin 1-β. If the patients show no improvement with this, they can try the health food product SUMA®, made from a Brazilian root, which induces production of large amounts of IL1-ra. The bottle directions are one 500 mg capsule three times a day, but most women cannot tolerate this dosage initially, and begin with one capsule a day after lunch. If they tolerate this, they can increase gradually to two a day and then to three a day after meals. Also, an injectable IL1-ra product is available that is approved for the treatment of rheumatoid arthritis (Kineret™). It is very expensive and not approved for the treatment of VVS, but theoretically it might help these women. This possibility awaits future study. Patients with this gene polymorphism should be advised that they are at increased risk to have arthritis, inflammatory bowel disease, and inflammatory eye disease as they get older. Pregnant women with this gene polymorphism, whose babies have the same polymorphism, are at risk for premature labor and delivery[18]. Amniocentesis with testing for this gene polymorphism may be indicated. Women whose fetuses have this gene polymorphism are candidates for low-dose acetylsalicylic acid and close observation during pregnancy.

The other gene polymorphism that is frequently found in women with VVS is the variant allele associated with a diminished production of MBL[12]. Patients with this polymorphism also have an increased rate of recurrent *Candida* vulvovaginitis[19]. Interestingly, they have a lower rate of tuberculosis, because the tubercle bacillus uses MBL to gain entrance into mammalian host cells. Knowledge of this patient's immune deficiency should indicate aggressive treatment of any infection in these patients. MBL has been isolated and patented by a company in Denmark, so that there may be therapeutic options available in the future.

Operative intervention for patients with VVS should be limited to a small cadre of patients who have failed all medical treatment. This requires physician discipline, because VVS patients are desperate and are anxious for a quick fix to their problem. Anyone who has dealt with patients who are operative failures becomes more selective in picking this therapeutic option. The best candidates are those with no gross vestibular inflammation (**153**) and whose symptoms are limited to those situations where vaginal penetration is attempted. In addition, a recent study from the Netherlands showed the best results after operations in women who were 30 years or younger at the time of the procedure[5]. In some cases, biopsy of the proposed operative site, sent to dermatopathology can yield an alternative dermatologic diagnosis that would negate an operative approach. Success requires more than operative skill. The operation removes the tender vestibular glands and the vulvar vestibular tissue, with the initial incision ranging from 2–10 o'clock, just superficial to the hymenal ring. The posterior vaginal tissue is mobilized and forms a new healthy tissue graft over the operative site. Post-operatively, these patients require a type of biofeedback exercise to increase the success rate of the operation. This is understandable. These women have had a pattern of months or years of painful intercourse, and naturally will 'flinch', i.e. contract the pelvic floor muscles when intercourse is attempted. They should use graduated dilators on their own with a larger size used after comfortable use of a smaller size. After they can tolerate the largest dilator, they can attempt intercourse and the success rate in these circumstances is around 75%[3], although the recent Netherlands study reported post-operative success in 93% of the patients[5].

This is the current state of the therapeutic armamentarium for the physician caring for the patient with VVS. As more information is obtained about the multiple etiologies of this condition, therapy will be directed and not empirical as it is at present.

Chapter 15

Dermatologic Disorders Causing Vulvar Disease

BACKGROUND

Women with vaginal and vulvar dermatologic disease represent difficult diagnostic and therapeutic challenges for physicians. These are socially disrupting medical problems that markedly diminish the quality of life for these vulvovaginal sufferers. Most have constant symptoms and have no semblance of the lifestyle they considered normal before being struck by these ailments. Uncomfortable, despairing patients with these chronic difficulties are a trial to themselves, to their families, and to the physician trying to care for them. There are no quick-and-easy solutions to their problems, no magic pill or salve that will immediately make their symptoms disappear.

These women present with complex clinical entities with the underlying dermatologic pathology often compounded by a secondary infection with either *Candida* or bacteria. Physicians, dealing with these patients, need to keep in mind that for these women, the prevention of present and future infection depends upon an intact epithelial barrier that consists of a few microns of keratin on the cornified squamous epithelium of the vulva or the thin coating of mucus on the sensitive membranes of the introitus and vagina. When these protective barriers become disrupted and remain so, an infection can occur. This complicated pathophysiology can be a source of frustration to the clinician. Successful detection and treatment of infection in these women with underlying dermatopathology will not restore the integrity of these compromised epithelial tissues, and the symptoms that have been diminished with treatment return rapidly and in full force.

Recognizing and treating the underlying skin pathology is the key to success. This is not easy. It often means repeated clinical observations of these lesions after attempts at treatment, keeping in mind that the clinical presentations of dermatologic disorders are often different on the vulva when compared to other body sites. The ultimate diagnostic test, the biopsy, requires physician time and patience, qualities often compromised by the demands of a busy office practice. In addition, the tissue obtained by biopsy often needs to be evaluated by a competent dermatopathologist, and these may not be readily available to all practitioners. Once the diagnosis is made, there are other problems. Understanding of disease mechanisms in these patients is still incomplete. In most cases, there will be no cure. Instead the focus will be on the use of the minimal amount of medication that will keep the patient free of symptoms without drug toxicity. Despite all of these concerns, there is a bright side, this is not an unending tale of medical toil and frustration! The physician who diagnoses and gives these women relief will have a thankful lifetime patient advocate. In that woman's household, you will be viewed as a miracle worker.

A clinical classification of these dermatologic disorders is the current basis for understanding and treatment of these women. This should be a familiar intellectual exercise for physicians. Because of the justifiable emphasis upon biologic science in medical training, physicians have become well versed in the discipline of classification. It removes the chaos of the multifaceted presentations of vulvovaginal dermatologic disease and replaces it with a recognizable, ordered scheme of distinctive individual clinical entities. This focus is needed, because the knowledge of the underlying pathophysiology is incomplete, and it will keep the physician's focus on the underlying skin pathology in these patients.

There are two broad classes of immune responses that influence the varied vulvovaginal epithelial pathology that can be encountered. The most common immune problem associated with vulvar pathology is the induction of a Th2 immune response. Stimulation of the Th2 subset of T helper lymphocytes results in an inhibition of cell-mediated immunity, manifested by a compromised epithelial barrier of atopic skin. With the flaking of the epithelium, these women are at great risk for developing a secondary *Candida* infection. The less common but more serious situation is the patients with an exaggerated pro-inflammatory Th1-directed immune response. Excessive and/or prolonged inflammation can result in epithelial erosion, so severe that it does not respond to local treatment, and sometimes requires systemic therapy for relief. All of these considerations must be part of the evaluation and care of these women. If and when an accurate diagnosis has been achieved, appropriate therapy can be prescribed.

IMMUNOLOGY

Many dermatological conditions can have vulvovaginal manifestations. In some cases, genital lesions may be the first indication of an underlying dermatological disorder that will eventually involve other body surfaces. Therefore, it is important for clinicians dealing with female genital tract disorders to recognize dermatologic pathology, to be able to differentiate it from infectious conditions, and to either initiate appropriate treatment or refer the patient to someone with more expertise in this area.

The etiology of dermatological conditions that affect the female genital tract remains incompletely understood. The prevailing evidence suggests an autoimmune pathology involving humoral and/or cell-mediated responses to components of the skin. The possible involvement of bacteria or viruses in initiating the original immune response leading to development of autoimmunity has also been postulated and associations with specific microorganisms have been inconsistently observed. However, no specific microorganisms have been definitively involved in the pathogenesis of a particular dermatological condition.

Lichen sclerosus, a chronic inflammatory skin disease predominately affecting the genital area, is believed to result from the interplay between environmetal and immune factors in genetically susceptible individuals. An association between lichen sclerosus and HLA DQ7 has been identified. The production of autoantibodies reactive with extracellular matrix protein 1 has been described. It has been suggested that an increase in oxidative stress, perhaps due to a decrease in anti-oxidant defense mechanisms in patients with lichen sclerosus, leads to the generation of unique antigenic determinants that become targets for an autoimmune response[1].

Unlike lichen sclerosus, vulvovaginal involvement is uncommon for the lesions caused by lichen planus. Lichen planus is a chronic inflammatory disease primarily confined to the oral mucosa. It appears to be due to the activation of CD8-positive cytotoxic T lymphocytes by a component of basal keratinocytes. The specific activating antigen on keratinocytes remains undetermined, but its autoantigenic nature leads to the classification of lichen planus as a probable autoimmune disease. Similar to the situation with aphthous ulcers (see below), heat shock protein expression has been observed in keratinocytes from lichen planus lesions. This suggests that heat shock protein-mediated autoimmunity might be involved in the pathogenesis of this disease. Alternatively, heat shock protein expression may merely be a consequence of the nonphysiological stress placed on these cells. In any event, the T lymphocyte activation triggers mast cell migration and degranulation in the lesions. This results in damage to the epithelial basement membrane, enhanced T cell migration, and further keratinocyte cell death[2].

Pemphigus vulgaris and pemphigus foliaceus are two pemphigoid disorders in which specific skin autoantigens have been identified. Autoantibodies from patients with these disorders specifically recognize two hemidesmosomal proteins, BP180 and BP230[3,4]. Antibody recognition of these proteins triggers neutrophil recruitment, activation of the complement cascade, and the release of proteases that initiate pathological changes in the epidermis. IgG and complement deposition in the basement membrane zone along with sub-epidermal blister formation are characteristic of these diseases. A subset of CD4-positive T lymphocytes, Th2 cells, may also recognize BP180 antigenic determinants and promote autoantibody production.

Recurrent aphthous ulcers is predominantly an oral ulcerative disease but painful single or multiple ulcers of the vulva can also occur. The pathogenesis of this painful disease has not been completely characterized, but an autoimmune response to a skin component appears to be involved. An intriguing mechanism, still to be proven, involves a primary infectious viral or bacterial trigger which results in the elicitation of antibodies and cell-mediated immunity to the highly conserved microbial 60 kD heat shock protein (hsp60). Since there is a human hsp60 with a 50% amino acid homology to the microbial hsp60, an autoimmune response to self-hsp60 can subsequently develop in genetically susceptible individuals. The human hsp60 is an inducible protein whose synthesis is greatly accelerated under nonphysiological conditions such as inflammation or elevated temperature. Thus, aphthous ulcer formation may be the result of a strong pro-inflammatory autoimmune response to self-hsp60[5]. The involvement of polymorphonuclear leukocytes as well as the Th1 subset of T lymphocytes, which induce production of pro-inflammatory cytokines such as tumor necrosis factor-α, interleukin-1β, and interferon-γ, in the induction of epithelial cell destruction and ulcer formation has also been documented[5,6]. A genetic association with HLA-B12 has also been demonstrated. A possible role for sex hormones in modulating the immune response in women with aphthous ulcers has been noted. In some affected women, ulcer formation is cyclical and is associated with menstruation or the luteal phase of the menstrual cycle. Most individuals with aphthous ulcers are otherwise healthy with no other pathological manifestations.

Aphthous ulcers are also a feature of Behçet's disease, a recurrent immuno-inflammatory small vessel vasculitis, mainly affecting young adults. It is characterized by endothelial cell dysfunction and can affect most areas of the body. The formation of genital aphthous ulcers is very common. The disease is rare in the Americas and Europe and is most common in Turkey, the Middle East, and the Far East. This geographic distribution strongly suggests a genetic component and carriage of HLA-B51 has been associated with development of Behçet's disease. The prevailing hypothesis is that when an individual with a genetic susceptibility to develop Behçet's disease is exposed to a viral (herpes simplex virus, HSV) or bacterial (*Streptococcus*) infection, an autoimmune response is triggered that results in the appearance of clinical symptoms. Interestingly, the concentration of a minor subset of T lymphocytes, gamma delta T cells, is increased in the circulation of individuals with either recurrent aphthous ulcers or Behçet's disease. Gamma delta T cells recognize, proliferate, and produce pro-inflammatory mediators in response to hsp60, lending support to the suggestion that hsp60 might be a target antigen in these conditions. Since pregnancy favors the predominance of a humoral immune response it was of interest to determine the effect of pregnancy on Behçet's disease manifestations[7]. No consistent response was observed. Symptoms improved in some women, became worse in others, and remained the same in a third group of patients.

DIAGNOSIS

Accurate diagnosis of the wide variety of skin disorders that can be seen in the vagina and on the vulva is a complex task for every physician. These women can present with more than one clinical problem, the underlying skin abnormality and a secondary infection of the affected area. Increasing the diagnostic difficulty further is the fact that some common dermatologic problems have a different gross appearance on the vulva than on other cutaneous sites on the body. Hints on the etiology of these skin disorders can come from examination of all other skin and mucous membrane surfaces. This is a clinical situation in which the physician's initial examination should not be limited to the vulva and vagina.

Flaking skin disorders

Atopic dermatitis (lichen simplex chronicus) is the most common of these skin afflictions. These patients are constantly uncomfortable and usually present with the chief complaint of vulvar itching. On questioning, most of these women have an allergic history, including seasonal allergies or skin allergies. Common triggers for the development of the disease or exacerbation of the symptoms include psychological stress and local environmental factors such as heat, sweating, or excessive dryness[8]. Patients under prior care have often been empirically treated for *Candida* with no established diagnosis, because the doctor has equated itching with a *Candida* infection. As might be expected, the result is minimum or no relief of symptoms. On examination, these women have an irritated vulva with demarcated thickened lesions as a result of frequent rubbing or scratching (**158**). Patients are often embarrassed by the reality that they might be scratching this private body area and often will deny it. They can be advised that their scratching can be involuntary while they sleep at night in the privacy of their bed. If there is a surface exudate and the thickened vulvar skin is inflamed, a scraping can be done and placed in a drop of 10% potassium hydroxide (KOH) to be examined under the microscope to see if hyphae are present. This altered surface tissue is prone to infection with the resulting inflammation exacerbating the itch–scratch cycle. If there are any questions about other possible etiologies on gross inspection of the lesions, a biopsy should be performed. Magnification of the lesions with a colposcope is an aid in evaluation, and an attached camera yields a visual record of the lesions before treatment. A portion of the biopsied tissue should be sent to a dermatopathologist. This helps establish the diagnosis of atopic dermatitis and on occasion other unexpected pathologies will be discovered.

Psoriasis, a common skin disorder, can also involve the vulva. This is a disease less commonly found in African-Americans than in the remainder of the United States' population and one in which the symptoms usually worsen in the winter and improve in the summer[9]. Some women complain of itching and all are aware that the vulvar skin does not look or feel normal. The first hints to the physician that this is a possibility are the patient's past history of psoriasis or the finding of psoriatic plaques on other areas of the body while doing the general physical examination, which is a 'must' in these patients. On the vulva, the lesions usually do not have the prominent plaques that are seen elsewhere on the body (**159**). This is a clinical situation in which a vulvar biopsy with the tissue sent to a dermatologist can be invaluable, eliminating all confusion about the diagnosis, setting the stage for appropriate therapy.

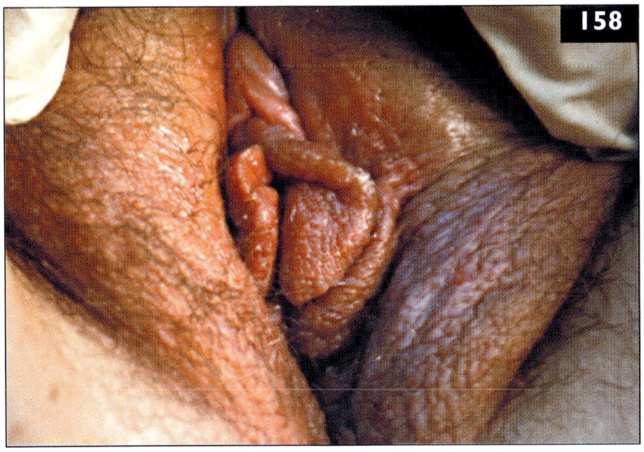

158 Lichen simplex chronicus of 6 years' duration. History was positive for asthma, hay fever, and eczema. Visible skin changes suggest chronic scratching, mainly in the left vulvar area. The condition responded to twice daily application of moderate strength steroid treatment. (Courtesy of Dr. Paul Sommers.)

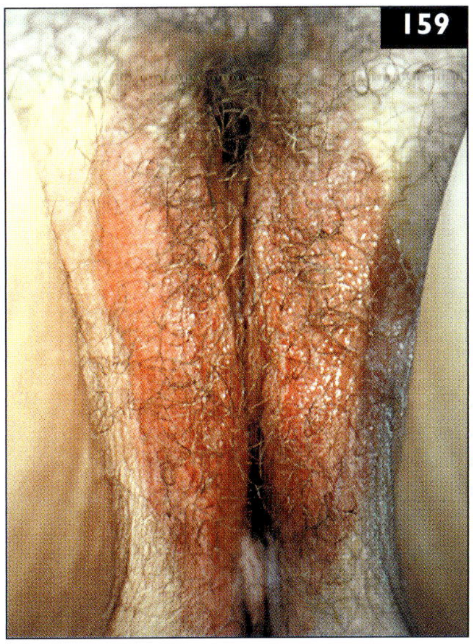

159 Asymptomatic vulvar psoriasis. The patient also had psoriasis involvement of the elbows. (Courtesy of Dr. Paul Sommers.)

Lichen sclerosis is a condition that has a bimodal peak in incidence from prepubertal children to menopausal women[10]. For the gynecologist, obviously this is a condition usually seen in women over the age of 50 years. Most women complain of itching, but a more serious concern is pain if there are erosions or fissures, and in these situations, dysuria, dyspareunia, or vulvar burning is common[11]. In contrast, some patients are asymptomatic[12]. Lichen sclerosis of the vulva has a variety of clinical presentations. Early on, the demarcated skin has an inflammatory appearance, but the lack of tissue flexibility is already present (**160**). Some symptomatic patients will have the vulva covered with a white exudate (**161**). On scraping these lesions, hyphae were seen in the microscopic examination of a KOH preparation (**162**), and the culture of this exudate was positive for *Candida albicans*. This patient was treated with four doses of 150 mg fluconazole every 4 days and when she returned for follow-up examination, she was free of infection (**163**). The underlying skin changes of early lichen sclerosis are still present. These early changes of lichen sclerosis can be reversed with the use of a local steroid. Figure **164** shows early pre-treatment vulvar lichen sclerosis. Figure **165** shows the same patient 4 weeks after twice daily treatment with a local ultrapotent steroid. The symptoms of dysuria and itching had disappeared. Over time, the untreated vulvar skin can become grossly white with a wrinkled appearance (**166**). There can be similar lesions in other body areas, but often the skin changes are limited to the vulva. The vagina is not involved with this cutaneous pathology. Without any local care, the white crinkled appearance becomes more prominent (**167**). This vulvar skin is less malleable and is prone to fissure formation (**168**). This is a clinical situation in which a biopsy is most helpful as it confirms the diagnosis, which is important in these women with a chronic skin problem. It is especially important in a woman who has failed to respond to prior treatment. Again, access to a dermatopathologist is very helpful in making the appropriate diagnosis.

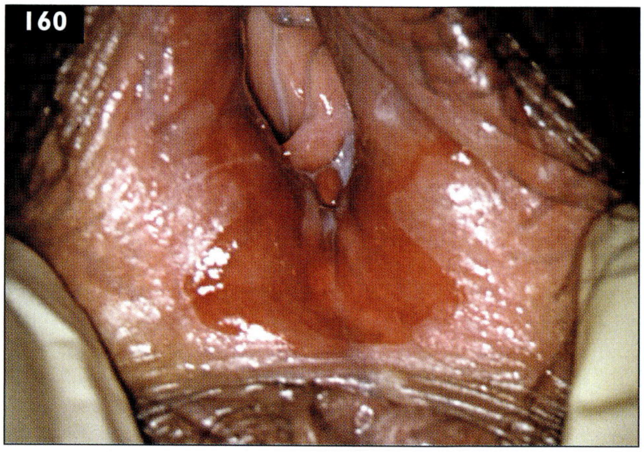

160 Patient with lichen sclerosis confirmed by biopsy, seen early in the course of the disease.

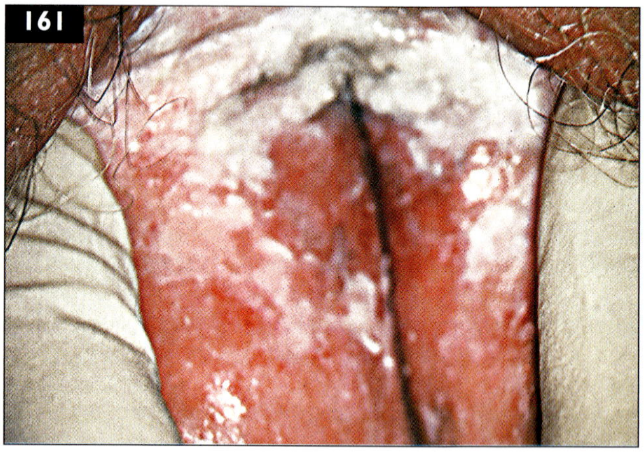

161 Patient with lichen sclerosis covered by a white exudate.

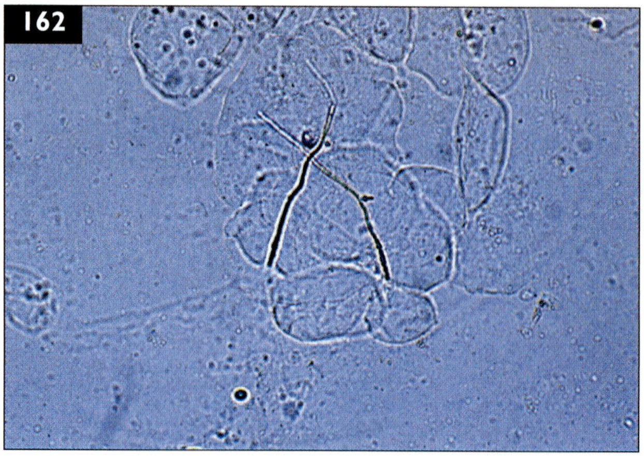

162 Scraping of vulvar lesion placed in 10% potassium hydroxide solution. Under the microscope, hyphae are seen. Culture grew *Candida albicans*.

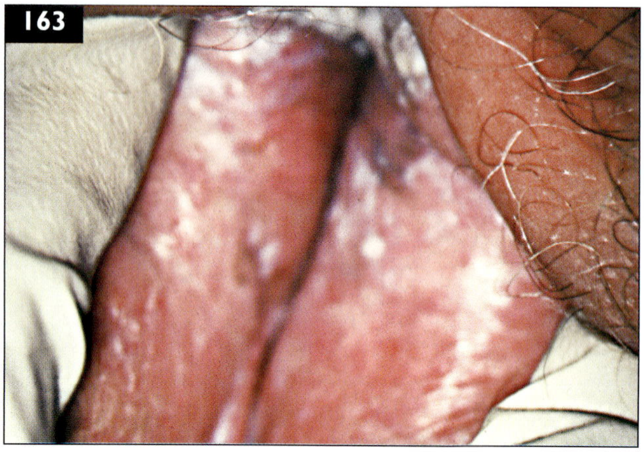

163 Same patient as in **162** after fluconazole treatment. No hyphae were seen on microscopic examination, and culture had no yeast. Underlying early changes of lichen sclerosis were identified.

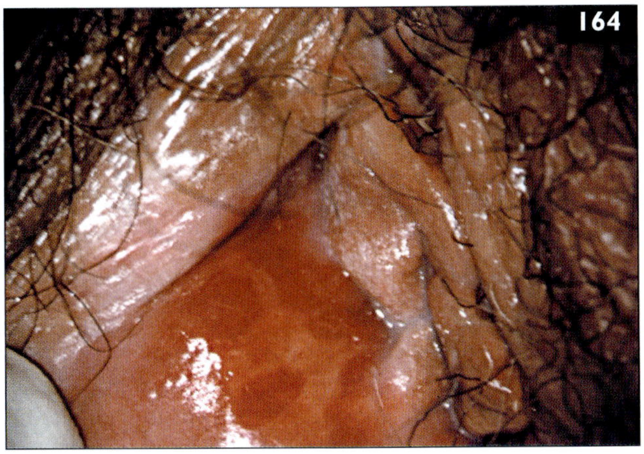

164 Pre-treatment stage of early lichen sclerosis with dysuria and vulvar itching.

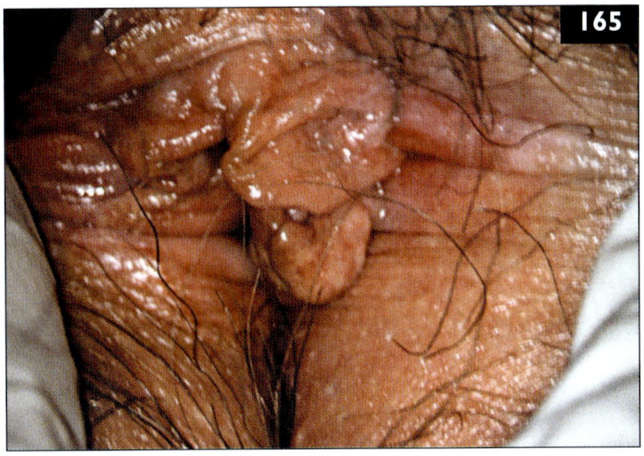

165 Post-ultrapotent steroid treatment of the patient in **164** taken at lower magnification. Symptoms are now absent.

166 Post-menopausal patient with lichen sclerosis. Note agglutination of labia minora in the midline. Generally the patient has atrophic parchment-like skin, but there are some areas of white thickened skin. These changes extend into the peri-rectal area. (Courtesy of Dr. Paul Sommers.)

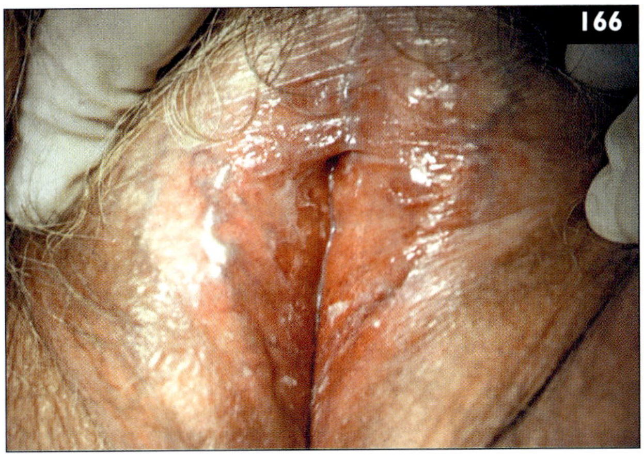

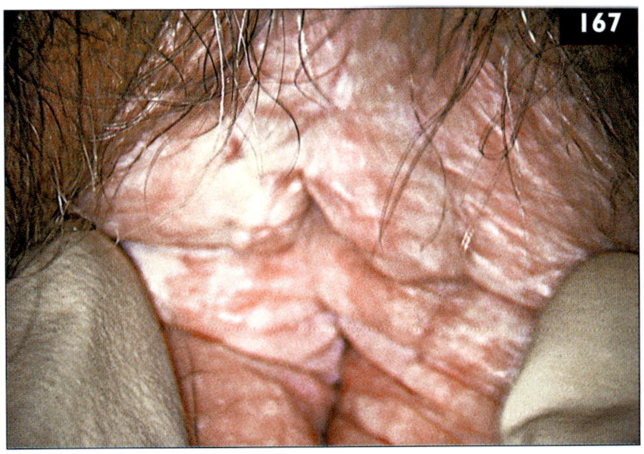

167 More advanced lichen sclerosis with grossly white crinkled skin.

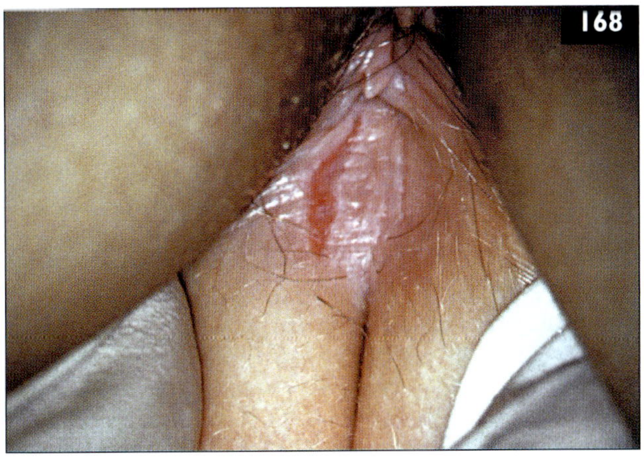

168 Vulvar fissure in a portion of the altered epithelium of lichen sclerosis.

Inflammatory and erosive skin disorders

The inflammatory skin disorder lichen planus has different clinical presentations, depending upon the clinical site. On keratinized skin, it presents as pruritic papules. On mucous membranes, it progresses from white plaques to erosive and ulcerative disease of the vulva. These ulcerations are painful, ending any attempts at intercourse because of pain and sometimes bleeding. These skin changes can involve other membranes, including the vagina and the oral mucosa. Again, a general physical examination is necessary to pick out these other lesion sites. If untreated, these lesions can result in labial scarring and atrophy with extreme narrowing of the introitus (**169**). This is a clinical situation in which the biopsy sent to a dermatopathologist can be invaluable. If there is an erosion, the biopsy should be obtained from the edge. In some cases, when the vulvar biopsy does not provide an answer, a biopsy of gingival lesions will be definitive.

Biopsy is also important, for it will detect a rare disease of genital skin, plasma cell mucositis or Zoon's vulvitis. Patients can present with vulvar pain, itching, a stinging sensation, and labial ulcers[13]. Grossly, it may not be distinguishable from lichen planus, psoriasis, or squamous cell carcinoma (**170**). In these cases, a biopsy is needed to determine the diagnosis and should be taken from the edge of an ulcer if present. The dermatopathologist is invaluable in these cases to evaluate the massive plasma cell infiltrate.

Patients with pemphigus initially relate periods of vulvar itching that precede the presentation of a vulvar blister[14]. Subsequently, these affected areas develop into thickened hyperkeratotic skin. When blisters are present, traction on the skin will allow the blister to extend (Nikolsky's sign). This reflects the underlying pathology of the loss of adhesion of the epidermal cells. This diagnosis is confirmed by biopsy with routine microscopy and direct immunofluorescence. Again, a general examination is important. Very often, these women will have oral mucosal lesions as well.

An uncommon but clinically confusing patient is the one presenting with aphthous ulcers. These necrotizing ulcers are painful and recurrent, mimicking the clinical presentation of a woman with genital herpes (**171**). Many of these women will have oral lesions as well. These ulcerations can be differentiated from herpes with the failure to isolate the virus on repeated attempts to culture the recurrent lesions. The absence of HSV-1 and -2 antibodies in blood testing is a confirmatory finding, but some patients may have antibodies from a prior exposure to herpes not related to these lesions. When ulceration recurs in a patient with these negative laboratory findings, a biopsy of the edge of the ulcer should be obtained and sent to a dermatopathologist, who can perform immunohistopathology on the specimen.

The diagnosis of Behçet's disease is a difficult task for gynecologists. For most practitioners in northern Europe and the United States, it will be a rare presentation. Since it is an endemic disease in the native populations of the Mediterranean areas, the Middle East, and Far East, it can be encountered in those patient populations. Also, this disease is not limited to the genital tract. It is a multisystematic, chronic, relapsing inflammatory disease classified among the vasculitides[15]. There are no distinctive laboratory tests that confirm the diagnosis. Instead, it is based upon clinical findings and criteria have been established[16] (*Table 20*). This diagnosis should be considered in a patient whose family

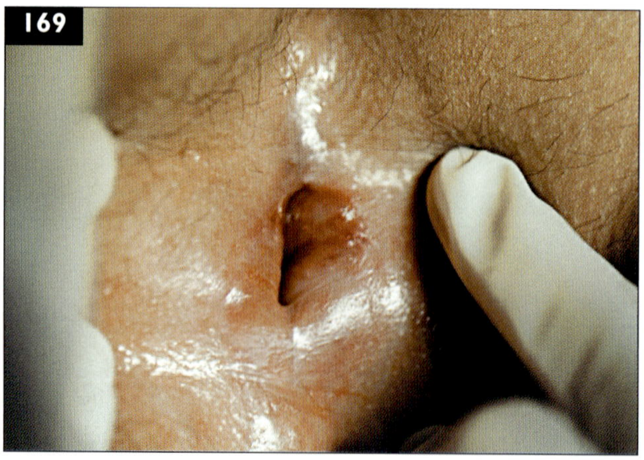

169 Erosive lichen planus of long duration resulting in severe vaginal stenosis with loss of normal external genital anatomy and pubic hair. The patient also had a painful chronic buccal erosion with a white lacy margin and a line of erythema at the base of her teeth. Three months of full dose azathioprine (Imuran) restored normal anatomy and pubic hair with significant varicosities on the perineum as the only residual. Pathology gradually recurred when Imuran was stopped. (Courtesy of Dr. Paul Sommers.)

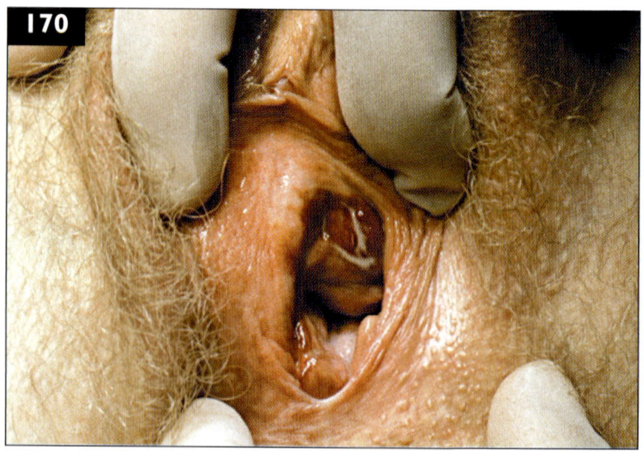

170 Vestibulitis due to Zoon's disorder. There was acute onset and then many months of persistent entry dyspareunea in a peri-menopausal patient. Patches of erythema circumferentially in the area of the vestibule were painful to contact with a swab. Associated purulent vaginal discharge, characterized by numerous white blood cells and parabasal cells, has accumulated in the urethal meatus. The patient responded slowly to medium strength topical steroid ointment. Excision of one patch for pathology healed with resolution of pain at that site. (Courtesy of Dr. Paul Sommers.)

roots are from the areas noted. In the genital area, recurrent ulcers are noted with subsequent scarring. These women will have no laboratory evidence of genital herpes, and the vulvar biopsies show no evidence of any other vulvar disease. The pathergy test, cited in *Table 20*, evaluates cutaneous hypersensitivity. A positive test consists of a sterile pustule that develops in 24–48 hours at the site of a needle-prick to the skin[16]. In addition to the importance of a general physical examination of the patient, a team evaluation with an internist and an ophthalmologist is very helpful.

TREATMENT

The treatment of these women requires physician inquisitiveness and patience. There can be multiple layers of disease which are detected only by physician contemplation and appropriate testing, particularly with the use of biopsy. Patience is needed to determine the diagnosis and for treatment. For most of these women, the underlying skin pathology cannot be cured, but it can be improved with proper care.

The treatment of atopic dermatitis (lichen simplex chronicus) requires a discipline that runs counter to most gynecologists' standard medical practice. Unlike infectious disease emphasis upon the bug and the drug, the diagnostic process is complex, with more than one factor involved, and the course of treatment is usually prolonged. The first focus in the care of these women is to remove the irritant triggers that contribute to the recurring cycle of inflammation itching, scratching, and then more itching. This requires careful attention to the history and a tight focus upon the physical findings at the time of examination. Infection can be an irritant and this altered skin surface is a favorable growth site for the growth of organisms. Vulvovaginal candidiasis is a frequently encountered problem and, when detected, is best treated by the oral azole fluconazole. This avoids any possible sensitive skin reaction to an azole-containing cream applied locally, which will worsen the patient's symptoms. More than one dose of oral fluconazole is usually necessary and these should be given no more frequently than at 4-day intervals. Attention to the patients' personal genital hygiene care is important. Most women with persistent chronic itching feel it due to a lack of personal cleanliness and will compensate by a sometimes compulsive ritual of repeated washing. Soap is an irritant and usually is inadequately removed with a residual remaining on the affected skin despite frequent rinsing with water. Other local irritants need to be eliminated, such as over-the-counter creams, marketed as panaceas for irritated skin.

Dr. Lynch has identified three additional steps to improve the health of this altered vulvar skin[8]. First, improve barrier layer function with soaks, either plain water or Burrough's solution. He advises the use of hand creams rather than lotions, gels, or lubricants, which all contain substances that can irritate the skin. Second, reduce local inflammation by the use of mid-potency (triamcinolone 0.1%) or high-potency (clobetasol propionate 0.05%) steroids. Third, break the itch–scratch cycle by the use of hydroxyzine, or a tricyclic. In the Cornell vaginitis clinic, the tricyclic of choice is amitriptyline 10–25 mg at bedtime. Despite an apparent cure, recurrences are common, particularly when the patient is exposed to such triggers as psychological stress, heat, sweating, or the excessive dryness

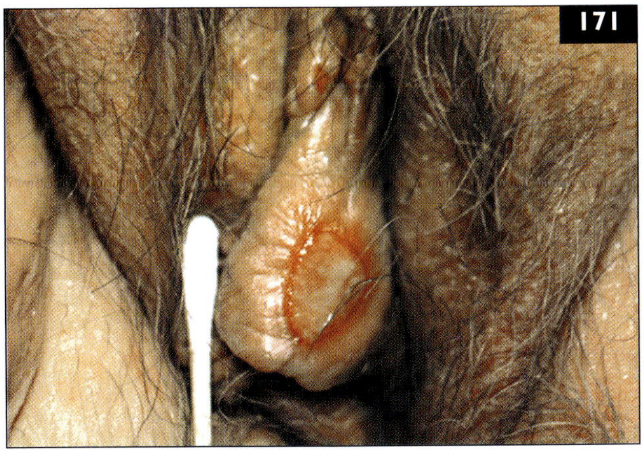

171 Painful labial aphthous ulcer with significant associated labial edema. This may be distinguished from vulvar pemphigoid and Behçet's disease by biopsy, with a segment of skin tissue sent for immune staining. Ophthalmologic evaluation may reveal posterior chamber inflammation in cases of Behçet's disease.

Table 20 Diagnosis of Behçet's disease: International Study Group Guidelines

Required:

- Recurrent oral ulceration: minor aphthous, major apthous, or herpetiform ulceration observed by physician or patient, which recurred at least three times in one 12-month period

Plus two of the following:

- Recurrent genital ulceration: aphthous ulceration or scarring, observed by physician or patient
- Eye lesions: anterior uveitis, posterior uveitis, or cells in the vitrous on slit lamp examination; or retinal vasculitis observed by ophthamologist
- Skin lesions: erythema nodosum observed by physician or patient, pseudofolliculitis, or papulopustular lesions; or acneiform nodules observed by physician in post-adolescent patients not on corticosteroid treatment
- Positive pathergy test: read by physician at 24–48 hours

(Findings applicable only in the absence of other clinical explanations)

encountered in the winter months of colder climates, when it is cold and dry outside and warm and dry in centrally heated buildings. There have been attempts to use alternative agents to steroids in the care of these women. Tacrolimus ointment (0.1%), a pro-inflammatory cytokine inhibitor, showed equivalent results when compared to 0.1% hydrocortisone butyrate[17]. An alternative to hydroxyzine or tricyclics is the use of a selective serotonin uptake inhibitor (SSRI) such as celexa[8].

There are new options in the treatment of genital psoriasis. This is important, for the genital skin is sensitive and often cannot tolerate the long-term treatments of psoriasis that have been employed for this skin disorder in other areas of the body. Topical coal tar, retinoids, and ultraviolet light have little or no place in the treatment of genital psoriasis, because of this. Initial therapy with a potent topical steroid such as clobetasol propionate is helpful, and the long-term intermittent use of a steroid combined with vitamin D analogue calciprotriene is often effective[9]. Since this is a chronic skin disease that affects other areas of the body, treatment in conjunction with a dermatologist is the rule rather than the exception. New systemic agents that target key mechanisms in the pathogenesis of psoriasis have been approved by the Food and Drug Administration (FDA) in the United States. These include alefacept, which induces apoptosis in circulating memory T cells; efalizumab, which interrupts the cutaneous recruitment of pathogenic leukocytes; and infliximab, which blocks TNF-α. Other medications under study should materially modify the treatment of patients with psoriasis in the future.

Lichen sclerosis treatment can be a source of confusion for practitioners, because of recent change in terminology and treatment. Older terms used to describe this skin condition including leukoplakia, kraurosis vulvae, and lichen sclerosis et atrophicus are no longer in vogue. The treatment has also changed. For older practitioners, the old dependence upon a testosterone-based cream made up in the pharmacy has been supplanted by more effective regimens. An excellent study demonstrated that superior results were obtained with the ultrapotent topical corticosteroid ointment, clobetasol propionate[18]. The regimen currently recommended for new cases is clobetasol ointment (0.05%) initially once a night for 4 weeks, then on alternate nights for 4 weeks, and in the third month twice weekly[11]. If the treatment is successful, there will be resolution of the hyperkeratosis ecchymoses, fissuring, and erosions, but the atrophy and color changes will remain. Since this is a chronic condition, the clobetasol propionate is used when needed. Women should also be advised to avoid soap in this area. There can be problems in individual patients. In the United States, the clobetasol propionate cream and ointment both contain propylene glycol and some women will react to this. A compounding pharmacy can make up a propylene glycol-free preparation or a potent steroid ointment free of propylene glycol can be substituted. These women need to be closely evaluated over time with biopsies taken of any suspicious areas. Squamous cell carcinoma of the vulva has been reported in this patient population.

Patients with lichen planus are a therapeutic trial for most gynecologists. They have a chronic painful ulcerative disease that with scarring can markedly diminish the size of the entrance of the vagina and the vagina itself (**169**). They need to be aware that to date, there is no cure, such as an antifungal or an antibiotic, but appropriate therapies can be very helpful. Local soaks can be soothing, and the use of a local lubricant like the foodstore solid white shortening Crisco® can be helpful in maintaining skin surface moisture. Erosive disease usually requires a potent steroid, fluocinoside 0.05%, or ultrapotent steroid, clobetasol propionate 0.05%. These can be applied to the vulva once a day. Unfortunately, there are no vaginal steroid preparations available in the United States. Rectal steroid suppositories or a rectal steroid foam can be substituted. Some women are sensitive to propylene glycol in these preparations and will need a steroid preparation compounded that does not contain this preservative. These agents may prevent progression, but are not restorative. This is a condition that can respond to a systemic immunomodulating agent like Immuran (azathioprine). Joint care with either a rheumatologist or dermatologist is usually beneficial for these women.

Plasma cell vulvitis or Zoon's disease has been successfully treated with a variety of agents. It is such a rare condition, to date only 31 cases have been reported worldwide[13], that there are no comparative studies or treatment strategies. Success has been reported with topical ultrapotent steroid application, intralesional steroid injection, retinoid therapy, and interferon[13]. The use of the ultrapotent steroid, clobetasol propionate 0.05%, twice a day for 4 weeks seems to be a logical first course.

There is limited information available to guide the treatment of the patient with vulvovaginal pemphigus. Only a handful of randomized controlled trials has been performed, and these have looked at small numbers of patients. Since there is evidence of skin autoantigens in this disorder[3,4], a variety of local and systemic agents have been tried in these patients. These include the topical ultrapotent steroid, clobetasol propionate 0.05%, systemic corticosteroids, antibiotics and nicotinamide, azathioprine, and other immunomodulatings agents[14]. Since this is a chronic, relapsing disease initial local therapy can be tried with dermatologic consultation for long-term immunosuppressive care.

Patients with aphthous ulcers present a therapeutic challenge to the physician caring for them. Untreated, the outcome will be pain, recurrences, self-limitation of the condition, and eventual destruction of the epithelium[5]. Local steroids have proven helpful. In more serious cases, systemic therapy with steroids or other immunomodulating agents have been tried. These include the immunosuppressive agent azathioprine, an immunopotentiating agent levamisole, or thalidomide, which inhibits the production of some cytokines. This is another situation in which joint therapeutic care with a dermatologist or rheumatologist will yield the best results for the patient.

REFERENCES

PREFACE

1 Ledger WJ, Polaneczky MM, Yih MC, *et al.* Difficulties in the diagnosis of Candida vaginitis. *Infect Dis Clin Prac* 2000;**9**:66–69.

2 Ross RA, Lee M-L T, Onderdonk AB. Effect of Candida albicans infection and clotrimazole treatment on vaginal microflora in vitro. *Obstet Gynecol* 1995;**86**:925–930.

3 Allen-Davis JT, Beck A, Parker R, *et al.* Assessment of vulvovaginal complaints: accuracy of telephone triage and in-office diagnosis. *Obstet Gynecol* 2002;**99**:18–22.

4 McClelland RS, Lavreys L, Katingima C, *et al.* Contributions of HIV-1 infection to acquisition of sexually transmitted disease: a 10-year prospective study. *J Infect Dis* 2005;**191**:333–338.

5 Rottingen JA, Cameron DW, Garnett GP. A systemic review of epidemiologic interactions between classic sexually transmitted diseases and HIV: how much is really known? *Sex Trans Dis* 2001;**28**:579–597.

CHAPTER 1

1 Barton PT, Gerber S, Skupski DW, Witkin SS. Interleukin-1 receptor antagonist gene polymorphism, vaginal interleukin-1 receptor antagonist concentrations, and vaginal *Ureaplasma urealyticum* colonization in pregnant women. *Infect Immunol* 2003;**71**:271–274.

2 Genc MR, Vardhana S, Delaney ML, *et al.* Relationship between a toll-like receptor-4 gene polymorphism, bacterial vaginosis-related flora and vaginal cytokine responses in pregnant women. *Eur J Obstet Gynecol Reprod Biol* 2004;**116**:152–156.

3 Verstraelen H, Verhelst R, Claeys G, Temmerman M, Vaneechoutte M. Culture-independent analysis of vaginal microflora: the unrecognized association of *Atopobium vaginae* with bacterial vaginosis. *Am J Obstet Gynecol* 2004;**191**:1130–1132.

4 Antonio MAD, Hawes SE, Hillier SL. The identification of vaginal *Lactobacillus* species and the demographic and microbiologic characteristics of women colonized by these species. *J Infect Dis* 1999;**180**:1950–1956.

5 Priestley CFJ, Jones BM, Dhar J, Goodwin L. What is normal vaginal flora? *Genitourin Med* 1997;**73**:23–28.

6 Eschenbach DA, Thwin SS, Patton DL, *et al.* Influence of the normal menstrual cycle on vaginal tissue, discharge, and microflora. *Clin Infect Dis* 2000;**30**:901–907.

7 Schwebke JR, Richey CM, Weiss HL. Correlation of behaviors with microbiologic changes in vaginal flora. *J Infect Dis* 1999;**180**:1632–1636.

8 Eschenbach DA, Patton DL, Hooton TM, *et al.* Effects of vaginal intercourse with and without a condom on vaginal flora and vaginal epithelium. *J Infect Dis* 2001;**183**:913–918.

9 Pabich WL, Fihn SD, Stamm WE, Scholes D, Boyko EJ, Gupta K. Prevalence and determinants of vaginal flora alterations in post-menopausal women. *J Infect Dis* 2003;**188**:1054–1058.

CHAPTER 2

1 Quayle AJ. The innate and early immune response to pathogen challenge in the female genital tract and the pivitol role of epithelial cells. *J Repro Immunol* 2002;**57**:61–79.

2 Janeway CA Jr, Medzhitov R. Innate immune recognition. *Ann Rev Immunol* 2002;**20**:197–216.

3 Zhang D, Zhang G, Hayden MS, *et al.* A toll-like receptor that prevents infection by uropathogenic bacteria. *Science* 2004;**303**:1522–1526.

4 Cole AM, Ganz T. Human antimicrobial peptides: analysis and application. *Biotechniques* 2000;**29**:822–831.

5 Hancock REW. Cationic peptides: effectors in innate immunity and novel antimicrobials. *Lancet Infect Dis* 2001;**1**:156–164.

6 Babovic-Vuksanovic D, Snow K, Ten RM. Mannose-binding lectin (MBL) deficiency: variant alleles in a Midwestern population of the United States. *Ann Allergy Asthma Immunol* 1999;**82**:134–143.

7 Babula O, Lazdane G, Kroica J, Ledger WJ, Witkin SS. Relation between recurrent vulvovaginal candidiasis, vaginal concentrations of mannose-binding lectin, and a mannose-binding lectin gene polymorphism in Latvian women. *Clin Infect Dis* 2003;**37**:733–737.

8 Wallin RPA, Lundqvist A, More SH, von Bonin A, Kiessling R, Ljunggren HG. Heat-shock proteins as activators of the innate immune system. *Trends Immunol* 2002;**23**:130–135.

9 Vilches C, Parham P. KIR: diversity, rapidly evolving receptors of innate and adaptive immunity. *Ann Rev Immunol* 2002;**20**:217–252.

10 Mestecky J, Russell MW. Induction of mucosal immune responses in the human genital tract. *FEMS Immunol Med Microbiol* 2000;**27**:351–355.

CHAPTER 3

1 Ledger WJ, Monif GRG. A growing concern: inability to diagnose vulvovaginal infections correctly. *Obstet Gynecol* 2004;**103**:782–784.

2 Musher DM, Montoya R, Wanahita A. Diagnostic value of microscopic examination of Gram-stained sputum and sputum cultures in patients with bacteremic pneumococcal pneumonia. *Clin Infect Dis* 2004;**39**:165–169.

3 Bartlett JG. Decline in microbial studies for patients with pulmonary infections. *Clin Infect Dis* 2004;**39**:170–172.

4 Nugent RP, Krohn MA, Hillier SH. Reliability of diagnosing bacterial vaginosis is improved by a standardized method of Gram stain interpretation. *J Clin Micro* 1991;**29**:297–301.

5 Amsel R, Totten PA, Spiegel CA, *et al.* Nonspecific vaginitis: diagnostic criteria and microbial and epidemiologic associations. *Am J Med* 1983;**74**:14–22.

6 Ledger WJ, Polaneczky MM, Yih MC, *et al.* Difficulties in the diagnosis of *Candida* vaginitis. *Infect Dis Clin Pract* 2000;**9**:66–69.

7 CDC, Sexually transmitted diseases. Treatment guidelines 2002. *MMWR* 2002;**51**:RR-6:1–80.

8 Witkin SS, Jeremias J, Toth M, *et al.* Detection of *Chlamydia trachomatis* by the polymerase chain reaction in the cervices of women with acute salpingitis. *Am J Obstet Gynecol* 1993;**168**:1438–1442.

9 Jeremias J, Draper D, Ziegert M, *et al.* Detection of *Trichomonas vaginalis* using the polymerase chain reaction in pregnant and nonpregnant women. *Infect Dis Obstet Gynec* 1994;**2**:16–19.

10 Hugenholtz P, Goebel BM, Pace NR. Impact of culture independent studies on the emerging phylogenetic view of bacterial diversity. *J Bacteriol* 1998;**180**:4765–4774.
11 Zhou X, Bent SJ, Schneider MG, *et al.* Characteristics of vaginal microbial communities in adult health women as determined by sequencing clones and terminal restriction fragment length polymorphism (T-RFLP) analyses. *Microbiology* 2004;**150**:2565–2573.
12 Ferris MJ, Masztal A, Aldridge KE, *et al.* Association of *Atopobium vaginae*, a recently describe metronidazole-resistant anaerobe, with bacterial vaginosis. *MMC Infectious Disease* 2004;**4**:1–8.
13 Jeremias J, Ledger WJ, Witkin SS. Interleukin 1 receptor antagonist gene polymorphism in women with vulvar vestibulitis. *Am J Obstet Gynecol* 2000;**182**: 283–285.
14 Babula O, Lazdane G, Kroica J, *et al.* Relation between recurrent vulvovaginal candidiasis, vaginal concentrations of mannose-binding lectin, and a mannose-binding lectin gene polymorphism in Latvian women. *Clin Infect Dis* 2003;**37**:733–737.

CHAPTER 4

1 Spinillo A, Zara F, Gardella B, *et al.* The effect of vaginal candidiasis on the shedding of human immunodeficiency virus in cervicovaginal secretions. *Am J Obstet Gynecol* 2005;**192**:774–779.
2 Mardh P-A. Facts and myths on recurrent vulvovaginal *Candidosis*: a review on epidemiology, clinical manifestations, diagnosis, pathogenesis, and therapy. *Int J STD AIDS* 2002;**13**:522–539.
3 Giraldo P, Von Nowaskonski A, Gomes FA, Linhares IM, Neves NA, Witkin SS. Vaginal colonization by *Candida* in asymptomatic women with and without a history of recurrent vulvovaginal candidiasis. *Obstet Gynecol* 2000;**95**:413–416.
4 Soll DR, Pujol C. *Candida albicans* clades. *FEMS Immunol Med Microbiol* 2003;**39**:1–7.
5 Babula O, Lazdane G, Kroica J, *et al.* Relation between recurrent vulvovaginal candidiasis, vaginal concentrations of mannose-binding lectin, and a mannose-binding lectin gene-polymorphism in Latvian women. *Clin Infect Dis* 2003;**27**:733–737.
6 Witkin SS. Immunology of recurrent vaginitis. *Am J Reprod Immunol Microbiol* 1987;**15**:34–37.
7 Steele C, Fidel PL. Cytokine and chemokines production by human oral and vaginal epithelial cells in response to *Candida albicans. Infect Immun* 2002;**70**:577–583.
8 Little CH, Georgiou GM, Marceglia A, Ogedgebe H, Cone RE, Mazza D. Measurement of T-cell derived antigen binding molecules and immunoglobulin G specific to *Candida albicans* mannan in sera of patients with recurrent vulvovaginal candidiasis. *Infect Immun* 2000;**68**:3840–3847.
9 Witkin SS, Hirsch J, Ledger WJ. A macrophage defect in women with recurrent *Candida* vaginitis and its reversal *in vitro* by prostaglandin inhibitors. *Am J Obstet Gynecol* 1986;**155**:790–795.
10 Kalo-Klein A, Witkin SS. Prostaglandin E_2 enhances and gamma interferon inhibits germ tube formation in *Candida albicans. Infect Immun* 1990;**58**:260–262.
11 Noverr MC, Phare SM, Toews GB, Coffey MJ, Huffnagle GB. Pathogenic yeasts *Cryptococcus neoformans* and *Candida albicans* produce immunomodulatory prostaglandins. *Infect Immun* 2001;**69**:2957–2963.
12 Witkin SS, Jeremias J, Ledger WJ. A localized vaginal allergic response in women with recurrent vaginitis. *J Allergy Clin Immunol* 1988;**81**:412–416.
13 Witkin SS, Jeremias J, Ledger WJ. Recurrent vaginitis as a result of sexual transmission of IgE antibodies. *Am J Obstet Gynecol* 1988;**159**:32–36.
14 Ledger WJ, Polaneczky MM, Yih MC, *et al.* Difficulties in the diagnosis of *Candida* vaginitis. *Infect Dis Clin Pract* 2000;**9**:66–69.
15 Ross RA, Lee M-LT, Onderdonk AB. Effect of *Candida albicans* infection and clotrimazole treatment on vaginal microflora *in vitro. Obstet Gynecol* 1995;**86**:925–930.
16 Sobel JD, Faro S, Force RW, *et al.* Vulvovaginal candidiasis: epidemiologic, diagnostic, and therapeutic considerations. *Am J Obstet Gynecol* 1998;**178**:203–211.
17 Dismukes WE, Wade JS, Lee JY, *et al.* A randomized, double-blind trial of nystatin therapy for the candidiasis hypersensitivity syndrome. *N Engl J Med* 1990;**323**:1717–1723.
18 Pirotta M, Gunn J, Chondros P, *et al.* Effect of lactobacillus in preventing post-antibiotic vulvovaginal candidiasis: a randomized controlled trial. *BMJ* doi: 10.1136/bmj. 38210.494977.DE (published 27 August 2004).
19 Sobel JD, Wisenfeld HC, Martens M, *et al.* Maintenance fluconazole therapy for recurrent vulvovaginal candidiasis. *N Engl J Med* 2004;**351**:876–883.
20 Guaschino S, De Seta F, Sartore A, *et al.* Efficacy of maintenance therapy with topical boric acid in comparison with oral itraconzaole in the treatment of recurrent vulvovaginal candidiasis. *Am J Obstet Gynecol* 2001;**184**:598–602.
21 Wang CC, McClelland RS, Reilly M, *et al.* The effect of treatment of vaginal infections on shedding of human immunodeficiency virus type 1. *J Infect Dis* 2001;**183**:1017–1022.
22 Singh S, Sobel JD, Bhargava P, *et al.* Vaginitis due to *C. krusei*: epidemiology, clinical aspects, and therapy. *Clin Infect Dis* 2002;**35**:1066–1070.
23 Valdes-Dapena MA, Arey JB. Boric acid poisoning. *J Pediatrics* 1962;**61**:531–546.
24 Sobel JD, Chaim W, Nagappan V, *et al.* Treatment of vaginitis caused by *Candida glabrata*: use of topical boric acid and flucytosine. *Am J Obstet Gynecol* 2003;**189**:1297–1300.

CHAPTER 5

1 Fitzpatrick M. The tyranny of health: doctors and the regulation of lifestyle. *Electronic J. Spike* 2000.
2 Ness RB, Hillier SL, Kip KE, *et al.* Bacterial vaginosis and risk of pelvic inflammatory disease. *Obstet Gynecol* 2004;**104**:761–769.
3 Sha BE, Zariffard MR, Wang QJ, *et al.* Female genital-tract HIV load correlates inversely with *Lactobacillus* species, but positively with bacterial vaginosis and *Mycoplasma hominis. J Infect Dis* 2005;**191**:25–32.
4 Ferris MJ, Masztal A, Aldridge KE, *et al.* Association of *Atopobium vaginae*, a recently described metronidazole resistant anaerobe, with bacterial vaginosis. *BMC Infect. Dis.* 2004;**41**:1–8.
5 Amsel R, Totten PA, Spiegel CA. Nonspecific vaginitis: diagnostic criteria and microbiologic and epidemiologic associations. *Am J Med* 1983:**74**:14–22.

6 Sewankambo N, Gray RH, Wawer MJ, *et al.* HIV-1 infection associated with abnormal vaginal flora morphology and bacterial vaginosis. *Lancet* 1997;**350**:546–550.
7 Donders GG, Bosmans E, Dekeermaecker A, *et al.* Pathogenesis of abnormal vaginal bacterial flora. *Am J Obstet Gynecol* 2000;**182**:872–878.
8 Hillier SL, Nugent RP, Eschenbach DA, *et al.* Association between bacterial vaginosis and pre-term delivery of a low birth-weight infant. *N Engl J Med* 1995;**333**:1737–1742.
9 Carey JC, Klebanoff MA, Hauth JC, *et al.* Metronidazole to prevent pre-term delivery in pregnant women with asymptomatic bacterial vaginosis. *N Engl J Med* 2000;**342**:534–540.
10 Guaschino S, Ricci E, Franchi M, *et al.* Treatment of asymptomatic bacterial vaginosis to prevent pre-term delivery: a randomized trial. *Eur J Obstet Gynecol Reprod Biol* 2003;**110**:149–152.
11 Hoyme UB, Möller U, Saling E. Results and consequences of the Thuringia prematurity prevention campaign 2000. *Geburtsh Frauenheilk* 2002;**62**:257–263.
12 McGregor JA, French JI, Seo K. Adjunctive clindamycin therapy for pre-term labor: results of a double-blind, placebo-controlled trial. *Am J Obstet Gynecol* 1991;**165**:867–875.
13 Diniz CG, Arantes RM, Cara DC, *et al.* Enhanced pathogenicity of susceptible strains of the *Bacteroides fragilis* group subjected to low doses of metronidazole. *Microbes Infection* 2003;**5**:19–26.
14 Schwebke JR, Richey CM, Weiss HL. Correlation of behaviors with microbiological changes in vaginal flora. *J Infect Dis* 1999;**180**:1632–1636.
15 Berger BJ, Kolton S, Zenilman JM, *et al.* Bacterial vaginosis in lesbians: a sexually transmitted disease. *Clin Infect Dis* 1995;**21**:1402–1405.
16 Pavlova SI, Kilic AO, Mou SM, *et al.* Phage infection in vaginal lactobacilli: an in vitro study. *Infect Dis Obstet Gynecol* 1997:**5**:36–44.
17 Cauci S, Driussi S, DeSanto D, *et al.* Prevalence of bacterial vaginosis and vaginal flora changes in peri- and post-menopausal women. *J Clin Microbiol* 2002;**40**:2147–2152.
18 Cauci S, Guaschino S, de Aloysio D, *et al.* Interrelationships of interleukin-8 with interleukin-1β and neutrophils in vaginal fluid of healthy and bacterial vaginosis positive women. *Molec Human Reprod* 2003;**9**:53–58.
19 Cauci S, Guaschino S, Driussi S, *et al.* Correlation of local interleukin-8 with immunoglobulin A against *Gardnerella vaginalis* hemolysin and with prolidase and sialidase levels in women with bacterial vaginosis. *J Infect Dis* 2002;**185**:1614–1620.
20 Cauci S, Thorsen P, Schendel DE, *et al.* Determination of immunoglobulin A against *Gardnerella vaginalis* hemolysin, sialidase, and prolidase activities in vaginal fluid: implications for adverse pregnancy outcomes. *J Clin Microbiol* 2003;**41**:435–438.
21 Donders GG, Vereecken A, Salembier G, *et al.* Assessment of vaginal lactobacillary flora in wet mount and fresh or delayed Gram's stain. *Infect Dis Obstet Gynecol* 1996;**4**:2–6.
22 Schwebke JR, Hillier SL, Sobel JD, *et al.* Validity of the vaginal Gram stain for the diagnosis of bacterial vaginosis. *Obstet Gynecol* 1996;**88**:573–576.
23 CDC, Sexually transmitted diseases. Treatment guidelines 2002. *MMWR* 2002;**51**:RR-6:1–80.
24 Leaman D, Sobel J. Suppressive maintenance therapy of recurrent bacterial vaginosis utilizing 0.75% metronidazole vaginal gel. *Int J Gyn & Obstet* 1999;**67**:Abstract 010,S41.
25 Witkin SS, Jeremias J, Ledger WJ. A localized vaginal allergic response in women with recurrent vaginitis. *J Allergy Clin Immunol* 1988;**81**:412–416.
26 Witkin SS, Jeremias J, Ledger WJ. Recurrent vaginitis as a result of sexual transmission of IgE antibodies. *Am J Obstet Gynecol* 1988;**159**:32–36.
27 Kiss H, Petricevic L, Husslein P. Prospective randomized controlled trial of an infection screening programme to reduce the rate of preterm delivery. BMJ,doi: 10.1136/bmj.3869.519653.EB.

CHAPTER 6

1 Witkin SS, Inglis SR, Polaneczky M. Detection of *Chlamydia trachomatis* and *Trichomonas vaginalis* by polymerase chain reaction in introital specimens from pregnant women. *Am J Obstet Gynecol* 1996;**175**:165–167.
2 Van Der Pol B, Williams JA, Orr DP, *et al.* Prevalence, incidence, natural history, and response to treatment of *Trichomonas vaginalis* infection among adolescent women. *J Infect Dis* 2005;**192**:2039–2044.
3 Hobbs M, Kazembe P, Reed AW, *et al. Trichomonas vaginalis* as a cause of urethritis in Malawian men. *Sex Transm Dis* 1999;**26**:381–387.
4 Cotch MD, Pastorek JG II, Nugent RP, *et al. Trichomonas vaginalis* associated with low birth weight and pre-term delivery. *Sex Transm Dis* 1997;**24**:353–360.
5 Kigozi GG, Brahmbhatt H, Wabwire-Mangen F, *et al.* Treatment of *Trichomonas* in pregnancy and adverse outcomes of pregnancy: a subanalysis of a randomized trial in Rakai, Uganda. *Am J Obstet Gynecol* 2003;**189**:1398–1400.
6 Klebanoff MA, Carey C, Hauth JC, *et al.* Failure of metronidazole to prevent pre-term delivery among pregnant women with asymptomatic *Trichomonas vaginalis* vaginitis. *N Engl J Med* 2001;**345**:487–493.
7 Sorvillo F, Smith L, Kerndt P, Ash L. *Trichomonas vaginalis*, HIV, and African-Americans. *Emerg Infect Dis* 2001;**7**:927–932.
8 Heine P, McGregor JA. *Trichomonas vaginalis*: a reemerging pathogen. *Clin Obstet Gynecol* 1993;**36**:137–144.
9 Graves A, Gardner WA. Pathogenicity of *Trichomonas vaginalis*. *Clin Obstet Gynecol* 1993;**36**:145–152.
10 Krieger JN, Jenny C, Verdon M, *et al.* Clinical manifestations of trichomoniasis in men. *Ann Intern Med* 1993;**118**:844–849.
11 Benchimol M, Chang TH, Alderete JF. *Trichomonas vaginalis*: observation of coexistence of multiple viruses in the same isolate. *FEMS Microbiol Lett* 2002;**215**:197–201.
12 Paintlia MK, Kaur S, Gupta I, *et al.* Specific IgA response, T-cell subset and cytokine profile in experimental intravaginal trichomoniasis. *Parisitol Res* 2002; **88**:338–343.
13 Heine RP, Wiesenfeld HC, Sweet RL, Witkin SS. Polymerase chain reaction analysis of distal vaginal specimens: a less invasive strategy for detection of *Trichomonas vaginalis*. *Clin Infect Dis* 1997;**24**:985–987.

14 Crowell AL, Sanders-Lewis KA, Secor WE. *In vitro* metronidazole and tinidazole activities against metronidazole-resistant strains of *Trichomonas vaginalis*. *Antimicrob Agents Chemother* 2003;**47**:1407–1409.
15 CDC, Sexually transmitted diseases. Treatment guidelines 2002. *MMWR* 2002;**51**:RR-6:1–80.
16 Wendel KA, Erbelding EJ, Gaydos CA, *et al.* *Trichomonas vaginalis* polymerase chain reaction compared with standard diagnostic and therapeutic protocols for detection and treatment of vaginal trichomoniasis. *Clin Infect Dis* 2002;**35**:576–580.
17 du Bouchet L, McGregor JA, Ismail M, *et al.* A pilot study of metronidazole vaginal gel versus oral metronidazole for the treatment of *Trichomonas vaginalis* vaginitis. *Sex Transm Dis* 1998;**25**:176–179.
18 Lossick JG, Müller M, Gorrell JE. *In vitro* drug susceptibility and doses of metronidazole required for cure in cases of refractory vaginal trichomoniasis. *J Infect Dis* 1986;**153**:948–955.
19 Sobel JD, Nyirjesy P, Brown W. Tinidazole therapy for metronidazole-resistant vaginal trichomoniasis. *Clin Infect Dis* 2001;**33**:1341–1346.
20 Nyirjesy P, Sobel JD, Weitz MV, *et al.* Difficult-to-treat trichomoniasis: results with paromomycin cream. *Clin Infect Dis* 1998;**29**:986–988.
21 Gorlero F, Bosco P, Barbieri M, *et al.* Fenticonazole ovules in the treatment of vaginal *Trichomonas* infections. A double blind randomized pilot clinical trial. *Curr Ther Res Clin Exp* 1992;**51**:367–376.

CHAPTER 7

1 Sobel JD. Desquamative inflammatory vaginitis: a new subgroup of purulent vaginitis responsive to topical 2% clindamycin therapy. *Am J Obstet Gynecol* 1994;**171**:1215–1220.
2 Donders GGG, Vereecken A, Bosmans E, *et al.* Definition of a type of abnormal vaginal flora that is distinct from bacterial vaginosis: aerobic vaginitis. *Br J Obstet Gynecol* 2002;**109**:1–10.
3 Scheffey LC, Rakoff AE, Lang WR. An unusual case of exudative vaginitis (hydrorrhea vaginalis) treated with local hydrocortisone. *Am J Obstet Gynecol* 1956;**72**:210–211.
4 Sobel JD. Erosive vulvovaginitis. *Curr Infect Dis Rep* 2003;**5**:494–498.
5 Gardner HL. Desquamative inflammatory vaginitis: a newly defined entity. *Am J Obstet Gynecol* 1968;**102**:1102–1106.
6 Murphy R. Desquamative inflammatory vaginitis. *Derm Ther* 2004;**17**:47–49.
7 Newbern EC, Foxman B, Leaman D, Sobel JD. Desquamative inflammatory vaginitis: an exploratory case-control study. *Ann Epidemiol* 2002;**12**:346–352.
8 Raz R, Stamm WE. A controlled trial of intravaginal estriol in post-menopausal women with recurrent urinary tract infection. *N Engl J Med* 1993;**329**:753–756.
9 Pearlman MD, Pierson CL, Faix RG. Frequent resistance of clinical group B streptococci isolates to clindamycin and erythromycin. *Obstet Gynecol* 1998;**92**:258–261.
10 Jeremias J, Ledger WJ, Witkin SS. Interleukin-1 receptor antagonist gene polymorphism in women with vulvar vestibulitis. *Am J Obstet Gynecol* 2000;**182**:283–285.
11 Babula O, Lazdane G, Kroica J, *et al.* Relation between recurrent vulvovaginal candidiasis, vaginal concentrations of mannose-binding lectin and a mannose-binding lectin gene polymorphism in Latvian women. *Clin Infect Dis* 2003;**35**:733–737.

CHAPTER 8

1 Fleming DT, McQuillan GM, Johnson RE, *et al.* Herpes simplex virus type 2 in the United States, 1976–1994. *N Engl J Med* 1997;**337**:1105–1111.
2 Gottlieb SL, Douglas JM, Jr, Schmid DS, *et al.* Seroprevalence and correlates of herpes simplex virus type 2 infection in five sexually transmitted disease-clinics. *J Infect Dis* 2002;**186**:1381–1389.
3 Wald A, Zeh J, Selke S, Warren T, Ryncarz AJ, *et al.* Reactivation of genital herpes simplex virus type 2 infection in asymptomatic seropositive persons. *N Engl J Med* 2000;**342**:844–850.
4 Benedetti JK, Corey L, Ashley R. Recurrence rates in genital herpes after symptomatic first-episode infection. *Ann Intern Med* 1994;**121**:847–854.
5 Brown ZA, Selke S, Zeh J, *et al.* The acquisition of herpes simplex virus during pregnancy. *N Engl J Med* 1997;**337**:509–515.
6 Brown ZA, Benedetti J, Ashley R, *et al.* Neonatal herpes simplex virus infection in relation to asymptomatic maternal infection at the time of labor. *N Engl J Med* 1991;**324**:1247–1252.
7 Gutierrez KM, Falkovitz Halpern MS, Maldonado Y, Arvin AM. Epidemiology of neonatal herpes simplex virus infections in California from 1985 to 1995. *J Infect Dis* 1999;**180**:199–202.
8 Tookey P, Peckham CS. Neonatal herpes simplex virus infection in the British Isles. *Paediatr Perinat Epidemol* 1996;**10**:432–442.
9 Roberts CM, Pfister JR, Spear SJ. Increasing proportion of herpes simplex virus type 1 as a cause of genital herpes infection in college students. *Sex Transmiss Dis* 2003;**30**:797–800.
10 Brown ZA, Wald A, Morrow RA, Selke S, Zeh J, Corey L. Effect of serologic status and cesarean delivery on transmission of herpes simplex virus from mother to infant. *J Am Med Assoc* 2003;**289**:203–209.
11 Duerst RJ, Morrison LA. Innate immunity to herpes simplex virus type 2. *Viral Immunol* 2003;**16**:475–490.
12 Watts DH, Brown ZA, Money D, *et al.* A double-blind, randomized, placebo-controlled trial of acyclovir in late pregnancy for the reduction of herpes simplex virus shedding and cesarean delivery. *Am J Obstet Gynecol* 2003;**188**:836–843.
13 CDC, Sexually transmitted diseases. Treatment guidelines 2002. *MMWR* 2002;**51**:RR-6:1–80.
14 Brown ZA. HSC-2 specific serology should be offered routinely to antenatal patients. *Rev Med Virol* 2000;**10**:141–144.
15 Rouse DJ, Stringer JSA. An appraisal of screening for maternal type-specific herpes simplex virus antibodies to prevent neonatal herpes. *Am J Obstet Gynecol* 2000;**183**:400–406.
16 Wilkinson D, Barton S, Cowan F. HSV-2 specific serology should not be offered routinely to antenatal patients. *Rev Med Virol* 2000;**10**:145–153.
17 Corey L, Wald A, Patal R, *et al.* Once daily valacyclovir to reduce the risk of transmission of genital herpes. *N Engl J Med* 2004;**350**:11–20.
18 Stanberry LR, Spruance SL, Cunningham AL, *et al.* Glycoprotein D-adjuvant vaccine to prevent genital herpes. *N Engl J Med* 2002;**347**:1652–1661.

CHAPTER 9

1 Ho GYF, Bierman R, Beardsley NP, *et al.* Natural history of cervicovaginal papillomavirus infection in young women. *N Engl J Med* 1998;**338**:423–428.
2 Ho GYF, Studentsou Y, Hall CB, *et al.* Risk factors for subsequent cervicovaginal human papillomavirus (HPV) infection and the protective role of antibodies to HPV 16 virus-like particles. *J Infect Dis* 2002;**186**:737–742.
3 Kirwan JMJ, Herrington CS. Human papillomavirus and cervical cancer: where are we now? *Brit J Obstet Gynaecol* 2001;**108**:1204–1213.
4 Schiffman M, Castle PE. Human papillomavirus. Epidemiology and public health. *Arch Pathol Lab Med* 2003;**127**:930–934.
5 Hildesheim A, Schiffman MH, Gravitt PE, *et al.* Persistence of type-specific human papillomavirus infection among cytologically normal women. *J Infect Dis* 1994;**169**:235–240.
6 Stoler MH, Rhodes CR, Whitbeck A, Wolinsky SM, Chow LT, Broker TR. Human papillomavirus type 16 and 18 gene expression in cervical neoplasias. *Hum Pathol* 1992;**23**:117–228.
7 Anttila T, Saikku P, Koskela P, *et al.* Serotypes of *Chlamydia trachomatis* and risk for development of cervical squamous cell carcinoma. *J Am Med Assoc* 2001;**285**:47–51.
8 Tindle RW. Immune evasion in human papillomavirus-associated cervical cancer. *Nature Rev Cancer* 2002;**2**:59–64.
9 Koutsky LA, Ault KA, Wheeler CM, *et al.* A controlled trial of a human papillomavirus type 16 vaccine. *N Engl J Med* 2002;**347**:1645–1651.
10 Federschneider JM, Yuan L, Brodsky J, *et al.* The borderline or weakly positive hybrid capture II HPV test: a statistical and comparative (PCR) analysis. *Am J Obstet Gynecol* 2004;**191**:757–761.
11 Tyring SK, Arany I, Stanley MA, *et al.* A randomized, control molecular study of condyloma acuminata clearance during treatment with imiquimod. *J Infect Dis* 1998;**178**:551–555.
12 Silverberg MJ, Thorson P, Lindeberg H, *et al.* Condyloma in pregnancy is strongly predictive of juvenile onset recurrent respiratory papillomatosis. *Obstet Gynecol* 2003;**101**:645–652.
13 Watts DH, Koutsky LA, Holmes KK, *et al.* Low risk of perinatal transmission of human juvenile papillomavirus: results from a prospective cohort study. *Am J Obstet Gynecol* 1998;**178**:365–373.
14 CDC. Sexually transmitted diseases. Treatment guidelines 2002. MMWR 2002;**51**:RR-6;1–80.
15 Kaufman RH, Adam E. Is human papillomavirus testing of value in clinical practice? *Am J Obstet Gynecol* 1999;**180**:1049–1053.
16 Ledger WJ, Gee R, Genç M, Bongiovanni AM, Witkin SS. Human papillomavirus testing in women with an abnormal Pap smear. *Int J Gynaecol Obstet* 2004;**16(3–4)**:103–109.
17 Nobbenhuis MAE, Walboomers JMM, Helmerhorst TJM, *et al.* Relation of human papillomavirus status to cervical lesions and consequences for cervical cancer screening. *Lancet* 1999;**354**:20–25.
18 Robinson WR, Hamilton CA, Michaels SH, *et al.* Effect of excisional therapy and highly active anti-retroviral therapy on cervical intra-epithelial neoplasia in women infected with human immunodeficiency virus. *Am J Obstet Gynecol* 2001;**184**:538–543.
19 Schuman P, Ohmit SE, Klein RS, *et al.* Longitudinal study of cervical squamous intraepithelial lesions in human immunodeficiency virus (HIV)-seropositive and at-risk HIV-seronegative women. *J Infect Dis* 2003;**188**:128–136.

CHAPTER 10

1 La Guardia KD, White MH, Saigo PE, *et al.* Genital ulcer disease in women infected with human immunodeficiency virus. *Am J Obstet Gynecol* 1995;**172**:553–562.
2 Curran JW, Rendtorff RC, Chandler RW, *et al.* Female gonorrhea. Its relation to abnormal uterine bleeding, urinary tract symptoms, and cervicitis. *Obstet Gynecol* 1975;**45**:95–98.
3 Cates W Jr., Joesoef MB, Goldman MR. Atypical pelvic inflammatory disease: can we identify clinical predictors? *Am J Obstet Gynecol* 1993;**169**:341–346.
4 Wolner-Hanssen P. Silent pelvic inflammatory disease: is it overstated? *Obstet Gynecol* 1995;**86**:321–325.
5 CDC, Sexually transmitted diseases. Treatment guidelines 2002. *MMWR* 2002;**51**:RR-6:1–80.
6 Katz AR, Effler PV, Ohye RG, *et al.* False-positive gonorrhea test results with a nucleic acid amplification test: the impact of low prevalence on positive predictive value. *Clin Infect Dis* 2004;**38**:814–819.
7 Moss B, Shisler JL, Xiang Y, Senkevich TG. Immune-defense molecules of *Molluscum contagiosum* virus, a human poxvirus. *Trends Microbiol* 2000;**8**:473–477.
8 Ganem D, Prince AM. Hepatitis B virus infection: natural history and clinical consequences. *New Eng J Med* 2004;**350**:1118–1129.
9 Salazar JC, Hazlett KRO, Radolf JD. The immune response to infection with *Treponema pallidum*, the stealth pathogen. *Microbes Infection* 2002;**4**:1133–1140.
10 Salzman RS, Kraus SJ, Miller RG, *et al.* Chancroidal ulcers that are not chancroid. Cause and epidemiology. *Arch Dermatol* 1984;**120**:636.
11 Peipert JF, Boardman L, Hogan JW, *et al.* Laboratory evaluation of acute upper genital tract disease. *Obstet Gynecol* 1996;**87**:730–736.
12 Brunham RC, Paavonen JA, Stevens CE, *et al.* Mucupurulent cervicitis: the ignored counterpart in women of urethritis in men. *N Engl J Med* 1984;**311**:1–6.
13 Ness RB, Soper DE, Holley RL, *et al.* Effectiveness of inpatient and outpatient treatment strategies for women with pelvic inflammatory disease: results from the pelvic inflammatory disease evaluation and clinical health (PEACH) randomized trial. *Am J Obstet Gynecol* 2002;**186**:929–937.
14 Ledger WJ. Selection of antimicrobial agents for treatment of infections of the female genital tract. *Rev Infect Dis* 1983;**5**:S98–S104.

CHAPTER 11

1 Todd J, Fishaut M, Kapral F, *et al.* Toxic shock syndrome associated with phage group I staphylococci. *Lancet* 1978;**2**:1116–1118.
2 CDC. Summary of notifiable diseases, United States 1996. *MMWR* 1997;**45**:1–86.
3 CDC. Toxic shock syndrome. United States. *MMWR* 1980;**29**:441–445.
4 Wagner G, Bohr L, Wagner P. Tampon-induced changed in vaginal oxygen and carbon dioxide tension. *Am J Obstet Gynecol* 1984;**148**:147–150.

5 Demers AE, Simor AE, Vellen PM, *et al.* Severe invasive group A streptococcal infections in Ontario, Canada, 1987–1991. *Clin Infect Dis* 1993;**16**:792–800.
6 Caudros J, Mazon A, Martinez R, *et al.* The aetiology of paediatric inflammatory vulvovaginitis. *Eur J Pediatr* 2004;**163**:105–107.
7 Mead PB, Winn WC. Vaginal–rectal colonization with group A streptococci in late pregnancy. *Infect Dis Obstet Gynecol* 2000;**8**:217–219.
8 Donders GG, Vereecken A, Bosmans E, Dekeersmaecker A, Salembier G, Spitz B. Definition of a type of abnormal vaginal flora that is distinct from bacterial vaginosis: aerobic vaginitis. *BJOG* 2002;**109**:34–43.
9 Mitchell TJ. The pathogenesis of streptococcal infections: from tooth decay to meningitis. *Nature Reviews Microbiology* 2003;**1**:219–230.
10 Banks MC, Kamel NS, Zabriskie JB, Larone DH, Ursea D, Posnett DN. *Staphylococcus aureus* express unique superantigens depending on the tissue source. *J Infect Dis* 2003;**187**:77–86.
11 The Working Group on severe streptococcal infections. Defining the Group A streptococcal toxic shock syndrome. *JAMA* 1993;**269**:390–391.
12 Miller LG, Perdreau-Remington F, Rieg G, *et al.* Necrotizing fasciitis caused by community-associated methicillin resistant *Staphylococcus aureus* in Los Angeles. *N Engl J Med* 2005;**352**:1445–1453.
13 Eagle H, Musselman AD. The slow recovery of bacteria from the toxic effects of penicillin. *J Bacteriol* 1949;**58**:475–490.
14 Ledger WJ, Headington JT. Group A betahemolytic streptococcus. An important cause of serious infections in obstetrics and gynecology. *Obstet Gynecol* 1972;**39**:474–482.
15 Kaul R, McGeer A, Norrby-Teglund A, *et al.* Intravenous immunoglobulin therapy for streptococcal toxic shock syndrome. A comparative observational study. *Clin Infect Dis* 1999;**28**:800–807.

CHAPTER 12

1 Ledger WJ, Kessler A, Leonard GH, *et al.* Vulvar vestibulitis: a complex clinical entity. *Infect Dis Obstet Gynecol* 1996;**4**:269–275.
2 Witkin SS, Jeremias J, Ledger WJ. A localized vaginal allergic response in women with recurrent vaginitis. *J Allergy & Clin Immun* 1988;**81**:412–416.
3 Witkin SS. Immunology of recurrent vaginitis. *Am J Reprod Immunol Microbiol* 1987;**15**:34–37.
4 Witkin SS, Roth DM, Ledger WJ. Papillomavirus infection and an allergic response to *Candida* in women with recurrent vaginitis. *J Am Med Assoc* 1989;**261**:1584.
5 Haye KR, Mandal D. Allergic vaginitis mimicking bacterial vaginosis. *Int J STD & AIDS* 1990;**1**:440–442.
6 Snijdewint FGM, Kalinski P, Wierenga EA, Bos JD, Kapsenberg ML. Prostaglandin E_2 differentially modulates cytokine secretion profiles of human T helper lymphocytes. *J Immunol* 1993;**150**:5321–5329.
7 Roper RL, Brown DM, Phipps RP. Prostglandin E_2 promotes B lymphocyte Ig isotype switching to IgE. *J Immunol* 1995;**154**:162–170.
8 Witkin SS, Kalo-Klein A, Galland L, Teich M, Ledger WJ. Effect of *Candida albicans* plus histamine on prostaglandin E_2 production by peripheral blood mononuclear cells from healthy women and women with recurrent candidal vaginitis. *J Infect Dis* 1991;**164**:396–399.
9 Witkin SS, Jeremias J, Ledger WJ. Recurrent vaginitis as a result of sexual transmission of IgE antibodies. *Am J Obstet Gynecol* 1988;**159**:32–36.
10 Witkin SS, Jeremias J, Ledger WJ. Vaginal eosinophiles and IgE antibodies to *Candida albicans* in women with recurrent vaginitis. *J Med and Vet Mycol* 1989;**27**:57–58.
11 Moraes PSA. Recurrent vaginal candidiasis and allergic rhinitis: a common association. *Ann Allergy Asthma Immunol* 1998;**81**:165–169.
12 Bernstein JA, Herd ZA, Bernstein DI, *et al.* Evaluation and treatment of localized vaginal immunoglobulin E-mediated hypersensitivity to human seminal plasma. *Obstet Gynecol* 1993;**82**:667–673.
13 Summers P. Allergic yeast vulvovaginitis is the most prevalent genital *Candida* syndrome. *Abstr Int Infec Dis Soc Obstet-Gynecol Meeting* 30 April–2 May 2004, Philadelphia, PA.

CHAPTER 13

1 Writing group for the Women's Health Initiative Investigators. Risks and benefits of estrogen plus progestin in healthy post-menopausal women. *JAMA* 2002;**288**:321–333.
2 Raz R, Stamm WE. A controlled trial of intravaginal estriol in post-menopausal women with recurrent urinary tract infection. *N Engl J Med* 1993;**329**:753–756.
3 Hillier SL, Lau RJ. Vaginal microflora in post-menopausal women who have not received estrogen replacement therapy. *Clin Infect Dis* 1997;**25(Suppl 2)**:S123–126.
4 Burton JP, Reid G. Evaluation of the bacterial vaginal flora of 20 post-menopausal women by direct (Nugent score) and molecular (polymerase chain reaction and denaturing gradient gel electrophoresis) techniques. *J Infect Dis* 2002;**186**:1770–1780.
5 Cauci S, Driussi S, De Santo D, *et al.* Prevalence of bacterial vaginosis and vaginal flora changes in peri- and post-menopausal women. *J Clin Microbiol* 2002;**40**:2147–2152.
6 Pabich WL, Fihn SD, Stamm WE, Scholes D, Boyko EJ, Gupta K. Prevalence and determinants of vaginal flora alterations in post-menopausal women. *J Infect Dis* 2003;**188**:1054–1058.
7 Pfeilschifter J, Koditz R, Pfohl M, Schatz H. Changes in pro-inflammatory cytokine activity after menopause. *Endocr Rev* 2002;**23**:90–119.
8 Kamada M, Irahara M, Maegawa M, *et al.* Transient increase in the levels of T-helper 1 cytokines in post-menopausal women and the effects of hormone replacement therapy. *Gynecol Obstet Invest* 2001;**52**:82–88.
9 Manson JE, Hsia J, Johnson KC, *et al.* Estrogen plus progestin and the risk of coronary heart disease. *N Engl J Med* 2003;**349**:523–534.
10 Rymer J, Wilson R, Ballard K. Making decisions about hormone replacement therapy. *BMJ* 2003;**326**:322–326.
11 Davis G, Wentworth J and Richard J. Self-administered topical imiquimod treatment of vulvar intraepithelial neoplasis: a report of four cases. *J Reprod Med* 2000;**45**:619–623.
12 Loombes RC, Hall E, Gibson LJ, *et al.* A randomized trial of exemestane after two to three years of tamoxifen therapy in post-menopausal women with primary breast cancer. *N Engl J Med* 2004;**350**:1081–1092.

13 Raz R, Cologner R, Rohanna Y, *et al.* Effectiveness of estriol-containing vaginal pessaries and nitrofurantoin microcrystal therapy in the prevention of recurrent urinary tract infection in post-menopausal women. *Clin Infect Dis* 2003;**36**:1362–1368.

CHAPTER 14

1 Haefner HK, Collins ME, Davis GD, *et al.* The vulvodyna guideline. *J Lower Gen Tract Dis* 2005;**9**:40–51.
2 Friedrich EG. The vulvar vestibule. *J Reprod Med* 1983;**38**:773–777.
3 Ledger WJ, Kessler A, Leonard GH, Witkin SS. Vulvar vestibulitis – a complex clinical entity. *Infect Dis Obstet Gynecol* 1996;**4**:269–275.
4 Goetsch MD. Vulvar vestibulitis: prevalence and historic features in a general gynecologic practice population. *Am J Obstet Gynecol* 1991;**164**:1609–1616.
5 Traas MAF, Bekkers RLM, Dony JMJ, *et al.* Surgical treatment for the vulvar vestibulitis syndrome. *Obstet Gynecol* 2006;**107**:256–262.
6 Witkin SS, Gerber S, Ledger WJ. Differential characterization of women with vulvar vestibulitis syndrome. *Am J Obstet Gynecol* 2002;**187**:589–594.
7 Westrom LC, Willen R. Vestibular nerve fiber proliferation in vulvar vestibulitis syndrome. *Obstet Gynecol* 1998;**91**:572–576.
8 Sarma AV, Foxman B, Bayirli B, Haefner H, Sobel JD. Epidemiology of vulvar vestibulitis syndrome: an exploratory case-control study. *Sex Transm Inf* 1999;**75**:320–326.
9 Smith EM, Ritchie, Galask R, Pugh EE, Jia J, Ricks-McGillan J. Case-control study of vulvar vestibulitis risk associated with genital infections. *Infect Dis Obstet Gynecol* 2002;**10**:193–202.
10 Morin C, Bouchard C, Brisson J, Fortier M, Blanchette C, Meisels A. Human papillomaviruses and vulvar vestibulitis. *Obstet Gynecol* 2000;**95**:683–687.
11 Asahman RB, Ott AK. Autoimmunity as a factor in recurrent vulvovaginal candidosis and the minor vestibular gland syndrome. *J Reprod Med* 1989;**34**:264–266.
12 Babula O, Danielsson I, Sjoberg I, *et al.* Altered distribution of mannose-binding lectin alleles at exon I codon 54 in women with vulvar vestibulitis syndrome. *Am J Obstet Gynecol* 2004;**191**:762–766.
13 Foster DC, Hasday JD. Elevated tissue levels of interleukin-1β and tumor necrosis factor-α in vulvar vestibulitis. *Obstet Gynecol* 1997;**89**:291–296.
14 Jeremias J, Ledger WJ, Witkin SS. Interleukin-1 receptor antagonist gene polymorphism in women with vulvar vestibulitis. *Am J Obstet Gynecol* 2000;**182**:283–285.
15 Gerber S, Bongiovanni AM, Ledger WJ, Witkin SS. Interleukin-1β gene polymorphism in women with vulvar vestibulitis syndrome. *Eur J Obstet Gynecol Reprod Biol* 2003;**107**:74–77.
16 Gerber S, Bongiovanni AM, Ledger WJ, Witkin SS. Defective regulation of the pro-inflammatory immune response in women with vulvar vestibulitis syndrome. *Am J Obstet Gynecol* 2002;**186**:696–700.
17 Babula O, Bongiovanni AM, Ledger WJ, Witkin SS. IgE antibodies to seminal fluid in women with vulvar vestibulitis syndrome: relation to onset and timing of symptoms. *Am J Obstet Gynecol* 2004;**190**:663–667.
18 Geneç MR, Gerber S, Nesin M, *et al.* Polymorphism in the interleukin-1 gene complex and spontaneous preterm delivery. *Am J Obstet Gynecol* 2002;**187**:157–163.
19 Babula O, Lazdane G, Kroica J, *et al.* Relation between recurrent vulvovaginal candidiasis, vaginal concentrations of mannose-binding lectin and a mannose-binding lectin gene polymorphism in Latvian women. *Clin Infect Dis* 2003;**35**:733–737.

CHAPTER 15

1 Sander CS, Ali I, Dean D, *et al.* Oxidative stress is implicated in the pathogenesis of lichen sclerosus. *Br J Dermatol* 2004;**151**:627–635.
2 Sugarman PB, Savage NW, Walsh LJ, *et al.* The pathogenesis of oral lichen planus. *Crit Rev Oral Biol Med* 2002;**13**:350–365.
3 Giudice GJ, Emery DJ, Diaz LA. Cloning and primary structural analysis of the bulbous pemphigoid autoantigens, BP180. *J Invest Dermatol* 1992;**99**:243–250.
4 Mueller S, Klaus-Kovtun JR, Stanley A. A 230-kD basic protein is the major bullous pemphigoid antigen. *J Invest Dermatol* 1989;**92**:33–38.
5 Natah SS, Konttinen YT, Enattah NS, *et al.* Recurrent aphthous ulcers today: a review of the growing knowledge. *Int J Oral Maxillofac Surg* 2004;**33**:221–234.
6 Lewkowicz N, Lewkowicz P, Kurnatowska A, *et al.* Innate immune system is implicated in recurrent aphthous ulcer pathogenesis. *J Oral Pathol Med* 2003;**32**:475–481.
7 Uzun S, Alpsoy E, Durdu M, *et al.* The clinical course of Behçet's disease in pregnancy: a retrospective analysis and review of the literature. *J Dermatol* 2003;**30**:499–502.
8 Lynch PJ. Lichen simplex chronicus (atopic/neurodermatitis) of the anogenital region. *Derm Ther* 2004;**17**:8–19.
9 Schön MP, Boehncke WH. Psoriasis. *N Engl J Med* 2005;**352**:1899–1912.
10 Tasker GL, Wajnarowska F. Lichen sclerosis. *Clin Exp Derm* 2003;**28**:128–133.
11 Neill SM, Tatnall FM, Cox NH. Guidelines for the management of lichen sclerosis. *Brit J of Derm* 2002;**147**:640–649.
12 Funaro D. Lichen sclerosis: a review and practical approach. *Derm Ther* 2004;**17**:28–37.
13 David L, Massey K. Plasma cell vulvitis and response to topical steroids: a case report. *Int J STD & AIDS* 2003;**14**:568–569.
14 Wojnarowska F, Kirtschig G, Highet AS, *et al.* Guidelines for the management of bullous pempligoid. *Brit J Derm* 2002;**147**:214–221.
15 Sfikakis PP. Behçet's disease: a new target for anti-tumor necrosis factor treatment. *Ann Rheum Dis* 2002;**61**:ii51–ii53.
16 International Study Group for Behçet's Disease. Criteria for diagnosis of Behçet's disease. *Lancet* 1990;**335**:1078–1080.
17 Reitamo S, Rustin M, Ruzicke T, *et al.* Efficacy and safety of tacrolimus ointment compared with that of hydrocortisone butyrate ointment in adult patients with atopic dermatitis. *J Allergy Clin Immunol* 2002;**109**:547–555.
18 Dalziel K, Millard PR, Wojnarowska F. The treatment of vulvar lichen sclerosis with a very potent corticosteroid (clobetasol propionate 0.05%) cream. *Br J Dermatol* 1991;**124**:461–464.

INDEX

Note: page numbers in *italics* refer to figures and tables.

acyclovir *57*
alefacept 118
allergens 87, 90–92, 105, 106
allergic response amplification 88
allergic vulvovaginitis 86–92
  diagnosis 86, 88, *89*, 90
  immunology 87–8
  microbiology 87
  treatment 90–2
amitriptyline 109, 117
Amsel criteria 23, 39, 40
antibody production 15
antihistamines 91, 92
anti-sperm antibodies 15
anti-viral immune defense mechanisms 54
aphthous ulcers 112, 116, *117*, 118
atopic dermatitis 113, 117
Atopobium vaginae 24, 36, 39
azathioprine 118
azithromycin 78, 79
azoles 32–34, 90

B lymphocytes 15, 88
bacilli *9*
  Gram-negative 93
bacterial vaginosis 16, *17*, 22, 35–42
  asymptomatic patients 41, 42
  diagnosis 24, 37–40
  HIV infection 36, 42
  post-menopausal women 94, 102
  recurrence 37, 41
  screening tests 40, 42
  sexual transmission 37
  treatment 40–2
  vaginal discharge *45*
  vulvar vestibulitis 104
  white blood cells 36, 38
Bacteroides 36
Bartholin's abscess 72, 76, 79
basophils 87
Behçet's disease 56, 112–13, 116–17
bichloracetic acid (BCA) 67, 68
boric acid 34, 52
breast-feeding post-partum 50, *51*

calciprotriene 118
Calymmatobacterium granulomatis 72, 74
Candida
  hyphae 20, *28*, *30*, *31*
  spores 30, *31*, 32
Candida albicans 10, 11, 24, 25–6
  allergic response 88, 90, 92
  post-menopausal women 102
  vulvar vestibulitis 96, 105, 108, 110
Candida glabrata 22, 32, 34, 102
Candida krusei 34, 102
Candida vaginitis 16, *17*, 52
Candida vulvovaginitis 21–2, 25–34
  cultures 23
  diagnosis 24, 27–8, *29*, 30, *31*, 32, 33
  menopausal 100
  treatment 32–4, 117
  vulvar vestibulitis 110
candidiasis, recurrent vulvovaginal (RVVC) 26, 33, 87
cefixime 79
cefoxitin 80
ceftriaxone 78, *79*
celecoxib 109
cervical cancer 62, 63
cervical intra-epithelial neoplasia (CIN) 69
cervicitis 77
chancre 71, 76, 79
chancroid 71, 74, *75*, 78
Chlamydia trachomatis 24, 71–2, 76, 79–80
  HPV malignancy progression 63
  ingestion by *T. vaginalis* 44
  lymphogranuloma venereum 74
ciprofloxacin 78, 79
clindamycin 41, 42, 49–50, 52, 80
clobetasol propionate 101, 117, 118
cocci *9*, 11, 49
conception, vaginal flora 11
condoms 91
condyloma acuminate 19, 61, 63–8, 87
cotton fibers 19–20, 28, *29*
cultures 23–4
cyclobenzaprine 109
cytokines, pro-inflammatory 94, 106
cytomegalovirus (CMV) 70, 74, 77

defensins 12–13, 27
dendritic cells 14–15
dermatologic disorders 111–18
  diagnosis 113–14, *115*, 116–17
  erosive 116–17
  flaking 113–14, *115*
  immunology 112–13
  inflammatory 116–17
  treatment 117–18
desquamative inflammatory vaginitis (DIV) 49–52
  diagnosis 50, *51*, 52
  immunology 50
  microbiology 49–50
  treatment 49–50, 52
diagnosis of vulvovaginal disease 16–24
  equipment 17–18
  laboratory tests 22–4
  pelvic examination 18–22
  physical examination 18
diet 33–4, 109
Digene HPV testing 61, 64
DNA fingerprinting 26
DNA probe testing 24
Donovan bodies 74, *75*
doxycycline 79, 80

efalizumab 118
ejaculate, male 91
endometrial polyp 99–100
endomyometritis 42, 85
epithelial cells 12–13, 88, *89*, 90, 111
equipment for diagnosis 17–18
erythromycin 78, 79
Escherichia coli, vaginal colonization 11, 94
estradiol, intravaginal cream 52, 102, 108
estrogen 11, 91, 93, 94, 101, 102
ethnic factors 10–11, 41, 106

famciclovir *57*
fenticonazole 47
fetus, genital herpes transmission 59
fever of undetermined origin (FUO) 84
fluconazole 32, 33, 34, 101, 117
5-fluorouracil 67, 68

gabapentin 109
Gardnerella vaginalis 23–4, 35, 36, 39, 40
gene polymorphism testing 24
genetic factors 10, 52
gentamicin 78, 80
gentian violet 34
glycogen, vaginal 11
gonorrhea 72–3
Gram stain 22–3
granuloma inguinale 71, 74, *75*, 78

Haemophilus ducreyi 72, 74
heat shock proteins 13–14, 112
hepatitis B 72, 77
herpes, genital 53–60
  asymptomatic patients 57
  diagnosis 55–7
  immunology 54–5
  microbiology 54
  pathophysiology 53–4
  perineal lesions 55
  post-menopausal 101
  primary infection 58
  recurrence 53–4, 58–9
  screening 60
  sexual partner 58–9, 60
  treatment 57–60
  vaccines 60
herpes, neonatal 54, 57, 60
herpes simplex virus 1 (HSV-1) 18, 24, 53–60
  antibody testing 56–7, 60
  microbiology 54
  screening 60
  vulvar ulcerations 74

herpes simplex virus 2 (HSV-2) 18, *19*, 24, 53–60
antibody testing 56–7, 60
microbiology 54
screening 60
vaccine 55
vulvar ulcerations 74
highly active anti-retroviral therapy 69
histamine *87*, 88
history taking 17
HIV infection
bacterial vaginosis 36, 42
Candida vulvovaginitis 25, 34
genital herpes 54, 59
human papillomavirus 62, 68, 69
testing 77, 79
Trichomonas vaginalis vaginitis 43
hormone replacement therapy (HRT) 11, 94
human papillomavirus (HPV) 61–9
allergic vaginal reaction 87
cervical cancer 62
diagnosis 63–6, *67*, 77
elimination of virus 61–2
high-risk types 61, 63, 66, 69
malignancy progression 63
microbiology 62–3
Pap smears 62, 68–9, 94, 101, 102
post-menopausal women 94, 101, 102
transmission 62–3
treatment 67–9, 101
vaccines 69
see also warts, genital
Hybrid Capture test 66
hydrocortisone 101
hydrogen peroxide 10, 11
hydroxyzine 109, 117

imiquimod 60, 68, 69, 101
immune defense mechanisms 26–7
immune responses 111
immunity 12–14, 15, 26
immuno-enhancers 60
immunoglobulin A (IgA) 15, 37
immunoglobulin E (IgE) 87–8
allergic vulvovaginitis 86, 90
anti-*Candida* 92
male ejaculate 91
vulvar vestibulitis 106
immunoglobulin G (IgG) 15
immunology of vagina 12–15
infections, vulvar vestibulitis 105–6
infliximab 118
interferon αβ 67, 109
interferon therapy 118
interleukin 1β (IL-1β) 37, 106, 108
interleukin 2 (IL-2) 15, 88
interleukin-1 receptor antagonist (IL1-ra) gene 24, 106, 108, 109–10
interleukin-8 (IL-8) 37
itraconazole 32, *33*, 34

ketoconazole 32, *33*, 34
killer cell immunoglobulin-like receptors (KIR) 14
KOH preparations 19–20, 21, 22

laboratory tests 22–4
Lactobacillus/lactobacilli *9*, 10–11, 34, 36, 37, 49, 94
hydrogen-peroxide producing 10, 11, 36, 37
lactoferrin 13
latex allergy 91
levamisole 118
levofloxacin 79
lice, pubic 73
lichen planus 49, 50, 52, 112, 116, 118
lichen sclerosus *28*, 101, 112, 114, *115*, 118
lichen simplex chronicus 113, 117
lindane 78
lymphogranuloma venereum 71, 72, 74, *75*, 79
lysozyme 13

macrophages 14, 88
major histocompatibility complex (MHC) 14, 15
mannose-binding lectin (MBL) 13, 24, 26
vulvar vestibulitis 105–6, 108, 110
mast cells 87
menopausal vulvovaginitis 93–102
diagnosis 94–6, *97*, 98–100
treatment 101–2
menopause 11, 93–4, 96, *97*
desquamative inflammatory vaginitis 50, *51*
menstrual cycle 11
metronidazole 36, 48, 80
bacterial vaginosis 40–1, 42
Trichomonas vaginalis treatment 43, 47, 48
microorganisms 9–11
micropapillomatosis labialis 66
microscopy 20–2
molecular analysis 24
molluscum contagiosum 72, 73, 77
mood-elevator drugs 109
Mycoplasma hominis 11, 24, 35, 36
mycoplasmas *9*

natural killer cells 14
necrotizing fasciitis 85
Neisseria gonorrhoeae 44, 72–3, 76, 79–80
diagnosis 23, 24
neonates *see* herpes, neonatal
Nikolsky's sign 116
nonoxynol nine contact allergy 91
Nugent criteria 23, 39–40, 42, 94

ofloxacin 79, 80
oral contraceptives 11
oral–genital syndrome 50
oxalates 109

Pap smears 62, 68–9, 94, 101, 102
paromomycin 47
pediculosis pubis 73, 78
pelvic examination 18–22
pelvic infection, bacterial vaginosis 40
pemphigus 112, 116, 118
penicillin 79, 85
peptides, antimicrobial 12–13
permethrin 78
phagocytic cells 14
Phthirus pubis 73
PKR protein kinase 14
plasma cell mucositis 116, 118
podophyllin 68
polymerase chain reaction (PCR) 24
pregnancy
bacterial vaginosis 40, 41
Candida vulvovaginitis 33
genital herpes 54, 57, 59–60
human papillomavirus 68
Trichomonas vaginalis 43, 48
vulvar vestibulitis 105, 110
pre-term labor 40, 41, 48
propylene glycol 90–1, 118
prostaglandin E_2 (PGE_2) 15, 26–7, 33, 88, 106
protein kinase 14
psoriasis 113, 118
puberty, vaginal flora 11

retinoids 118
RVVC *see* candidiasis, recurrent vulvovaginal (RVVC)

Sarcoptes scabiei (scabies) 73, 78
secretory leukocyte protease inhibitor (SLPI) 12
selective serotonin reuptake inhibitors (SSRIs) 118
seminal fluid 15, 27, 90
sexual intercourse 11, 15
sexual partner, genital herpes 58–9, 60
sexually transmitted diseases 70–80
bacterial vaginosis 37
diagnosis 73–4, *75*, 76–7
immunology 72–3
menopausal women 94
microbiology 72–3
treatment 77–80
see also herpes, genital; human papillomavirus (HPV)
skin pathology *see* dermatologic disorders
spermatozoa 22, *23*
spermicides, contraceptive 87
squamous cell cancer, vulval 98, *99*, 118
Staphylococcus aureus 23, 81–5
steroids 92, 118
streptococci
aerobic 10
Group A 23, 81–5
Group B 23, 50, 52
Streptococcus pneumoniae 23
Streptococcus pyogenes 82
SUMA® 109–10
superantigens 82
syphilis 71, 72, 76, 79

T cell-derivedantigen binding
molecules (TABM) 26
T lymphocytes 15, 26, 88
tacrolimus ointment 118
tamoxifen 102
Th1 and Th2 immune responses 111
thalidomide 118
tinidazole 43, 47
toll-like receptors (TLRs) 12, *13,* 14, 26
toxic shock syndrome 81–2, 83–4, 85
Treponema pallidum 71, 72, 74, 76, 79
triamcinolone 117
trichloracetic acid (TCA) 67, 68
Trichomonas vaginalis 24, 44, 47, 105
  vaginitis 16, 22, 43–8, 102
trimethoprim–sulfamethoxazole 79
tumor necrosis factor α (TNF-α) 106

ulcers, genital 70–1, 72, 74, *75,* 76
  post-menopausal women 101
  see also aphthous ulcers
Ureaplasma urealyticum 11, 24
urethral caruncle 95–6
urinary tract infection 11
  misdiagnosis 104, 105
  post-menopausal women 93, 94

vagina
  immunology 12–15
  microbiology 9–11
vaginal burning 101, 102
vaginal discharge 101, 102
vaginal pH 10, 11, 19
  Candida vulvovaginitis 32
  menopausal 102
  sexually transmitted infections *77*
vaginal secretion collection 19–20
valacyclovir *57,* 58, 59
viruses *9*
virus-like particles (VLPs) 63, 69
vulvar intraepithelial neoplasm (VIN) 66, *67,* 98, *99,* 101
vulvar irritation 18, *19*
vulvar nerve activity moderation 108–9
vulvar vestibulitis 19, 24, 96, *97,* 98
  diagnosis 106, *107,* 108
  frequency 104
  genetic factor 52
  immunology 106
  inappropriate treatment 105
  infections 105–6
  microbiology 105–6
  pregnancy 105
  surgical treatment 110
  symptomatology 105
vulvar vestibulitis (*continued*)
  syndrome 103–10
  treatment 101, 108–10
  urinary tract symptoms 104
vulvodynia 103–10

warts, genital
  cervical 61, 64, *65,* 68
  diagnosis 63–6
  squamous cell carcinoma 68
  treatment 67–8
  vaginal 61, 64–6
  vulval 63–4
white blood cells
  bacterial vaginosis 36, 38
  desquamative inflammatory vaginitis 50, *51,* 52
  endometrial polyp 99–100
  sexually transmitted infections *77*
  streptococcal vaginitis 83
  Trichomonas infection 45, 46

yeasts *9*

Zoon's vulvitis 116, 118